Assessment and Treatment of Sexual Offenders with Intellectual Disabilities

Assessment and Treatment of Sexual Offenders with Intellectual Disabilities: A Handbook

Edited by

**Leam A. Craig, William R. Lindsay
and Kevin D. Browne**

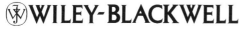

A John Wiley & Sons, Ltd., Publication

Registered Office
John Wiley & Sons Ltd, The Atrium, Southern Gate, Chichester, West Sussex, PO19 8SQ, UK

Editorial Offices
The Atrium, Southern Gate, Chichester, West Sussex, PO19 8SQ, UK
9600 Garsington Road, Oxford, OX4 2DQ, UK
350 Main Street, Malden, MA 02148-5020, USA

For details of our global editorial offices, for customer services, and for information about how to apply for permission to reuse the copyright material in this book please see our website at www.wiley.com/wiley-blackwell.

Library of Congress Cataloging-in-Publication Data

Assessment and treatment of sexual offenders with intellectual disabilities : a handbook / edited by Leam A. Craig, William R. Lindsay and Kevin D. Browne.
    p. cm.
  Includes bibliographical references and index.
  ISBN 978-0-470-05838-1 (cloth) – ISBN 978-0-470-05839-8 (pbk.) 1. Sex offenders–Rehabilitation. 2. Offenders with mental disabilities–Rehabilitation. 3. Sex offenders–Psychology. 4. Sex offenders–Mental health services.
I. Craig, Leam. II. Lindsay, William R. III. Browne, Kevin D. (Kevin Dominic)
  HV6556.A774 2010
  364.3'8–dc22

                                                                                        2009052110

ISBN: 978 0 470-05838-1 (cloth : alk. paper)

A catalogue record for this book is available from the British Library.

Set in 10/12 pt Times Roman by Thomson Digital, Noida, India

First Impression   2010

Dedication

Leam A. Craig: For my parents and family

William R. Lindsay: For the colleagues, staff and clients who have helped me in my work over the years

Kevin D. Browne: For children with disabilities, I hope the time I have invested in this book will offer better care and protection from the problems they suffer

Contents

About the Editors

Leam A. Craig, BA (Hons), MSc, PhD, CSci, AFBPsS, EuroPsy, C.Psychol (Forensic) is a consultant forensic psychologist and partner at Forensic Psychology Practice Ltd. He is a chartered psychologist, a chartered scientist and holder of the European Certificate in Psychology. His current practice includes direct services to forensic National Health Service Adult Mental Health Trusts and consultancy to Prison and Probation Services. He acts as an expert witness to civil and criminal courts in the assessment of sexual and violent offenders. He coordinates community-based treatment programmes for sexual offenders with intellectual disabilities in National Health Service, community forensic units and probation settings. He has published numerous chapters and research articles in a range of research and professional journals. He has recently completed an authored book with Professors Kevin Browne and Anthony Beech entitled *Assessing Risk in Sex Offenders: A Practitioners Guide* (Wiley-Blackwell, 2008), and an edited book entitled *Assessment and Treatment of Sex Offenders: A Handbook* (Wiley-Blackwell, 2009). He is currently working on *Assessments in Forensic Practice: A Handbook* (Wiley-Blackwell) with Kevin Browne and Anthony Beech. He is an Honorary Senior Research Fellow at the Centre for Forensic and Criminological Psychology, University of Birmingham, UK.

Forensic Psychology Practice Ltd, The Willows Clinic, Boldmere, Sutton Coldfield, UK. Email: LeamCraig@forensicpsychology.co.uk

William R. Lindsay, PhD, C.Psychol, FBPsS is Consultant Forensic Clinical Psychologist and Lead Clinician in Scotland for Castlebeck Care. He was previously Head of Psychology (LD) in National Health Service Tayside and a consultant with the State Hospital, Carstairs. He is Professor of Learning Disabilities and Forensic Psychology at the University of Abertay, Dundee and Visiting Professor at the University of Northumbria, Newcastle. He has published over 200 research articles and book chapters and given many presentations and workshops on cognitive therapy and the assessment and treatment of offenders with intellectual disabilities. His recent publications include a workbook entitled *The Treatment of Sex Offenders with Developmental Disabilities: A Practice Workbook* (2009) and an edited book entitled *Offenders with Developmental Disabilities* (Lindsay, Taylor & Sturmey, 2004) both by Wiley.

Lead Clinician in Scotland and Head of Research for Castlebeck Care, Darlington, UK. Email: BillLindsay@castlebeck.com

Kevin D. Browne, BSc, MSc, MEd, PhD, MI.Biol, AFBPsS, C.Psychol (Forensic) is both a chartered biologist and chartered psychologist employed by the University of Nottingham as Chair of Forensic Psychology and Child Health. In 2008 re-established the Centre of Forensic and Family Psychology within the Institute of Work, Health and Organisation at Nottingham, after he originally set it up at the University of Birmingham in 1998. He has been researching family violence and child maltreatment for 30 years and has published extensively on the prevention of violence to children. After 12 years as an executive councillor of the International Society for the Prevention of Child Abuse and Neglect (ISPCAN), he is currently Consultant to the European Commission, UNICEF and heads the World Health Organization Collaborating Centre on Child Care and Protection based in the UK. His research interests are concerned with the development of aggression, antisocial and criminal behaviour in children and teenagers, in particular the role of family violence, child abuse and neglect. Nationally, he is involved in the professional training of applied psychologists and he has developed the first professional doctorates in forensic psychology at the Universities of Birmingham and Nottingham.

His most recent books are *A Community Health Approach to the Assessment of Infants and their Parents: the CARE Programme* (Browne, Douglas, Hamilton-Giachritsis & Hegarty, 2006) and *Assessing Risk in Sex Offenders* (Craig, Browne & Beech, 2008), both published by Wiley.

Institute of Work, Health & Organisations (I-WHO), University of Nottingham, International House, Jubilee Campus, Nottingham, NG8 1BB. Email: Kevin.browne@nottingham.ac.uk

Contributors

Douglas P. Boer, BSc, MSc, PhD, R.Clin.Psych (Canada and New Zealand) is an associate professor in the Department of Psychology at The University of Waikato, Hamilton, New Zealand and an adjunct professor of the Royal Melbourne Institute of Technology, Melbourne, Australia. Prior to going to New Zealand in 2006, he worked for 15 years in the Correctional Service of Canada in a variety of roles, including sex offender programme therapist, sex offender programme director and supervising/regional psychologist. He currently is the Director of the Clinical Psychology Programme at The University of Waikato, New Zealand. He also provides community-based treatment programmes for sexual offenders with intellectual disabilities and acts as an expert witness for criminal courts in Canada and the USA in the assessment of violent and sexual offenders. He has authored or co-authored a number of publications in the field of forensic correctional psychology including the Sexual Violence Risk – 20.

Eleanor Brewster, MD is a specialist registrar training in the Psychiatry of Learning Disabilities and General Adult Psychiatry. She has a particular interest in the treatment of severe mental illness affecting people with learning disabilities, and learning disability in the forensic population. Research interests include improving patient assessment tools and the interface between psychiatry and the legal system.

Kevin D. Browne, BSc., MSc., PhD., M.Ed., C. Biol., C.Psychol (Forensic) is Chair of Forensic Psychology and Child Health at the University of Nottingham and Director of the Centre of Forensic and Family Psychology within the Institute of Work, Health and Organisation, Nottingham. He also heads the World Health Organization Collaborating Centre on Child Care and Protection based in the UK. See 'About the Editors' section for more information about this author/editor.

Leam A. Craig, BA (Hons), MSc, PhD, CSci, AFBPsS, EuroPsy, C.Psychol (Forensic) is a consultant forensic psychologist and Partner at Forensic Psychology Practice Ltd. He is an Honorary Senior Research Fellow at the Centre for Forensic and Criminological Psychology, University of Birmingham, UK. See 'About the Editors' section for more information about this author/editor.

Lynne Eccleston, BA, BA (Hons), PhD is a consultant forensic psychologist, and Director of Myndscape Consulting. She was formerly Director of the Forensic Psychology Program, the University of Melbourne. She is currently a guest lecturer and Fellow of the University of Melbourne. She has experience in the assessment, treatment and rehabilitation of male and female offenders, specialising in sexual and violent offenders including intellectually disabled offenders. She has designed and implemented programmes that address offenders' behaviours and psychopathology, and focus on rehabilitation and reducing criminogenic needs. Lynne's research interests and publications include the prediction of risk and dangerous behaviour in violent and sexual offenders and the assessment, treatment and rehabilitation of offenders.

Paul Fedoroff, MD is Vice Chair of the Royal Ottawa Research Ethics Committee, Director of the Integrated Forensic Program Sexual Behaviours Clinic, and Director of the Forensic Research Unit at the University of Ottawa Institute of Mental Health Research. He is also Associate Professor of Psychiatry in the Department of Medicine at the University of Ottawa in Canada. Dr Fedoroff's primary clinical and research interests are in the assessment and treatment of men and women with problematic sexual behaviours, especially those with intellectual disabilities. He has published extensively in these areas and provided consultation internationally. His publications support the proposition that, with modern methods, many criminal sexual problems can not only be treated but also prevented.

Hannah Ford, **BSc (Hons), MPhil, ClinPsyD** is a clinical psychologist working in the West Midlands with young people in care, including those who are involved in offending. Before moving to this role, Hannah worked for the Lucy Faithfull Foundation, contributing to the assessment and treatment of perpetrators of sexual offences against children and completing a Home Office commissioned evaluation of national need for residential treatment provision for sex offenders (with Anthony Beech). She has a particular interest in women who commit sexual offences and has written a book about this topic, published in 2006 by Wiley, entitled *Women Who Sexually Abuse Children*. She also has an interest in sex offenders with intellectual disabilities and completed her doctoral research in this area.

Matthew Frize is a registered psychologist in New South Wales (NSW), Australia and a member of the Australian Psychological Society. He works as a Senior Clinical Consultant in NSW's Department of Ageing Disability & Home Care's Criminal Justice Program - the state's community forensic disability service. In this role he provides assessment and intervention to people with an intellectual disability with a history of serious offending behaviours across NSW. He holds a Master's in Developmental and Educational Psychology and is currently completing a doctorate in Clinical Psychology.

Dorothy M. Griffiths is the Associate Dean of the Faculty of Social Sciences, a professor in the Child and Youth Studies Department and the Centre for Applied Disabilities Studies and the Co-Director of the International Dual Diagnosis Certificate Programme. Dr Griffiths has worked in the area of sexuality and behaviour challenges with persons with intellectual disabilities for more than 30 years. Among her many books, chapters and articles is the groundbreaking book *Changing Sexually Inappropriate Behaviour* (1989, Brookes

Publishing) and the revised *Socio-Sexual Knowledge and Attitude Assessment Tool* (2003, Stoelting Company).

Fabian Haut is a consultant psychiatrist with responsibility for the Tayside forensic learning disability (LD) service. Additionally, he has Responsible Clinician responsibility for a generic LD community team. He holds a CCST for general adult psychiatry and learning disability and has an interest in dual diagnosis. His research interests lie in the area of dual diagnosis, particularly diagnostic criteria and their applicability to people with learning disability and forensic learning disability issues.

Susan C. Hayes, **AO, PhD, FIASSID** is Professor of Behavioural Science in Medicine and Head of the Centre for Behavioural Sciences in the Faculty of Medicine at the University of Sydney, Australia, where she teaches in the USyd Medical Program. She has been practising as clinical forensic psychologist with victims and offenders with intellectual disabilities for over 20 years, as well as undertaking research. A current research project is examining the prevalence of people with the dual diagnoses of intellectual disability and psychiatric disorder, presenting before NSW Magistrates Courts. In 2006 she was appointed as Benjamin Meaker Visiting Professor at the Norah Fry Research Centre at the University of Bristol, UK. She has previously acted as a consultant to the Australian and NSW Law Reform Commissions in the area of the person with intellectual disability and the law. She was a member of the NSW Guardianship Tribunal. In 2004 she was made a Fellow of the International Association for the Scientific Study of Intellectual Disability (IASSID). She has published extensively in the field of rights of people with intellectual disabilities. She is a member of the editorial board of the *Journal of Intellectual and Developmental Disability* and was recently guest editor for a special edition of the *British Journal of Learning Disability*, focussing on offenders with learning (intellectual) disabilities. In 2007, she was appointed to the post of Academic Advisor and Consultant for the Secure Specialised Commissioning Team for North West National Health Service (UK), to interact with various academic establishments in the UK and take the lead role in the formulation of research specifications and contracts, as well as monitoring the quality of commissioned research and advising about new research areas.

Frank Lambrick, D Psych (Forensic) is a registered psychologist with over 20 years experience working within the forensic disability field. He currently works as a practice leader with the Office of the Senior Practitioner, in the Victorian Department of Human Services, Australia. He also conducts lectures on forensic disability issues at the University of Melbourne. His research interests include assessment and treatment approaches for offenders with intellectual disability, including risk assessment and management.

Peter E. Langdon, BSc, D.Clin.Psy, C.Psychol, AFBPsS is a chartered clinical and forensic psychologist who is employed as a clinical lecturer within the School of Medicine, Health Policy and Practice, University of East Anglia (UEA). He has been involved in clinical psychology training for a number of years, and is part of the Doctorate in Clinical Psychology course team at UEA. His clinical sessions take place the Broadland Clinic, Hertfordshire Partnership National Health Service Foundation Trust in Norwich, which is a National Health

Service medium secure unit for offenders with intellectual and developmental disabilities. Among other areas, his research and clinical interests involve sexual offenders and other offenders with intellectual disabilities. He is a founder member of SOTSEC-ID, and has been involved in running sex offender treatment programmes for men with ID for a number of years.

William R. Lindsay, PhD, C.Psychol, FBPsS is Consultant Psychologist and Lead Clinician in Scotland for Castlebeck Care. He is Professor of Learning Disabilities and Forensic Psychology at the University of Abertay, Dundee and Visiting Professor at the University of Northumbria, Newcastle. See 'About the Editors' section for more information about this author/editor.

Michelle McManus, MSc completed her MSc in Investigative and Forensic Psychology, at the University of Liverpool in 2009 and is now completing her PhD at the Centre of Forensic and Family Psychology within the Institute of Work, Health and Organisation, University of Nottingham on Juvenile offenders and the court system.

Ruth E. Mann, PhD, C.Psychol is a chartered forensic psychologist and works for the National Offender Management Service, England and Wales, where she has overall responsibility for the national Sex Offender Treatment Programme, cognitive skills programmes and interventions research. She has been involved with the treatment of imprisoned sexual offenders for over 20 years.

Amanda M. Michie, PhD is Head of Clinical Psychology Services in Lothian NHS Learning Disability Service. She has completed research in the assessment and treatment of social and community living skills and in the last 10 years has worked with offenders with learning disabilities. Her clinical and research interests include sex offenders, anger management and cognitive behavioural therapy.

Catrin Morrissey, PhD, C.Psychol is a chartered forensic psychologist and lead psychologist in the National High Secure Learning Disability service at Rampton Hospital, one of three high secure hospitals in England. She has more than twenty years experience of working with sexual offenders and clinical and research interests in assessment and treatment of personality disorder in intellectual disability.

Shawn Mosher qualified in Canada before beginning his career in the UK with Partnerships in Care at Kneesworth House in Cambridgeshire, working with persons with ID in settings of medium security. He now works at Castlebeck Care in the north east of England. He has developed interests in working with persons with ID and sex offending and other challenging behaviours, as well as with staff, particularly around staff training and how it can affect direct work with this client group. Other interests include risk assessments of sexual and physical violence for both adolescents and adults as well as assessment of parents with ID.

Glynis H. Murphy, PhD, C. Psychol, FBPsS is a chartered clinical and forensic psychologist, Fellow of the British Psychological Society and President of the International Association of the Scientific Study of Intellectual Disabilities (IASSID). She is is a joint Chair of Clinical Psychology and Learning Disability at the Tizard Centre, University of Kent and at Oxleas National Health Service Trust. She is coeditor of *Journal of Applied Research in Intellectual Disabilities* and now works at the Tizard Centre, University of Kent. For many years, she has had research interests in challenging behaviour, abuse, forensic issues and the law in learning disabilities, and she has published widely on these topics. Among other activities, she is currently running a multi-site trial of cognitive-behavioural treatment for people with learning disabilities at risk of sexual offending (the SOTSEC-ID project).

Ruth Pappas is a senior clinical consultant with the NSW Dept of Ageing Disability and Homecare – Statewide Behaviour Intervention Service a specialist service that provides clinical support to those working with individuals with challenging and or offending behaviour. She has worked in the area of intellectual disability for over 25 years. Over the past eight years she has been specifically involved in resource development, training and group work with sex offenders and offenders with an intellectual disability.

Deborah Richards, BA, CHMH is a manager of specialised services for Community Living Welland Pelham as well as a Professor in Disability Studies at Niagara College Canada in Welland, Ontario. She is an author, lecturer, clinician and sex educator. She designs and teaches sexuality and social skills training curriculum for people with intellectual disabilities.

John Rose, PhD is Academic Director of the Clinical Psychology Training Course at The University of Birmingham and Divisional Psychologist in the Learning Disability Service for Dudley Primary Care Trust. Prior to this he worked on the Cardiff Clinical Psychology Training Course and as a clinical psychologist in a number of different services. He has written over 80 articles in academic and professional journals on issues related to cognitive therapy, service design, offenders with learning disabilities and staff and organisational issues in intellectual disability services. He continues to work clinically and apply his academic interests in practice.

John L. Taylor, BSc (Hons), MPhil, DPsychol, CPsychol, CSci, AFBPsS is a chartered clinical and forensic psychologist, Professor of Clinical Psychology at Northumbria University, Newcastle upon Tyne, and Consultant Clinical Psychologist and Psychological Services Professional Lead with Northumberland, Tyne & Wear NHS Foundation Trust, UK. Since qualifying as a clinical psychologist from Edinburgh University he has worked mainly in intellectual disability and forensic services in high and medium secure hospitals, prison and community settings in the UK. He has published widely on the assessment and treatment of offending and mental health problems associated with intellectual disabilities. He is currently President of the British Association for Behavioural and Cognitive Psychotherapies (BABCP) and Chair of the British Psychological Society's Mental Health Act Working Party.

Marleen Verhoeven completed her training in the Netherlands and moved to New Zealand 17 years ago. She is a consultant clinical psychologist at the Dual Disability Service (DDS), Auckland. DDS is a tertiary mental health service specialising in treating people with an intellectual disability and complex needs. Marleen has an interest in working with people with severe behavioural challenges and personality disorder and has worked extensively in both intellectual disability and in general mental health and is a guest lecturer on issues related to DBT and intellectual disability at Massey, Auckland and Waikato Universities. She has published on Asperger's Syndrome and psychological assessment and interventions for people with an intellectual disability.

Tony Ward, PhD, MA. (Hons), DipClinPsyc is Professor of Clinical Psychology and Clinical Director at Victoria University of Wellington, New Zealand. He was previously director of the Kia Marama Programme for sexual offenders at Rolleston Prison, Christchurch, New Zealand and has taught clinical and forensic psychology at Canterbury and Melbourne Universities. His research interests include the offense process in offenders, cognitive distortions and models of rehabilitation. He has published over 235 research articles, chapters and books. These include *Theories of Sexual Offending,* Wiley (2006), *Rehabilitation: Beyond the Risk Paradigm,* Routledge (2007), and *Morals, Rights and Practice in the Human Services,* Jessica Kingsley (2008). School of Psychology, Victoria University of Wellington, PO Box 600, Wellington, New Zealand. Email: Tony.Ward@vuw.ac.nz

Barry Watermam, Bach. Appl. Sci. (Hon), Dpsych (Forensic) is the currently Manager of the Disability Pathways Program, Corrections Victoria, Australia. He is also an honorary fellow of Deakin University. His research and clinical work has been in the assessment of offenders with a cognitive impairment and the development and implementation of offence specific treatment programs, particularly for violence and sex offenders with an intellectual disability.

Fiona Williams is responsible for the Adapted Sex Offender Treatment Programme in Prisons in England and Wales. She has lead on the treatment of ID sexual offenders since work on the ASOTP first started in 1995. She is currently developing a revised version of the ASOTP to enable seamless treatment options for intellectually disabled sexual offenders in custody and in the community.

Foreword

Historically, the sexual behaviour of individuals with intellectual disabilities has been viewed as reflective of their underlying mental health issues, criminality, sexual dangerousness and lack of common moral standards. In fact, studies, conducted by Hubert Goddard (Goddard, 1912) in the United States, following the turn of the century, led him to conclude that intellectual delay was the cause for persons becoming prostitutes, criminals, perverts and whorehouse madams. As a result, he proposed a systematic solution of separating these individuals from society and barring them from reproduction. These 'scientific' conclusions, and others like them, led to sterilisation laws and a movement to institutionalise individuals with intellectual disabilities that persisted into the late 1970s and early 1980s within the United States and beyond. Institutionalisation allowed for complacency and an 'out of sight, out of mind' attitude in addressing their sexually challenging behaviours. At the same time, reproductive laws were viewed as making the world safer for future generations. It was not until the 'deinstitutionalisation' movement of the 1960s that attention was finally directed to the rights and needs of intellectually disabled individuals. While the steps were small and going was slow, this marked the beginning of a recognition that intellectually disabled individuals' sexuality could be supported in a positive manner with a combination of social skills training, behavioural interventions and sexual education. Winifred Kempton, a therapist, said that by the 1970,s without precedents to follow, resources to use, research or experts to consult, we had to try to convince the public that persons with intellectual disabilities were sexual human beings with rights and, also, that we had to address sexually challenging behaviours of this population (Griffiths, Quinsey & Hingsburger, 1989). Still, in the early 1980s there were no theoretical models to give direction to the treatment of intellectually disabled sex offenders. It was not until the 1990s that there was a significant emphasis on developing sexual offender treatment programming for persons with intellectual disabilities that was tailored to their unique characteristics, rather than 'simplified' versions of adult offender treatment strategies.

Despite the phenomenal increase in attention focused on sex offender assessment and treatment since the 1980s, relatively little effort has gone into developing parallel programming for intellectually disabled sex offenders. A variety of barriers have limited work in this area. Initially professionals in the field were limited by their own isolation, which slowed the development of theories and tailored strategies for working with disabled sex offenders. Further, professionals had serious concerns that focusing attention on sexual offending behaviour with this population would further label them as dangerous and increase their rejection by members of the wider community. A central and significant barrier to addressing sexual offending was the reluctance associated with viewing intellectually disabled individuals as 'sexual beings'. It was not uncommon, even among professionals, for there to be considerable apprehension and discomfort in advocating for intellectually disabled individuals' rights to sexual expression. This matter was complicated by our longstanding historical propensity to treat these individuals as perpetual children who are asexual or, conversely, are sex crazed, lacking any ability to control themselves. These barriers have contributed to societal and professional norms that have made it easy to put the needs of this population on the 'back burner'.

The success of the deinstitutionalisation movement created its own set of challenges.

As community integration became the norm, we were forced to address the complexities of intervening in sexually challenging behaviour perpetrated by intellectually disabled individuals in a broad array of community settings. The greater the integration of these individuals into the community the higher the stakes and the greater the challenge. One might argue that our earlier forays into the treatment of this population were based on a certain degree of naivety and that we were guilty of minimising the potential risks to the community as well as to other individuals with intellectual deficits. In the late 1970s and the 1980s the watch words in working with this population were 'close supervision' and 'containment'. The focus on public safety and the creation of group living environments in the community drove the development of intervention and supervision strategies, which were inextricably linked to the characteristics of these settings. As a result, one of the greatest dilemmas we currently face in working with this population is the unwitting development of 'institutions' for housing offenders with intellectual disabilities in the community. The institutional nature of these settings and the tight controls provided by the containment model have reduced community safety concerns. However, they have also obviated the need to develop more effective self-management approaches that can be used by intellectually disabled offenders. In essence, this combination of forces runs the risk of perpetuating a new era of 'institutionalisation' for this group of individuals.

As the field has devoted more attention to the sexual offending behaviour of persons with intellectual disabilities it has relied heavily on research and intervention strategies based on non-intellectually disabled adult sex offenders. Not surprisingly, there has been considerable debate in the field as to the merits of this approach. Does it make sense to adapt research findings and programmatic materials from non-disabled offenders, or would we be best served by encouraging the separate development of a research foundation specifically related to the characteristics, needs and nuances of the intellectually disabled sex offender? While it has been expedient to borrow from an existing literature, certainly the answer lies in a comprehensive understanding of the characteristics, nature and development of offending by persons with intellectual disabilities. This will likely require patience as we strive to strengthen both the theoretical foundation for our work with this population and the strategies that flow from these conceptualisations. At the same time, the need for strongly grounded, evidence-based approaches to therapeutic interventions with this population offers the promise of more effective treatment programming.

Drs Craig, Lindsay and Browne have created a book that critically considers the progression of work in this field, recognises the complexities of the tasks associated with treating intellectually disabled sex offenders, and incorporates promising research in the development of interventions tailored to the needs and characteristics of this population. This book provides critical information on how we can improve the quality of life for individuals with intellectual disabilities who exhibit sexually challenging behaviours, without compromising community safety. This book offers strategies for increasing the disabled offender's ability to actively participate in their treatment, without losing a victim centered focus. It also encourages the judicious use of containment and supervision strategies where indicated. It does, however, point out that using containment as the primary method to manage sexual offending behaviour is costly and does not lend itself to long-term offender change. Similarly, the authors suggest that supervision should be prescriptively used where risk dictates its value. In contrast, by using 'blanket' containment approaches as an overall primary management strategy is unnecessary and financially burdening.

The authors have also done an exceptional job of highlighting an exciting movement in the field that embraces the advantages of collaboration. Of particular note are the partnerships that involve experts who have previously published outside of the area of intellectual disability or outside the sex offender assessment and treatment arena. These collaborations brought new ideas to the area and led to an 'explosion' of publishing on issues related to the assessment and treatment of sexually disabled sex offenders. The inclusion of these individuals in this book brings with it the incorporation new paradigms and new perspectives. Moreover, it offers the opportunity to consider methods and interventions used previously in other fields and only recently utilised with intellectually disabled sex offenders. As such, work in this area will begin to inform the broader sex offender treatment literature.

Leam Craig, Bill Lindsay and Kevin Browne have done an impressive job of organising and editing this book around the issues most relevant and timely for addressing sexually offending issues with intellectually disabled individuals. They have gathered a 'who's who' of experts in the field to create a collection of chapters that covers theory, research and practical intervention approaches designed for the practitioner. This book provides an up-to-date review of the research literature pertaining to theories; prevalence; offender characteristics; sexual offending behaviour; and cutting edge assessment and treatment strategies appropriate for use in institutions and community settings. These approaches create a strong foundation for the development of effective interventions that are a better fit for our systems of care, that are cost effective and make sense for the intellectually disabled sex offender population that we serve. This book is destined to become a primary resource for practitioners committed to high quality treatment that promotes greater offender responsibility and autonomy, without compromising community safety.

James Haaven

Portland, United States
November 2009

REFERENCES

Goddard, H.H. (1912). *The Kallikak family*. New York: The MacMillan Company.
Griffiths, D., Quinsey, V. & Hingsburger, D. (1989). *Changing inappropriate sexual behaviour: A community based approach for persons with developmental disabilities*. Baltimore, MD: Paul H. Brookes.

Acknowledgements

The authors are privileged to have the intellectual companionship of a number of world renowned practitioners and researchers in the field of violent and sex offender assessment, treatment and research both in the UK and overseas. We are grateful to the contributors of this volume for sharing their experience and expertise and working tirelessly on this project alongside their hectic schedules.

We should like to thank all those at Wiley-Blackwell for allowing us the opportunity to produce this book; a special thank you to Karen Shield for all her hard work and patience.

We would also like to thank James Haaven for his valued and much appreciated contribution at short notice.

PART ONE

Introduction

1

Overview and Structure of the Book

LEAM A. CRAIG, WILLIAM R. LINDSAY AND KEVIN D. BROWNE

INTRODUCTION

The relationship between behavioural disturbance and forensic problems in people with intellectual disability (ID) is subtle. There is no doubt that many behaviour problems in people with severe and profound ID would be construed as offences in more able individuals. One of the determining characteristics of an 'offence' is that the perpetrator is aware of behaviour that is socially sanctioned or censured. Even when someone with mild ID may understand the nature of the offence, the criminal justice response and the response of carers is diverse across cases and situations (Clare & Murphy, 1998; Swanson & Garwick, 1990).

A problem encountered in researching the topic of sex offenders with ID is the range and interchange of terms used to describe individuals or groups of individuals with intellectual disabilities. Some authors use the term 'learning disability', 'learning impairment', 'learning disorders', 'learning difficulties', 'intellectual disabilities' and 'developmentally delayed'. This confuses and blurs the applicability of the research findings as sample sources vary, even though the aim is to encapsulate the same group. For the purpose of this chapter the term 'intellectual disability' will be used, which can be defined as:

- A significantly reduced ability to understand new or complex information, to learn new skills (impaired intelligence). A reduced ability to cope independently (impaired social functioning);
- Arising before adulthood (under 18 years of age) and having a lasting effect on development.

(Department of Health, 2001, p.14).

The Department of Health (2001) note that this encompasses a large range of disabilities, with a basic categorisation into four groups, based on IQ scores; which is the method most

---

Assessment and Treatment of Sexual Offenders with Intellectual Disabilities: A Handbook
Edited by Leam A. Craig, William R. Lindsay and Kevin D. Browne
© 2010 John Wiley & Sons, Ltd.

studies utilise: 50–70 – mild; 35–50 – moderate; 20–35 – severe; < 20 - profound. Assessments are usually conducted using the Wechsler Intelligence Scale for Children – Third Edition (WISC-III: Wechsler, 1991) or the Wechsler Adult Intelligence Scale – Third Edition (WAIS-III: Wechsler, 1999) with less than 70 indicating a level of intellectual disability. The assessment of social functioning causes more difficulty for research because of varying assessments and the inconsistent use of the term (O'Callaghan, 1999). Highlighting methodological problems with studies, Murphy, Harnett & Holland (1995) found none of the prison sample of sex offenders investigated had an IQ assessed under 70 but 21 percent had been referred to special schools, which may be an indication for some authors to classify these individuals as intellectually disabled.

General methodological difficulties with work in this area are that offenders with ID are only mentioned as part of larger offender cohorts. Where studies are specifically directed towards offenders with ID many studies are small in subject numbers (Johnston & Halstead, 2000). This is particularly true for sexual offenders with ID (Courtney, Rose & Mason, 2006; Craig, Stringer & Moss, 2006; Lindsay, Olley, Baillie & Smith, 1999). Under the auspices of The Prison Reform Trust (PRT), Loucks (2007) examined the attitudes and resources for people with ID within the criminal justice system in England and Wales. From this review it was estimated that 20–30 per cent of offenders have ID that interfere with their ability to cope within the criminal justice system. The Mottram (2007) research estimates that approximately 30 per cent of offenders within the prison system have an IQ less than 80. It is generally considered that the prevalence rates for offenders within the population of individuals with ID may be higher than those in the general population.

In his report, *The Incidence of Hidden Disabilities in the Prison Population*, Rack (2005) suggests that 20 per cent of the prison population has some form of hidden disability. Further research reported in the July 2006 edition of Community Care suggests that up to 7 per cent of the prison population is learning disabled and a further 23 per cent of prisoners are 'borderline' (PRT, 2006). On the other hand, Holland and Persson (in press) studied the prison population in Victoria, Australia and found a prevalence rate of around 1 per cent which is consistent with the prevalence of people with ID in the general population.

Many of the characteristics that are attributed to sexual offenders often overlap with those individuals categorised with ID. For example, research highlights the impulsive actions of individuals with ID, and this may increase the chances of them being involved in sex offences. However, these factors may also increase the likelihood of detection and give a biased picture of the relative prevalence of individuals with ID involved in sex offences.

The need for competent assessment and treatment of sexual offenders with ID has never been greater. The population in custody in England and Wales on 31 May 2008 was 82,822 (2 per cent more than a year earlier), with 82,372 in prison. In May 2009 this figure rose to 83,300 in custody, of which, 82,900 were in prison. Among the sentenced prison population, sexual offences saw an increase by 4 per cent from May 2007, rising to 7,573 sexual offenders (Ministry of Justice, 2008). In May 2009 this rose to 7, 907 sexual offenders (Ministry of Justice, 2009) a further increase of 4 per cent on the previous year. However, of these figures, it is not clear how many sexual offenders with ID are currently held in prison. While initial screening of prisoners at reception into prison or during induction may highlight problems, such testing is not systematic (Murphy, Harrold, Carey & Mulrooney, 2000) nor are these tools specific enough to identify intellectual disabilities (Williams & Atthill, 2005). The true estimate of the number of people with ID in prison remains unknown. Assuming an equal distribution in IQ scores across the prison sex offender sample, based on Mottram (2007) estimations, there could be as many as 2,271 sexual offenders with ID currently in prisons in England and Wales. Even taking the lower figures reported by Holland and Persson (in press) the estimate would be around 800, which remains a significant number of individuals requiring special procedures for assessment and treatment. If one includes those on probation and community orders (see Lindsay, Michie and Lambrick, Chapter 15), the figures rise considerably.

Since the 1980s there has been a growing interest in the assessment and treatment of sexual offenders with ID, and researchers and practitioners have developed a range of assessment protocols and treatment interventions for this client group. Specifically in relation to assessing sexual offenders with ID a range of psychometric measures have now been developed and standardised (Lindsay, Michie, Whitefield, Martin, Grieve & Carson, 2006; Murphy, Powell, Guzman & Hays, 2007) allowing for a more accurate assessment of risk and treatment need (Lindsay & Taylor, 2009). Similarly, clinicians and researchers have begun to address the problem of treatment for men with ID who have offended sexually. Without necessarily admitting clients for in-patient treatment, several reports have suggested the feasibility of such treatment (Craig, Stringer & Moss, 2006; Lindsay, Neilson, Morrison & Smith, 1998; Lindsay, Olley, Baillie & Smith, 1999; Murphy, 2007).

Clearly, this is rapidly developing area of interest where clinicians are experimenting intellectually and conceptually with how best to assess and improve treatment services for this client group. The PRT (2006) recently made a number of recommendations regarding the diagnostic assessment and management of offenders with ID. It is hope that this volume goes some way to addressing the assessment and treatment needs in sexual offenders with ID.

STRUCTURE OF THE BOOK

The book itself is divided into a number of sections as follows:

Introduction

The second chapter in the introductory section of the book is by Leam Craig and William Lindsay who explore the characteristics, prevalence, and assessment issues for sexual offenders with ID. It is important first of all to describe in detail the client group this book focuses on and aetiological theories of sexual offending by men with ID. They provide an up-to-date review of the theories of sexual offending by men with ID and argue that such behaviour is unlikely to be comprehensively described by a single theory but by a combination of several theories including tendencies toward sexual offending, personality traits and impulsiveness can be considered alongside the hypothesis of counterfeit deviance. Unlike non-ID sexual offenders, accurate estimations of prevalence of sexual offending by men with ID are often difficult to establish. In reviewing the prevalence and reconviction rates for this client group they note that, because of poorly controlled studies and methodological differences, it is extremely difficult to conclude that there are any characteristics which might be considered unique to the client group. Nevertheless, there is some consistency in the literature that sex offenders with ID pose a greater risk of sexual recidivism in a shorter time period than their non-ID counterparts. Craig and Lindsay explore the specific types of offending and re-offending as well as the familial and offence characteristics.

Part One: Background, Theory and Incidence

We begin this section with Susan Hayes (Chapter 3) who explores the developmental pathways in intellectually disabled sex offenders. This chapter reviews the developmental pathways from adverse childhood experiences to juvenile sex offending and adult sex crimes. As there is a dearth of research and the limitations of existing research on developmental characteristics of sexual offenders with ID, Hayes draws upon studies of non-disabled populations of offenders in order to extrapolate factors, conditions and events experienced by those with ID. The influence of a person having an ID in relation to these developmental pathways is specifically considered and this is compared to individuals with neuro-developmental deficits (such as ADHD) and young people without deficits or disabilities. She concludes that the earlier the investment in young people's lives, the more cost-effective the intervention to prevent sex offending.

This is followed by Chapter 4 from Kevin Browne and Michelle McManus, who seek to identify the characteristics of family sexual abuse committed by adolescents with ID and its relation to sibling abuse and incest. The role of parents/carers and the potential impact on the family are discussed with the aim of identifying opportunities for prevention of sex offences by adolescents and adult with ID.

Finally in this section, Lynne Eccleston, Tony Ward and Barry Waterman (Chapter 5) consider the application of the self-regulation model (SRM) (Ward & Hudson, 1998) to sexual offending in men with ID. The SRM has seen a great deal of research since 2000 as part of understanding the relapse prevention process in non-ID (Bickley & Beech, 2002) and ID sexual offenders. The SRM represents a breakthrough in understanding the relapse process and links to the Good Lives Model which has also been tested with sexual offenders with ID (Keeling, Rose & Beech, 2006; Langdon, Maxted & Murphy, 2007; Lindsay, Steptoe & Beech, 2008). Eccleston, Ward and Waterman describe the aetiology of the model and provide case examples of how the model can be applied to sex offenders with ID. They argue that ID sexual offenders are capable of explicit planning in addition to implicit planning and they can be less impulsive and opportunistic than previously considered. This has implications for treatment and management strategies, and they offer guidance on therapeutic approaches and techniques.

Part Two: Diagnostic Assessment and Comorbidity

This section of the book deals with issues of diagnostic assessment frameworks and comorbidity. In Chapter 6, Fabian Haut and Eleanor Brewster discuss the prevalence of mental illness in people with ID and the diagnosis and treatment of some of the more common diagnosed disorders. From reviewing the literature they suggest there are significant issues with mental illness for people with ID and that the prevalence of schizophrenia and other non-affective psychoses is considerably higher in people with ID than in the general adult population. They describe some of the difficulties in establishing dual diagnosis in people with ID and go on to consider different forms of pharmacological treatment for differing disorders. They then discuss pervasive developmental disorders – for example, autism, Asperger's syndrome and attention deficit hyperactivity disorder, which are often identified in people with ID – and describe the difficulties in dual diagnosing forms of mental illness. Finally, they discuss offending and sexual offending in people with autistic spectrum disorders. They conclude that although there is little to link specific psychiatric diagnoses with sexual offences, effective treatment of a comorbid psychiatric condition in people with an ID may help to reduce a person's offending behaviour, particularly if it is driven by mental illness.

In Chapter 7, Dorothy Griffiths, Paul Fedoroff and Deborah Richards discuss sexual and gender identity disorders identified within the DSM-IV-TR under three distinct sections: Sexual Dysfunctions, Gender Identity Disorders and Paraphilias. They review how these criteria are applied to persons with ID. The authors demonstrate how additional cautions should be applied when utilising the DSM-IV-TR criteria with persons with ID. Its application to this population requires knowledge of the nature of the disabling condition the person experiences and the impact of their life experiences on the commission of the offence. They make important but often overlooked points regarding the relationship between diagnosis of these disorders and sexual offences. As Seto (2008) points out, paedophilia (a psychiatric diagnosis) is an important factor in child molestation (a sexual offence) but the causal link between the two is not inevitable.

Part Three: Risk Assessment

In this section, three chapters consider issues around the assessment of risk and factors associated with sexual re-offending. William Lindsay and John Taylor (Chapter 8) begin this section and provide a comprehensive review of the risk factors associated with sexual offence recidivism within the mainstream literature and discuss how these risk factors can be applied to sexual offenders with ID.

Following on from this, in Chapter 9, Catrin Morrisey provides an overview of the relevant literature related to personality disorder and psychopathy in particular, both for forensic populations in general and for those with ID who offend sexually. Morrisey emphasises the importance of assessing for personality disorder in those referred to sex offender treatment in ID settings and that failing to recognise such disorder may result in a failure to provide appropriate treatment and management for the client. The chapter begins by describing the clinical symptomatology of personality disorder with particular reference to antisocial personal disorder and psychopathy associated with sexual offending. This is followed by a discussion on the problems in diagnosing personality disorder and psychoapthy in sexual offenders with ID. As an example of how this area is a new and developing area of research, Morrisey notes that no studies have thus far specifically examined the relationship between personality disorder and sexual offending in those who have ID. There seems little doubt that examination of personality disorder is likely to be relevant to some sexual offenders with ID. Morrisey goes on to provide a detailed analysis of the practical and ethical implications for assessing personality disorder and psychopathy in sexual offenders with ID and gives guidance on how to 'adapt' measures such as the Psychopathic Checklist-Revised (PCL-R) (Hare, 2003) when applied to offenders with ID. Morrisey highlights there are a number of intervention and management implications following a diagnosis of personality disorder in a person with ID who offends sexually and offers practical guidance to practitioners when working with this client group.

In Chapters 10 and 11, Douglas Boer, Matthew Frize, Ruth Pappas, Catrin Morrisey and William Lindsay review the use of the clinical structured risk assessment tools Historical Clinical Risk-20 (HCR-20: Webster, Douglas, Eaves & Hart, 1997) and Sexual Violence Risk-20 (SVR-20: Boer, Hart, Kropp & Webster, 1997) and provide alternative working definitions for sexual offenders with ID for both scales. Boer and colleagues make a number of suggestions to the items of both scales in an attempt to standardise the use of the scales when applied to people with ID. They propose that the principles and strategies elucidated in these chapters applied in risk assessment of offenders with ID could potentially be adapted to provide an assessment framework for people with ID who, though not ever (or at least not currently) involved in the criminal justice system, exhibit behaviours labelled as 'challenging'.

Part Four: Assessing Treatment Need and Deviancy

The focus of this section is the assessment of treatment need and sexual deviant interests in sexual offenders with ID. It has been well established that the identification and assessment of sexual deviancy is a central factor in terms of sexual recidivism risk and treatment targets. In Chapter 12 Leam Craig and William Lindsay consider the concept of measuring sexual deviancy in offenders with ID. The 'concept' of sexual deviancy is explored as part of the Structured Risk Assessment (SRA) model described by Thornton (2002). Following the recent development in the number of psychometric measures standardised on sexual offenders with ID, Craig and Lindsay organise the various psychometric measures within the SRA framework of assessment. It is argued that such an approach to assessment may help structure limited and valued resources based on the '*risk*, *need* and *responsivity*' principle in determining the course of treatment or management for a particular individual.

Following on from this, Peter Langdon and Glynis Murphy describe the process of assessing treatment need in sexual offenders with ID in Chapter 13. They argue that while the assessment of sexual offending by people with ID is no different from that used when assessing non-disabled sexual offenders some additional factors should be considered. They emphasise the importance of developing a functional analysis for the behaviour as part of a clinical assessment which can inform risk and treatment need. They review some of the risk assessment scales currently available and psychometric measures used to assess psychological constructs which may be used as an indicator of treatment amenability. They argue that when considering whether or not people with ID are likely to be amenable to psychological interventions it is important to challenge previous assumptions of amenability. They conclude that the process of assessing sexual offenders with ID is multifaceted, covering several areas of bio-psycho-social functioning. There is some emerging evidence to suggest that people with ID can complete some of the necessary tasks of cognitive-behavioural therapy, improving sexual knowledge and victim empathy as well as reducing the distorted cognitions.

Part Five: Provisions and Treatment

In this section four chapters review a range of different treatment approaches designed for sexual offenders with ID both within community and secure settings. Aside from the ongoing research and development into the assessment and treatment of sexual offenders with ID, the impact on staff and the support required in order to maintain a therapeutic environment with this challenging client group are all too often overlooked. In an attempt to address some of these issues, Shawn Mosher begins this section with Chapter 14 on a discussion of the staff support requirements when working with sexual offenders with ID. It is noted that working with a challenging client group can often have a number of effects on care staff including burnout, isolation and subtle shifts in the therapeutic milieu. Mosher highlights some of the effects on care staff and offers guidance in terms of staff training, supervision and support. It is crucial for all members of the care team to feel rewarded and valued, and issues around organisational structure, philosophy and staff isolation are also discussed. Equally important is the issue of security and managing the balance between client safety, staff safety and community safety. Here, Mosher describes a useful framework of the interplay between therapy and security. It is important to note that working with persons with an ID can be highly challenging but ultimately very rewarding employment and this chapter discusses several ways in which workers can be empowered to be good at their jobs, confident in their decisions and to build up a therapeutic and supportive rapport with the people they support.

In Chapter 15, William Lindsay, Amanda Michie and Frank Lambrick provide a review of the community-based treatment programmes currently available for sexual offenders with ID. They review the importance of placing treatment in the context of society and community. They go on to review the principles of treatment and its organisation, concentrating on cognitive behavioural methods. They also review research on characteristics of offenders and outcomes of treatment and management.

In Chapter 16, Fiona Williams and Ruth Mann describe Her Majesty's Prison Service 'Adapted' Sex Offender Treatment Programme (ASOTP). They begin by describing the development of the adapted programme using the same aims and objectives as those used in the mainstream programme based on the risk, need and responsiveness principle. They go onto describe the content and structure of the 14-block programme based on the Old Me/New Me model (Haaven, Little & Petre-Miller, 1990). They argue this approach is consistent with that of The Good Lives Model proposed by Ward (2002) because it is concerned with the enhancement of the offender's capabilities to improve their life. They highlight the importance of transitional care and maintenance when working with ID sex offenders and describe how the Adapted Better Lives Booster programme was designed to refresh, maintain and enhance the treatment gains made on the ASOTP. As is often the case in this area of research they highlight the difficulties of finding sufficient sample sizes in order to measure treatment efficacy. However, as part of a clinical evaluation of treatment effect they found evidence of positive cognitive shift by examining the pre- and post-treatment assessment measures. They note that the ASOTP is continually evolving to incorporate new ideas and as such a new adapted programme designed to meet the needs of those both in the community and in prison will be introduced in the coming years.

Finally in this section, in Chapter 17 Marleen Verhoeven discusses alternative approaches to working therapeutically with sexual offenders with ID and considers the application of dialectical behaviour therapy. She describes the complexities in the diagnosis of personality disorder for people with an ID and briefly describes psychological treatments for people who offend sexually. Dialectical Behaviour Therapy and various adaptations, both for offenders and for people with an ID are discussed in detail.

Part Six: Future Directions

In the final chapter of this book, Chapter 18, Hannah Ford and John Rose discuss improving service provisions for ID sexual offenders. Although offending by those with ID is not new, the detection and criminal justice response to offenders with ID is a developing area of debate. In this chapter Ford and Rose explore the possible pathways for ID sexual offenders through the criminal justice system, from reporting offences, police investigations and sentencing, to possible disposals such as prison, probation, mental health or specialist services. This is contrasted with the services offered in the United States and Australia. They go on to review the treatment, delivery and outcome across different service models and consider factors in intervening with ID offenders in these different settings. They offer practical suggestions on ways to improve service delivery for this client group. They highlight the need to improve education and training for staff and carers at all levels, particularly in relation to the recognition of ID in the criminal justice system and the need for further resources to develop treatment approaches and monitor the outcome of treatments. The importance of grounding the theoretical underpinnings of the treatment programme is discussed as well the relevance of specific aspects of treatment to ID offenders.

Summer 2009

Leam A. Craig
William R. Lindsay
Kevin D. Browne

REFERENCES

Bickley, J. & Beech, A. R. (2002). An empirical investigation of the Ward & Hudson self regulation model of the sexual offence process with child abusers. *Journal of Interpersonal Violence, 17* (371), 393.

Boer, D. P., Hart, S. D., Kropp, P. R. & Webster, C. D. (1997). *Manual for the Sexual Violence Risk – 20 Professional guidelines for assessing risk of sexual violence.* Vancouver, BC: The Mental Health, Law, and Policy Institute.

Clare, I. C. H. & Murphy, G. H. (1998). Working with offenders or alleged offenders with intellectual disabilities. In E. Emerson, C. Hatton, J. Bromley & A. Caine (Eds), *Clinical psychology and people with intellectual disabilities.* Chichester: J. Wiley.

Courtney, J., Rose, J. & Mason, O. (2006). The offence process of sex offenders with intellectual disabilities: A qualitative study. *Sexual Abuse: A Journal of Research and Treatment, 18* (2), 169–92.

Craig, L. A., Stringer, I. & Moss, T. (2006). Treating sexual offenders with learning disabilities in the community: A critical review. *International Journal of Offender Therapy and Comparative Criminology, 50,* 369–90.

Department of Health (2001). *Valuing people: A new strategy for learning disability for the 21st Century.* London: The Stationery Office.

Hare, R. D. (2003). *The Hare Psychopathy Checklist-Revised (PCL-R),* 2nd edn. Toronto, Canada: Multi-Health Systems.

Haaven, J., Little, R. & Petre-Miller, D. (1990). *Treating intellectually disabled sex offenders.* Orwell VT: Safer Society Press.

Holland, S. & Persson, P. (in press). Intellectual disability in the Victorian prison system: Characteristics of prisoners with an intellectual disability released from prison in 2003–2006. *Psychology, Crime and Law.*

Johnston, S. J. & Halstead, S. (2000). Forensic issues in intellectual disability. *Current Opinion in Psychiatry, 13,* 475–80.

Keeling, J. A., Rose, J. L. & Beech, A. R. (2006). A comparison of the application of the self-regulation model of the relapse process for mainstream and special needs offenders. *Sexual Abuse: A Journal of Research & Treatment, 18,* 373–82.

Langdon, P. E., Maxted, H. & Murphy, G. H. (2007). An exploratory evaluation of the Ward and Hudson Offending Pathways Model with sex offenders who have intellectual disabilities. *Journal of Intellectual & Developmental Disabilities, 32,* 94–105.

Lindsay, W. R., Michie, A. M., Whitefield, E., Martin, V., Grieve, A. & Carson, D. (2006). Response patterns on the Questionnaire on Attitudes Consistent with Sexual Offending in Groups of Sex Offenders with intellectual disabilities. *Journal of Applied Research in Intellectual Disabilities*, *19*, 47–53.

Lindsay, W. R., Neilson, Q. C., Morrison, F. & Smith, A. H. W. (1998). The treatment of six men with a learning disability convicted of sex offences with children. *British Journal of Clinical Psychology*, *37*, 83–98.

Lindsay, W. R., Olley, S., Baillie, N. & Smith, A. H. W. (1999). Treatment of adolescent sex offenders with intellectual disability. *Mental Retardation*, *37*, 201–11.

Lindsay, W. R., Steptoe, L. & Beech, A. T. (2008). The Ward and Hudson Pathways Model in sex offenders with intellectual disability. *Sexual Abuse: A Journal of Research & Treatment*, *4*, 379–92.

Lindsay, W. R. & Taylor, J. L. (2009). The assessment of treatment-related issues and risk in sex offenders and abusers with intellectual disability. In A. R. Beech, L. A. Craig & K. D. Browne (Eds), *Assessment and Treatment of Sex Offenders: A Handbook*. Chichester: Wiley-Blackwell.

Loucks, N. (2007). No one knows: Offenders with learning difficulties and learning disabilities: The prevalence and associated needs of offenders with learning difficulties and learning disabilities. Prison Reform Trust. Available from: Prison Reform Trust, 15 Northburgh Street, London, EC1V 0JR.

Ministry of Justice, (2008). Population in custody: Monthly tables May 2008. England and Wales. Retrieved January 2009. Available electronically from www.justice.gov.uk/publications/docs/population-in-custody-may08.pdf.

Ministry of Justice, (2009). Population in custody: Monthly tables May 2009. England and Wales. Retrieved July 2009. Available electronically from www.justice.gov.uk/publications/docs/population-in-custody-05-2009.pdf.

Mottram, P. G. (2007). *HMP Liverpool, Styal and Hindley study report*. Available from the author from the University of Liverpool, The School of Population, Community & Behavioural Sciences, Liverpool, UK. Available electronically from www.prisonreformtrust.org.uk/temp/StudyspReport2.pdf.

Murphy, G. H. (2007). Intellectual disabilities, sexual abuse and sexual offending. In A. Carr, G. O'Reilly, P. Noonan Walsh & J. McEvoy (Eds), *Handbook of intellectual disability and clinical psychology practice*. London: Routledge.

Murphy, G., Harnett, H. & Holland, A. J. (1995). A survey of intellectual disabilities among men on remand in prison. *Mental Handicap Research*, *8*, 81–98.

Murphy, M., Harrold, M., Carey, S. & Mulrooney, M. (2000). *A survey of the level of learning disability among the prison population in Ireland*. Dublin: Department of Justice, Equality and Law Reform.

Murphy, G., Powell, S., Guzman, A. M. & Hays, S. J. (2007). Cognitive-behavioural treatment for men with intellectual disabilities and sexually abusive behaviour: A pilot study. *Journal of Intellectual Disability Research*, *51* (11), 902–12.

O'Callaghan, D. (1999). Young abusers with learning disabilities: Towards better understanding and positive interventions. In M. C. Calder (Ed.), *Working with young people who sexually abuse: New pieces of the jigsaw puzzle* (pp. 225–50). Dorset: Russell House Publishing.

Prison Reform Trust (PRT) (2006). Memorandum submitted by the PRT. Retrieved 1 June 2009. Available electronically from www.parliament.the-Stationery-office.co.uk/pa/cm200607/cmselect/cmeduski/170/170we21.htm.

Rack, J. (2005). The incidence of disabilities in the prison population: Yorkshire and Humberside Research. Available from The Dyslexia Institute, Park House, Wick Road, Egham, Surrey TW20 0HH. Also available electronically from www.dyslexiaaction.org.uk/Administration/uploads/HiddenDisabilities.pdf.

Seto, M. C. (2008). *Pedophilia and sexual offending against children: Theory, assessment and intervention*. Washington DC, American Psychological Association.

Swanson, C. K. & Garwick, G. B. (1990). Treatment for low functioning sex offenders: Group therapy and interagency co-ordination. *Mental Retardation, 28,* 155–61.

Thornton, D. (2002). Constructing and testing a framework for dynamic risk assessment. *Sexual Abuse: A Journal of Research and Treatment, 14* (2), 139–53.

Ward, T. (2002). Good lives and the rehabilitation of offenders: Promises and problems. *Aggression and Violent Behaviour: A Review Journal, 7,* 513–28.

Ward, T. & Hudson, S. M. (1998). A model of the relapse process in sexual offenders. *Journal of Interpersonal Violence, 13,* 700–25.

Webster, C. D., Douglas, K. S., Eaves, D. & Hart, S. D. (1997). *HCR-20: Assessing risk for violence (Version 2).* Burnaby, British Columbia, Canada: The Mental Health, Law, and Policy Institute of Simon Fraser University.

Wechsler, D. (1991). *Wechsler intelligence scale for children – Third edition (WISC-III).* London: Psychological Corporation.

Wechsler, D. (1999). *Wechsler adult intelligence scale – Third edition (WAIS-III).* London: Psychological Corporation.

Williams, J. & Atthill, C. (2005). Learning difficulties and disabilities in prison: Setting the scene. Briefing paper for *No One Knows.* London: Prison Reform Trust.

2

Sexual Offenders with Intellectual Disabilities

Characteristics and Prevalence

LEAM A. CRAIG AND WILLIAM R. LINDSAY

INTRODUCTION

Assessment and treatment of sexual offenders has been the focus of considerable research in recent years (Beech, Craig & Browne, 2009; Marshall, Fernandez, Marshall & Serran 2006; Hanson *et al.* 2002), and the literature has witnessed the number of theoretical and clinical advances leading to increasingly effective risk assessment and treatment (Hanson & Thornton 2000, Marshall, Anderson & Fernandez, 1999; Thornton, 2002) and relapse prevention processes with sexual offenders (Ward & Hudson, 1998). However, while much of this research is based on mainstream sex offenders, it is only since the 1980s that researchers and clinicians have focused on sex offenders with intellectual disability (ID). Similarly, there is comparatively little research into the characteristics of men with ID and sexually abusive behaviour. The purpose of this chapter is to explore the aetiology of sexual offending and summarise the current literature in describing the characteristics of sexual offenders with ID. Before exploring some of the behavioural and psychological characteristics of sexual offenders with ID, it is important first of all to define the term 'Intellectual Disability' as this term is also used interchangeably with 'Learning Disability', 'Developmental Delay' and 'Mental Retardation'.

Defining Intellectual Disability

A major difficulty when reviewing the literature on sex offenders with ID is the variation of clinical diagnosis and descriptions of cognitive ability which makes making any direct comparison between studies problematic. For example, in their study of adolescent sexual offenders Gilby, Wolf and Goldberg (1989) described the sample as 'mentally retarded' who

Assessment and Treatment of Sexual Offenders with Intellectual Disabilities: A Handbook
Edited by Leam A. Craig, William R. Lindsay and Kevin D. Browne
© 2010 John Wiley & Sons, Ltd.

functioned in the moderate–mild range of intellectual disability. However, in his study, Day (1994) referred to his sample as moderate–mild intellectual disability, as well as those in the borderline range of learning disability. For the purposes of this chapter, the term 'intellectual disability' refers to the diagnostic criteria described by The Professional Affairs Board of The British Psychological Society (BPS) document, *ID: Definitions & Context* (2001), which recommends that a classification of ID should only be made on the basis of assessed impairments of both intellect and adaptive/social functioning. The document outlines the features that make up the definition of ID are consistent with that of The American Psychiatric Association (*Diagnostic & statistical manual of mental disorders, fourth edition, text revised* (DSM-IV-TR), 2000) and The Royal College of Psychiatrists (2001). They refer to three criteria for ID, all of which must be present for a person to be considered to have an intellectual disability:

1. a significant impairment of intellectual functioning with an Intelligence Quotient (IQ) of less than 70 – interpretation of IQ should take account of the standard error of the test.
2. significant impairment of adaptive and social functioning (i.e. the person's effectiveness in meeting the standards expected of his/her age and cultural group in at least two of the following: communication, self-care, home living, social and interpersonal skills, use of community resources, self-direction, functional academic skills, work, health and safety);
3. onset of impairment before the age of 18 years.

An individual is defined as having significant impairment of adaptive and social functioning when he or she 'requires significant assistance to provide for his/her own survival (eating and drinking needs, and to keep him/herself clean, warm and clothed), and/or with his/her social/ community adaptation (e.g., social problem solving and social reasoning)' (BPS Professional Affairs, Board, 2001, p. 6). Difficulties in assessing adaptive/social functioning have contributed to a tendency among clinicians to concentrate on assessment of intellectual functioning (BPS Professional Affairs, Board, 2001). This assumes that provided significant impairment of intellectual functioning has been established, similar deficits and adaptive/social functioning are likely (p. 4). The diagnosis of an ID is not solely related to intellect. It is a mistake to over emphasise the role of IQ as an indicator of appropriate treatment strategies since IQ alone does not adequately describe a person's ability (Coleman & Haaven, 2001).

The principal method for determining levels of intellectual functioning is the use of psychometric assessment. The most commonly used assessment is the Wechsler Adult Intelligence Scale – III Edition (WAIS III) (Wechsler, 1999) from which IQ can be calculated. The mean IQ Score is 100 with a standard deviation of 15. A score of 1 standard deviation below the mean would correspond to an IQ of 85 or lower, and 2 standard deviations below the mean would correspond to an IQ of 70 and/or lower. In addition to using formal assessments of intellectual functioning, the *International classification of diseases* – 10 (ICD-10) (WHO, 1992) and the Professional Affairs Board recommends the use of the *Vineland adaptive behaviour scales* (VABS) (Sparrow, Balla & Cicchetti 1984) as an assessment tool to measure impairment of adaptive/social functioning. The VABS assesses the developmental level of populations with ID and provides an estimate of the person's developmental level in each of the three areas of communication, daily living skills and socialisation as well as providing a general estimate of developmental functioning based on the aggregate level of the scores. In general terms, individuals with ID are likely to experience a range of important cognitive deficits including reduced capacity for and speed of processing information; difficulties in learning new information; concrete thinking styles that present difficulties in dealing with abstract information; difficulties with language; and limited education based knowledge and skills (Mackinnon, Bailey & Pink, 2004).

Before exploring the characteristics of sexual offenders with ID, the next section considers the various aetiological theories used to explain sexual offending in this population.

Aetiological Theories of Sexual Offending by Men with Intellectual Disabilities

In trying to explain sexual offending in people with ID, a number of hypotheses have been postulated. These are summarised as follows:

Counterfeit Deviance

This hypothesis was first outlined by Hingsburger, Griffiths and Quinsey (1991) and attempts to explain that inappropriate sexual behaviour in men with ID has been precipitated by factors such as a lack of sexual knowledge, poor social and interpersonal skills, limited opportunities to establish appropriate sexual relationships and sexual naivety rather than deviant sexual interests. Luiselli (2000) argues that the counterfeit deviance hypothesis was the most influential basis for the development of treatment services for offenders with ID. Based on this hypothesis, Griffiths, Quinsey and Hingsburger (1989) developed a comprehensive behavioural and educational programme to promote personal, social and sexual competence in men with ID who had behaved inappropriately sexually. This was an impressive rehabilitative programme employing a range of assessments and treatment approaches focussing on interpersonal relationships and interpersonal skills. The authors reported on a series of 30 cases in which they recorded no re-offending and described a number of successful cases to illustrate their methods. Others (e.g., Haaven, Little & Petra-Miller 1990; Grubb-Blubaugh, Shaire & Bausler, 1994) have also employed behavioural and social programmes to promote appropriate skills and reduce inappropriate sexual behaviour in similar cases.

More recently a number of studies have cast doubt on the validity of the counterfeit deviance hypothesis. Lambrick and Glasser (2004) reported that features of poor sexual knowledge and social skills have been found in mainstream sex offenders and that this may indicate a vulnerability to detection in those with ID rather than specific characteristics disposing them to commit offences. Similarly, Galea, Butler, Iacono and Leighton (2004) used the Assessment of Sexual Knowledge (ASK) and found that sexual offenders with ID had good sexual knowledge on the topics of parts of the body and public and private places. They found that participants had a relatively poor knowledge of sexually transmitted diseases and contraception, although these two areas of sexual knowledge have been shown to be poorer than others across a range of groups including non-sexual offenders with ID and college students (Lindsay, Bellshaw, Culross, Staines & Michie, 1992; Griffiths & Lunsky 2003). Several authors have reported increases in sexual knowledge following sex education programmes (Craig, Stringer & Moss, 2006; Lindsay, Bellshaw, Culross, Staines & Michie, 1992).

A number of research groups have now tested the counterfeit deviance hypothesis directly. Talbot and Langdon (2006) assessed the sexual knowledge of sex offenders with ID who had been in treatment, those who had not been in treatment and control participants who had not offended. They found no significant differences between the untreated sex offenders and the non-offenders and concluded that limited sexual knowledge was unlikely to be a factor placing men with ID at risk of committing sexual offences. Michie, Lindsay, Martin and Grieve (2006) used the Socio Sexual Knowledge & Attitudes Test (SSKAT) in a comparison of levels of sexual knowledge in people with ID who had committed sexual offences and others who had not. They found that the sexual offender cohort actually had a higher level of sexual knowledge than the non-sexual offenders, casting doubt on the causative effect of poor sexual knowledge on the commission of sexual offences. These authors then pooled the data for all 33 sex offenders and 35 control participants and found a significant positive correlation between the IQ and SSKAT total score for the control group but no significant relationship between IQ and SSKAT total score for the sex offender cohort. They suggested that the lack of correlation for the sex offender cohort may indicate both increased sexual interest for these participants, irrespective of intellectual ability, and prior sexual contact which, by definition, all those participants had experienced. These authors concluded that their results cast doubt on the counterfeit deviance hypothesis.

Lunsky, Frijters, Griffiths, Watson and Williston (2007) conducted a further, more detailed study comparing a cohort of men who had committed sexual offences with controls who had committed no sexual offences. They split the sexual offenders into those who had committed repeated and forced offences and those who had committed inappropriate sexual behaviours such as public masturbation or inappropriate touching. They found that the former (repeated and forceful offenders) had higher levels of sexual knowledge than the non-offenders. However, the inappropriate offenders had a level of knowledge and attitudes more consistent with non-offenders. They concluded that the counterfeit deviance hypothesis may continue to pertain to inappropriate offenders rather than persistent deviant offenders.

Taking these various studies into account, Lindsay (2009) has constructed a revision of the counterfeit deviance hypothesis. He has postulated that although sex offenders with ID may have a higher level of sexual knowledge and more liberal sexual attitudes than non-offenders, their sexual knowledge remains at a stage where it is considerably poorer than that required by non-handicapped men. In addition, although they may also understand something of the illegality of inappropriate sexual behaviour, they may not have a full comprehension of the extent of which such practices are condemned by society. This relative lack of understanding may interact with a wish or need for sexual contact or indeed a deviant sexual interest resulting in episodes of inappropriate sexual behaviour. Prolonged treatment may provide the opportunity to develop appropriate sexual knowledge and understanding of society's laws and conventions to the extent that the individual becomes motivated to learn a range of pro-social heterosexual skills and strategies for self-restraint that non-handicapped adult males adopt as part of their developmental experiences. Therefore, although in the early 2000s some doubt has been placed on the counterfeit deviance hypothesis, it remains an important partial explanation for inappropriate sexual behaviour in men with ID.

Tendencies toward Sexual Offending and Lack of Discrimination

This hypothesis assumes persistent sexual offending as a result of deviant sexual interests mediated by cognitive distortions and attention to selective cues that are interpreted in a sexual manner. Like sexual offenders without ID (Hanson & Bussière, 1998), sexual offenders with ID have been found to display deviant sexual arousal patterns and cognitive distortions (Murphy, Coleman & Haynes, 1983), as well as having low self-esteem (Lackey & Knopp, 1989). There is some anecdotal evidence related to the persistence of inappropriate sexual behaviour in some men with ID which would support the hypothesis of deviant sexual interest. In an early study, Scorzelli and Reinke-Scorzelli (1979) reported that 68 per cent of a mixed group of offenders with learning disability had previous offences. Lindsay *et al.* (2002) reported that 62 per cent of referrals of sex offenders with ID had a history of sexual offending. When one considers that it is fairly usual for a great deal of censure to be aimed at these individuals following an incident of inappropriate sexual behaviour, the fact that a significant percentage persist in the behaviour suggests a degree of inappropriate drive or sexual deviancy. It has also been suggested that sex offenders with ID tend to have low specificity for the age and sex of their victims (Gilby, Wolf & Goldberg, 1989; Griffiths, Hinsburger & Christian, 1985) and may have a greater tendency to offend against male children and younger children (Blanchard *et al.*, 1999).

    A series of studies by Blanchard and colleagues deserve further attention. Blanchard *et al.* (1999) investigated patterns of sexual offending in a large group of 950 participants. They reported that 'lower functioning' sexual offenders were significantly more likely to commit offences against younger children and male children. Although the proportion of variance was not high, they also reported that their results suggest that choices of male or female victims by offenders with ID were not primarily determined by accessibility or other circumstantial factors but by their relative sexual interest in male and female children. In a further study, Cantor, Blanchard, Robichaud and Christensen (2005) reported a detailed meta-analytic study of previous reports which have included reliable data on IQ and sexual offending. They reanalysed data on 25,146 sex offenders and controls and found a robust relationship between lower IQ and sexual offending. More specifically, the relationship was between lower IQ and paedophilia. They hypothesised that some organic perturbation may be the cause of both low IQ and sexual interest in children. For the purposes of this volume, it has to be said that although the difference in IQ between those participants who offended against children and those participants who have offended against adults was significant, the individuals who offended against children had a mean IQ which remained in the normal range. However, this information on the relationship between intellectual ability and sexual preference, coming as it does from a highly reliable research group, presents more persuasive evidence than the essentially anecdotal accounts of previous authors such as Lindsay *et al.* (2002, 2004). Therefore, sexual drive and sexual preference may be important considerations within a treatment programme and several treatment chapters in this volume (Eccleston, Ward & Waterman, Chapter 5; Lindsay, Michie & Lambrick, Chapter 15) argue that self-regulation and self-control of any inappropriate sexual drive or preference is an important aspect of treatment programmes.

Sexual Abuse

This hypothesis assumes that there may be an association with sexual abuse in childhood and sexual offending. There is no doubt that several authors have found a high incidence of childhood sexual abuse among samples of sex offenders with ID (Thompson & Brown 1997). However, Langevin and Pope (1993), with non-handicapped offenders, and Briggs and Hawkins (1996) note that not all sexual abusers will themselves have been abused and it is not the case that all individuals who have been sexually abused will become sexual abusers or offenders. Lindsay, Law, Quinn, Smart and Smith (2001) compared the physical and sexual abuse histories of 46 sexual and 48 non-sexual offenders with intellectual disabilities and found that 38 per cent of the sexual offenders and 12.7 per cent of the non-sexual offenders had experienced sexual abuse while 13 per cent of the sexual offenders and 33 per cent of the non-sexual offenders had experienced physical abuse. This study gave some support to the hypothesis that experience of sexual abuse in childhood will promote a cycle in which the individual 'acts out' their childhood experiences with others in the form of sexual abuse. However, even in this study, where the sex offenders with ID had significantly higher rates of sexual abuse in childhood, it was still the case that the majority of sexual offenders (62 per cent) did not report experiencing sexual abuse in childhood. Furthermore, the 12 per cent of non-sexual offenders who had been sexually abused in childhood did not go on to commit a sexual offence.

Another significant study presents pause for thought in relation to the 'abused to abuser' hypothesis. A major review of sexual abuse was conducted by the House of Representatives (General Accounting Office, 1996) in which they commissioned a retrospective/prospective study in relation to sexual abuse and sexual offending. The study involved a review of records from the early 1970s of boys who had attended the Emergency Department in two major United States hospitals. Information was collected on those boys who had attended for reasons of general injuries such as sports injuries and medical problems and a second cohort of boys who had attended for reasons of sexual abuse. As many as possible of these males were then followed up until the late1990s to ascertain the extent to which they differed in respect of the numbers who had recorded sexually abusive incidents. No difference was found between the group who had been sexually abused and the group who had not. Sequeira and Hollins (2003) note that the few existing studies on sexual abuse and people with ID, such as Beail and Warden (1995), suggest that behavioural problems such as sexual disinhibition may be a consequence of sexual abuse in childhood. However, lack of standardised assessments, lack of appropriate control and an absence of agreed criteria used to report sexual abuse make such conclusions speculative. In addition, the conclusions from the study commissioned by the House of Representatives would suggest that if sexual abuse is a variable which has salience in the commission of sexual offences then it remains far from a complete account.

Personality Characteristics and Impulsivity

In studies of mainstream sex offenders, there has been a growing awareness that personality considerations are an important variable when evaluating whether or not an individual is at risk of committing a sexual offence. Much of this evidence comes from the work on risk assessment in which personality measures have been included in assessments reviewing the risk of future sexual incidents. The Sex Offender Risk Appraisal Guide (SORAG), developed by Quinsey, Harris, Rice and Cormier (1998, 2006), has been found to be one of the best predictors of future sexual offences in cohorts of previous sexual offenders (e.g., Barbaree, Seto, Langton & Peacock 2001; Bartosh, Garby, Lewis & Gray 2003). The SORAG is based on its sister assessment The Violence Risk Appraisal Guide (VRAG) and includes four broad clusters of variables. These are variables related to childhood adjustment, those related to adult adjust- ment, those related to offence characteristics and assessment information. Items related to adult adjustment include sex offence history and the nature of victims while those related to offence characteristics review the relationship of the offender to the victim. However, included in the assessment information and in the adult adjustment variables are a number of items related to personality characteristics and anti-sociality, including any previous diagnosis of personality disorder, scores on the Psychopathy Check List Revised (PCL-R) and any criminal history for violent offending. Harris, Rice, Quinsey, Lalumiere, Boer and Lang (2003) found that the PCL-R (Hare, 1991) made significant, independent contributions to predictions for future offending in a large cohort of sexual offenders.

Several authors have used risk assessments which incorporate personality disorder measures and evaluations of antisociality and have found the predictive reliablity of these assessments with regard to future violent offences in offenders with ID to be equal that for mainstream offenders (Quinsey, Book & Skilling, 2004; Lindsay *et al.*, 2008). Morrissey *et al.* (2007) and Morrissey, Mooney, Hogue, Lindsay and Taylor (2007) found that the PCL-R scores were significantly associated with level of security and inversely associated with treatment progress in a mixed group of offenders with ID. Therefore, it is likely that personality correlates are an important factor in assessment and treatment of sex offenders with ID in that significant antisociality may be associated with high doses of treatment.

One specific personality characteristic has been singled out as potentially important for sex offenders with ID. Swartz and Masters (1983) argue that populations of adult sex offenders, both those with ID and those with normal intellectual functioning, exhibit complex cognitive and behavioural characteristics, various levels of denial, immature social skills (including lack of assertiveness), low self-esteem/high self-criticism, poor empathy and deficient processing and evaluation skills. They also state that sex offenders with and without ID all exhibit poor impulse control. Several authors have hypothesised that impulsivity is likely to be a feature of sexual offenders with ID (e.g., Caparulo, 1991; Hayes, 1991). However, observations based on clinical samples must be treated with caution since the characteristics may simply reflect the nature of the referral pattern in that area or to that clinician. Glaser and Deane (1999) looked at a total of 120 offenders with ID who had been admitted to an intensive residential treatment programme based in Victoria and Melbourne, as well as a unit within Victoria prison, between 1989 and 1994. Comparing the sexual and non-sexual offenders, they found no differences in variables such as age, marital status, educational history, family disruption, accommodation at time of index offence and contact with psychiatric services. What they did find, however, were significant differences relating to substance misuse and prior imprisonment. The sex offender group had a much lower rate (past and present) of abusing drugs or alcohol (21 per cent compared to 78 per cent in the non-sex offender group) and fewer sex offenders had served prior terms in prison (37 per cent compared to 74 per cent). Notably, there was a slightly higher, non-significant, proportion of non-sex offenders with a prior history of sexual offences. These authors found it to be 'a reasonable conclusion . . . that for some disabled offenders, sex crimes are part of a pattern of impulsivity and poorly controlled behaviour consistent with psychosocial disadvantage rather than with any inherent propensity for sexual deviation' (p. 349). Therefore, Glaser and Deane (1999) hypothesise that these offenders with ID are characterised by impulsivity which will lead them to a range of offending including sexual offences.

In a subsequent study, Parry and Lindsay (2003) compared 22 sex offenders with groups of non-sexual offenders and non-offenders, all with ID, using the Barratt Impulsiveness Scale (BIS). They found that sexual offenders reported significantly lower impulsiveness traits in all areas than their comparison groups. These authors noted that the high frequency of grooming behaviour by such offenders, albeit simple grooming behaviour, suggested that they were aware of the importance of gaining the victims' trust and friendship and also suggested an ability to delay gratification to some extent, which is exactly the opposite to the features of impulsiveness. However, it may also be the case that different categories of sexual offender may differ with regard to impulsiveness. For example, offenders against children may have a greater ability to plan and delay gratification than offenders against adults, who may have a greater tendency to act on the spur of the moment. Given the findings of Lunsky, Frijters, Griffiths, Watson and Williston (2007), reported above, one might also hypothesise that inappropriate offenders may have higher levels of impulsivity than persistent deviant offenders. Parry and Lindsay (2003) also made the important distinction between trait and state impulsiveness and agitation. They assessed trait impulsiveness whereas more transitory states of agitation and impulsiveness may have different effects. These transitory states may appear more frequently in different categories of sexual offenders with ID, such as the inappropriate, non-contact offences reported in the Lunsky, Frijters, Griffiths, Watson and Williston (2007) study. In this way concepts of personality traits and impulsiveness can be considered alongside the hypothesis of counterfeit deviance.

Mental Illness

This hypothesis assumes that sexual offenders with ID are more likely to have a dual diagnosis of mental illness acting as a disinhibitor for offending. Day (1994) and Lindsay *et al.* (2004) both reported that 32 per cent of sexual offenders with ID had been diagnosed with psychiatric illness. However, Lund (1990) reported on 274 offenders with ID most of whom were under care orders or restriction orders imposed by the legal system. A substantial 91.7 per cent of this cohort had a diagnosed mental illness, 87.5 per cent of which were categorised as behaviour disorders. This gives rise to questions about the inclusion criteria for mental illness across various studies. There have obviously been some methodological differences whereby challenging and behaviour disorder have been included as a mental illness or have been classified separately in different studies. In both the Day (1994) study and the Lindsay *et al.* (2002) study, behaviour disorders were classified separately. In addition, Lambrick and Glaser (2004) and Lindsay, Smith, Law (2004) compared cohorts of sexual offenders with cohorts of other types of male offenders. Both these studies reported no differences between the groups in terms of the incidence of recorded mental illness. This certainly suggests that mental illness is not a primary motivating factor in the commission of sexual offences since the cohorts of individuals in the group whose offences were non-sexual had similar rates of mental illness.

In studies on the prediction of offences in general and sexual offences in particular, mental illness has been an ever-present variable in the diverse analyses. Interestingly, different researchers have arrived at opposing conclusions on the influence of mental illness in relation to the perpetration of offences. In their classic study on variables predicting future violent recidivism, Harris, Rice and Quinsey (1993) included a number of assessment variables. They found that a diagnosis of schizophrenia was, significantly, negatively associated with recidivism with 12 per cent of re-offenders having such a diagnosis but 28 per cent of those who had not re-offended having a diagnosis of schizophrenia. Therefore, there was a significantly higher level of mental illness in those individuals who did not re-offend. The variable of mental illness was significant and robust enough in this and subsequent studies for these authors to include it as a protective factor in risk assessment for violence and risk assessment for future sexual offending. (SORAG, Quinsey, Harris, Rice & Cormier, 2006). Bonta, Law and Hanson (1996) carried out a meta-analysis of factors predicting recidivism in which they categorised a range of variables into deviant lifestyle, criminal history, personal demographic and clinical. In their study, static criminal history variables had the largest predictive effect. Some personal demographic variables (marital status, gender and age), substance abuse and deviant lifestyle variables were also significantly related to recidivism. However, a diagnosis of psychosis was negatively related to recidivism.

In a replication of the findings of Bonta *et al.* (1998), Phillips *et al.* (2005) conducted a similar study with a cohort of 315 mentally disordered offenders from secure hospital settings. They found that the variables related to previous offences and demographic variables were predictive of future recidivism but clinical diagnosis made no additive contribution to these predictions. In their study on a range of variables and their contribution to the prediction of future sexual offences in 52 sex offenders with ID, Lindsay, Elliot and Astell (2004) found that a previous diagnosis of mental illness did not correlate significantly with re-offending and made no contribution to the regression analysis.

While there is a body of research which does not support the contribution of mental illness to risk for future offending and sexual offending, in their important risk assessment, the HCR-20, Webster, Douglas, Eaves and Hart (1997) include major mental illness as a historical and current risk factor. They cite a range of research including the important study by Hodgins (1992) in which she conducted a large-scale piece of research on 15,117 individuals followed up over 30 years. She found that those who had been diagnosed with major mental disorder were 2.5 times more likely to commit crime than men with no disorder. However, the type of major mental disorder was not specified in this study. Swanson, Borum, Swartz and Monahan (1996) also found that there was an increased risk of future violence associated with those individuals who had an underlying mental disorder. They further investigated their cohort, separating them into different clusters of psychotic symptoms. Those who had symptoms associated with paranoid delusions and perceived threat were particularly at risk of future assaultive behaviour. They were around twice as likely to engage in assaults when compared to those who experienced hallucinations or other psychotic symptoms. Both groups were more likely to engage in assault than those with no mental disorder. In relation to general and sexual recidivism, in a review of 153 consecutive referrals of offenders with ID over an eight-year period, Smith, Quinn and Lindsay (2000) found that 22 per cent of the sample had a serious recorded mental illness. They noted that this rate was sevenfold higher than in non-offender populations with ID, suggesting that mental illness was a risk factor for offending in populations of individuals with ID.

There is, therefore, conflicting research on the importance of mental illness with regard to future risk of offending. There are excellent studies which have found a higher rate of mental illness in violent offenders (Hogdins 1992; Swanson, Borum, Swartz & Monahan, 1996) and equally good studies finding a lower rate of major mental illness in violent recidivists (Harris, Rice & Quinsey, 1993). Other studies again have found no relationship between mental illness and recidivism (Phillips *et al.* 2005; Lindsay, Elliot & Astell, 2004). In their review of the relationship between mental illness and offenders with ID, Smith and O'Brien (2004) concluded that 'pharmacological treatment of the illness is not sufficient for the effective management of most offenders, particularly sex offenders involving children and offenders convicted of arson' (p. 253). In addition, they make the important point that effective pharmacological treatment can allow an offender to become better organised when their psychosis is better controlled. As a result of this more effective personal organisation, certain individuals can become at greater risk of planning a future offence. In two important reviews on the relationship between psychotic symptoms violence towards others, Bjorkly (2002a, b) concluded that on the one hand the available evidence suggested that persecutory delusions appeared to increase risk for violence and the presence of persecutory delusions and emotional stress also increased the risk of violence, while, on the other hand, the evidence linking hallucinations and command hallucinations to violence was inconclusive.

Prevalence

Accurate estimations concerning the prevalence of sex offenders with ID are notoriously difficult to establish since sexually abusive behaviour by men with ID often goes unreported (Murphy, 2007). Indeed, a significant increase in research of sexual offenders with ID has led to an awareness that sexual offences by men with 'special needs' may be more prevalent than previously acknowledged (Dolan, Holloway, Bailey & Kroll, 1996; Timms & Goreczny, 2002). Many studies have highlighted ID as more prevalent among those who offend and those who offend sexually. Commonly cited evidence of relatively high or increasing incidents of sexual offending with ID populations include studies by Lund (1990), Gross (1985), and Walker and McCabe (1973). For example, in their classic study of secure hospitals in England, Walker and McCabe (1973) reviewed 331 men with ID who had committed offences and had been detained under hospital orders to secure provision in England and Wales. They found high rates of fire raising (15 per cent) and sexual offences (28 per cent) when compared with other groups in the secure hospital sample. However, as Lindsay, Hastings, Griffiths and Hayes (2007) have pointed out, studies conducted in different settings have produced different prevalences of offenders and types of offending. In a more recent study, which included offenders detained under hospital orders to secure provision, Hogue et al. (2006) reviewed a number of characteristics of offenders with ID across community, medium/low secure and high secure settings. He found that rates of arson in the index offence depended on the setting with lower rates in the community setting (2.9 per cent) and higher rates in the medium/low secure setting (21.4 per cent). This was a clear example of the fact that the setting in which the data was collected is very likely to influence the results and subsequent conclusions about the population.

Well controlled studies have found prevalence rates for individuals with ID to be slightly higher in offender populations than in the general population. MacEachron (1979) conducted a carefully controlled study in which she employed recognised intelligence tests in 436 adult male offenders in Maine and Massachusetts state penal institutions. She reported prevalence rates of ID of 0.6–2.3 per cent. These rates are broadly consistent with the rates of ID in the general population.

The methodological difficulties between studies make it extremely difficult to make sound estimates of offenders with ID in a range of criminal populations. These methodological differences continue to the present day as evidenced by two pieces of research finding markedly different rates of offenders with ID in prison settings. Crocker, Cote, Toupin and St-Onge (2007) attempted to assess 749 offenders in a pre-trial holding centre in Montreal.

For a number of reasons, including refusal to participate, administrative difficulties and technical problems, they were only able to assess 281 participants with three sub-scales of a locally standardised mental ability scale. They reported that 18.9 per cent were in the probable ID range with a further 29.9 per cent in the borderline range of intelligence. This study reported very high rates of people with ID in the prison system. On the other hand, in a study of prisoners in Victoria, Australia, Holland and Persson (in press) found a prevalence rate of less than 1.3 per cent using the Wechsler Adult Intelligence Scale (WAIS). In the latter study, all prisoners were assessed routinely by trained forensic psychologists while, in the former study, only around one-third of potential participants were included in the study. In the former study, three sub-scales of an intelligence test were used while, in the latter, a full WAIS was used for all participants. It is difficult to reconcile these two pieces of work but it is likely that the differences in assessment methods and comprehensiveness of the sample were significant contributors to the disparity of results.

In the study described previously, Cantor, Blanchard, Robichaud and Christensen (2005) conducted a meta-analysis of reports on sexual offending and IQ which included over 25,000 sexual offenders and controls. They found a significant relationship between low IQ and sexual offending and, in particular, low IQ and paedophilia. There was no comparable relationship between IQ and sexual offending against adults or sexual offending in juvenile populations. In a further study, Blanchard *et al.* (2007) reviewed the information on 832 adult sex offenders and found that those who offended against children had an IQ around 10 points lower than those who offended against adults. However, the offenders against children had an average IQ of 90, which is well in excess of the range of intellectual disability. Ho (1997) studied 288 subjects (including 82 sex offenders) from The Mentally Retarded Defendant Programme (MRDP), a secure forensic institution in Florida for offenders who are not considered competent to stand trial because of intellectual disability. He concluded, 'This study demonstrated that there were no significant differences in a variety of MRDP offender demographic, psychiatric, and legal characteristics between retarded sex offenders and other retarded offenders. Regardless of the type of criminal charges, mentally retarded sex offenders were indistinguishable from other retarded offenders in terms of offender mental retardation, deficit of adaptive behaviour and IQ' (p. 259). Therefore, in this study of offenders with ID, there were no systematic differences between those who had committed sex offences and others. Hayes (1991) reported findings on a comparison between offenders with and without ID. She found fairly similar and low (between 3 per cent and 4 per cent) figures of sexual conviction among both cohorts and concluded there seemed no clear evidence for either over-representation or under-representation of intellectual disability clients in the sex offender population.

Types of Offending and Re-offending

In a 10-month prospective study, Barron, Hassiotis and Banes (2004) followed up 61 offenders with ID referred to specialist mental health and criminal justice services. Although not specific to sexual offenders, they found that ID offenders started offending at an earlier age, had a history of multiple offences and that sexual and arson offences were over-represented and half re-offended at follow-up. While these authors found a higher rate of sexual and arson offences, it has to be remembered that Hogue *et al.* (2006), in their study across different settings, found that arson offences were significantly lower in a community forensic sample in low/medium secure setting. Thompson and Brown (1997) estimated that 6 per cent of the population of individuals with ID had severe sexual aggression while McBrien, Hodgetts and Gregory (2003) found that 41 per cent engaged in challenging behaviour defined as 'sex related', of which 17 per cent had had police contact and 4 per cent were convicted of sexual crimes. Therefore, it would seem that at least a proportion of inappropriate sexual behaviour in men with ID goes unreported to the authorities. Hawk, Rosenfield and Warren (1993) found the prevalence rate of sex offence charges was nearly twice as high among defendants with ID than among non-disabled defendants. Therefore, there is some evidence that sex offences may be more prevalent among individuals with ID than in the general population.

Having made this point, it is important to note that the higher prevalence rate may be, to some extent, an artefact of several sources. It has to be remembered that people with ID are generally under greater scrutiny from relatives and carers than those others in the general population. Men with ID who behave inappropriately sexually are more likely to be supervised and detected by significant others than normally able men in ordinary circums- tances. As a result, inappropriate sexual behaviour in men with ID may be more likely to be reported. Another factor is that a higher prevalence rate may be an artefact of misinterpreta- tion of certain behaviours by others. As has been noted, Hingsburger, Griffiths and Quinsey (1991) have argued that many instances of inappropriate sexual behaviour in men with ID are in fact the result of lack of knowledge and lack of understanding of the laws of society rather than deviant sexual interest. Craig and Hutchinson (2005) have also pointed out that when men with ID commit a sexual offence it is often less sophisticated than similar offences in mainstream populations, and this correspondingly increases the possibility of detection. Furthermore, in studies comparing rates of sexual offending and ID and non-ID groups, it is not clear whether those groups are matched on a range of socio-demographic variables.

These various sexual re-offence rates are somewhat high compared with the UK sexual re- conviction rate ranging from 2 per cent to 12 per cent in a four-year follow-up period, from 3 per cent to 14 per cent in a six-year follow-up period and from 18 per cent to 25 per cent in a 21-year follow-up period for mainstream sexual offenders without ID (Craig, Browne, Stringer & Hogue, 2008). A review of UK mainstream (non-ID) sex offender follow-up studies reported the mean sexual reconviction rate was 5 per cent at two years and 6 per cent at four years. Using Klimecki, Jenkinson and Wilson's (1994) re-offence rates of 34 per cent at two years and Lindsay et al.'s (2002) re-offence rate of 21 per cent at four years, Craig and Hutchinson (2005) calculated that the re-conviction rate for sex offenders with ID is 6.8 times and 3.5 times that of sex offenders without ID at two years and four years follow-up respectively. However, Lindsay and colleagues (Lindsay et al. 2002; Lindsay, Steele, Smith, Quinn & Allan 2006) have used different definitions as indications of offending, re-offending and inappropriate sexual behaviour, which may limit the extent to which the rates of recidivism of various studies can be compared. These authors reported a wide-ranging network of social and health care workers who reported any incident within a circumscribed and relatively stable geographical population. In this study, they felt that most, if not all, incidents of inappropriate sexual behaviour would be reported back to the forensic intellectual disability service and each of these reports was counted as an incident of re-offending, whether or not it had been prosecuted or received any criminal justice intervention. Depending on which definition was being used, and the method for recording offending behaviour, the base rate for sexual reconviction, re-arrest and recidivism will vary (Falshaw, Bastes, Patel, Corbett & Friendship

2003). The methodological differences associated with measuring the prevalence of sexual offending by people with ID also apply when estimating the sexual reconviction rates in this client group.

Lindsay (2002) argues that although some studies have suggested an increase in incidents of sexual offences among offenders with ID, there is no compelling evidence for the over- or under-representation of people with intellectual disabilities among sex offenders. Methodological differences between studies are so great that it is extremely difficult to draw any firm conclusions. As we have pointed out, these methodological differences continue until the time of writing in 2009. It would be inaccurate to take the figures from various stages in the criminal justice system at face value and not consider the filters involved at each stage (e.g., prior to arrest, at point of charging, when attending court or when receiving sentencing). Indeed Ho (1997) comments 'the coexistence of mental retardation and sex-related criminality among retarded criminal offenders creates substantial difficulties to the criminal justice system' (p. 251), both in terms of assessing criminal responsibility and designing treatment programmes. It may be that inappropriate sexual behaviour in convicted offender with ID results in a different profile of sentencing.

The information on recidivism is similarly difficult to assess. Several studies since the early 1960s have reported re-offending rates of around 50 per cent in mixed groups of offenders with ID (e.g., Gibbens & Robertson, 1983; Lund, 1990; Wildenskov, 1962). Some more recent studies reported recidivism rates of offenders with ID who have presumably been subject to the policies of deinstitutionalisation. Klimecki, Jenkinson and Wilson (1994) report re-offending rates in previous prison inmates with ID two years after their release. They found that overall, re-offending rates were 41.3 per cent with higher rates for less serious offences. However, the lower re-offending rates (around 31 per cent) for sex offences, murder and violent offences were artificially reduced because a number of those individuals were still in prison and therefore unable to re-offend. Linhorst, McCutchen and Bennet (2003) followed up 252 convicted offenders with ID who had completed a case management community programme found that 25 per cent who had completed the programme were rearrested within six months and 43 per cent of those who dropped out were re-arrested during the same period. A lack of controlled studies involving ID and mainstream offenders makes it is difficult to make direct comparisons of recidivism rates. However, it would appear that recidivism rated for offenders with ID are consistent with those for populations of mainstream offenders.

In one recent study, Gray, Fitzgerald, Taylor, MacCulloch and Snowden (2007) conducted a two-year follow-up of 145 offenders with ID and 996 offenders without ID, all discharged from independent sector hospitals in the UK. The ID group had a lower rate of reconviction for violent offences after two years (4.8 per cent) than the non-ID group (11.2 per cent). This trend also held true for general offences (9.7 per cent for the ID group and 18.7 per cent for the non-ID group). While this latter study is not specifically restricted to sexual offenders, its well-controlled design casts doubt on the hypothesis that offenders with ID have a higher reconviction rate than mainstream offenders. Clearly, there is a wide range of conflicting evidence on both the prevalence of offenders and sex offenders with ID in the criminal population and their relative rates of reconviction. However, it has to be said that all of the research studies agree that there is a significant proportion of men with ID in the sex offender population and that these individuals require treatment and service provision if we are to deal with their risk for future re-offending.

CHARACTERISTICS ASSOCIATED WITH SEXUAL OFFENDERS WITH INTELLECTUAL DISABILITIES

Sexual Offence Characteristics

In one of the first pieces of work reviewing the types of sexual offences committed by men with ID, Day (1994) reported that these men tended to offend equally against male and female victims. Gilby, Wolf and Goldberg (1989) also reported a tendency for men with ID to have low specificity for sex (males or females) and for victim age. They felt that these perpetrators may be more opportunistic in their offences and less focussed on particular types of victims. There was also some suggestion that sex offenders with ID may be less likely to be violent during their offences than mainstream sexual offenders and less likely to commit penetrative offences (Murrey Briggs & Davis, 1992). Day (1994) also found in his sample that sexual offenders with ID were more likely to offend against stranger victims, perhaps reflecting poor ability to form appropriate relationships or poor social skills development. Echoing the counterfeit deviance hypothesis (Hingsburger, Griffiths & Quinsey 1991), Day (1994) also reported evidence of sexual naivety, a poor understanding of normal sexual relationships, limited relationship skills, poor social skills and impulse control.

In the Lindsay *et al.* (2002) study reported earlier, the most common reported offence was an offence against children. However, when offences against adults were combined (sexual assault, attempted rape, rape and sexual harassment), offences against adults were more frequent than offences against children. These authors noted that this finding was consistent with Day (1994). Gillis, De Luca, Hume, Morton and Rennpferd (1998) studied the differences between 11 sex offenders and 11 non-offenders, both with ID. They found that the sex offenders scored significantly higher on the hostility towards women scale. These authors concluded that this finding supports clinical observations which claim sex offenders with ID view women in very negative and stereotypical ways. More recently, Lindsay, Whitefield and Carson (2007) compared four groups of participants, sex offenders with ID, other types of offenders with ID, non-offenders with ID and controls without ID on seven scales which reviewed attitudes towards sexual offending in different areas. Attitudes in cognitive distortions are reviewed in greater detail in Chapter 12 of Craig and Lindsay (in press). The authors found that sex offenders with ID endorsed significantly more cognitive distortions and attitudes consistent with sexual offending on every scale.

In the series of studies conducted by Blanchard and colleagues, reviewed earlier, a relationship was found between intelligence level and victim age orientation. Lower intelligence was associated with significantly greater interest in younger, male children. The authors concluded 'intellectual deficiency (or some factor it represents) decreases the likelihood of exclusive sexual interest in girls' (p. 124). In a later study (Blanchard *et al.*, 2007) they replicated this finding and provided further evidence that this bias was not determined by accessibility or circumstances and that it could not be accounted for by referral bias (the suggestion that those more serious offences were referred to a sex offender clinic).

Sexual Recidivism Characteristics

Much of the research on sexual recidivism has relied on data from prison populations and does not take into account individuals diverted from the criminal justice system (Ashman

& Duggan, 2003). In work we reported earlier, we noted that offenders with ID were five times more likely to commit a violent offence (Hodgins 1992) and that re-offending rates of untreated sexual offenders with ID were between 40 per cent and 70 per cent (Scorzelli & Reinkie-Scorzelli 1979; Klimecki, Jenkinson & Wilson, 1994). Thomas and Singh (1995) reported re-offending rates following treatment to be between 20 per cent and 55 per cent depending on the type of treatment and the offence. These authors found that in a three-year follow-up of 20 offenders treated in a community based service, 50 per cent of participants re-offended and appeared before a court. This is a very high figure indeed and may be a reflection of the small sample.

Lindsay, Steele, Smith, Quinn and Allan (2006) followed up 247 consecutive referrals of offenders with ID in their community forensic intellectual disability service. Of these referrals, 121 were for sexual offending or inappropriate sexual behaviour, and all of these individuals were followed up for a period of up to 13 years. The re-offending rates were high at 23.9 per cent, but the authors noted that all but a handful of participants had full access to the community and were not supervised. McGrath, Livingston and Falk (2007) followed 103 sexual offenders with ID in the state of Vermont over an average follow-up period of 5.8 years. In this sample 10.7 per cent were identified as committing a further act of inappropriate sexual behaviour or a sexual offence, although these authors noted that over 60 per cent received 24-hour supervision, which limited their access to potential victims. Most of the re-offences were non-contact, with most victims being staff members, relatives or housemates of the abuser.

Familial and Relationship Characteristics

There is little doubt that developmental experiences in families are related to conflict in childhood and to antisocial behaviour in adulthood. Patterson and Yoerger (1997) conducted an extensive series of studies reviewing a developmental model for the onset of delinquency and criminal behaviour. They found that in some families from as early as 18 months a child may experience negative reinforcement of coercive behaviour such as temper tantrums and hitting because these behaviours have functional value in terminating conflict. As these interactions are repeated, the behaviours are strengthened and firmly established. Such children are less well adjusted and antisocial behaviour patterns can be seen as early as age 6 or 7 (Snyder & Patterson 1995). Farrington (1995) found that delinquency in early adolescents was significantly associated with troublesome behaviours at 8 to 10 years, an uncooperative family at 8 years, poor housing at 8 to 10 years, poor parental behaviour at 8 and low IQ at 8 to 10 years. Clearly, family variables are significantly associated with the development of crime and deviance in later years. The cycle of delinquency and adult criminal behaviour begins with uncooperative families, poor parental behaviour, parental conviction, troublesome behaviour, poor housing and low IQ at 8 years. Wilson (2004) noted the importance of the links between family, parenting, poverty and education in the development of antisocial behaviour in teenagers and adults. He also notes that 55 per cent of those convicted between the ages on 10 and 16 are conviction free by the age of 25 and 32. However, this means that 45 per cent of those convicted will persist in their criminal behaviour over that period.

There has been little research on the effects of family interaction on sex offenders with ID but several authors have reported on the nature of the families of sex offenders with

ID referred to the clinic. Caparullo (1991), Day (1994) and Hayes (1991) all noted that sex offenders with ID come from homes which are characterised by multiple family pathology, marital discord or parental separation, negative early sexual experience, abuse, neglect and violence, a lack of power and control, school adjustment and behavioural problems and relationship and peer difficulties. Similarly, there is some suggestion that the families of sex offenders with ID are more often violent and neglectful if the parents themselves have criminal histories (Day 1994, Fortune & Lambie, 2004; Gilby, Wolf & Goldberg, 1989). However, Lindsay (2004) commented that although many of these observers are highly experienced in the field of offenders with ID, 'one cannot help but notice that their identification of characteristics is comprehensive and inclusive ... it may be that an appropriate control comparison would find several or all of these features in men with intellectual disability who have offended in other ways or have not offended at all' (p. 164).

One study investigated the quality of relationships in sex offenders and non-sexual offenders. Steptoe, Lindsay, Forrest and Power (2006) investigated the perceived quality of life and relationships of 28 sex offenders with ID in comparison with a control group of 28 individuals with ID matched for IQ and age. Both groups completed a significant others scale (SOS) which assesses self-perceptions of potential and ideal support from significant others in the individual's life, and the life experience check list (LEC) which assesses experiences and opportunities across five living domains: home, leisure, freedom, relationships and opportunities. Steptoe, Lindsay, Forrest and Power (2006) found no differences on the SOS in the number of times each significant other was reported. Actual and ideal levels of support from both mother and father were lower for sexual offenders than the control group. On the LEC, sex offenders reported lower scores on the relationships and leisure sections. They argued that poorer relationships and little inclination of any wish to change that, may indicate lower levels of integration and identification with society for sex offenders in comparison with the control group. In relation to mainstream sex offenders without ID, lower levels of integration and lower levels of perceived social support have been associated with sexual recidivism.

CONCLUSIONS

It is only since the 1980s that research and literature has developed to investigate the various characteristics of sex offenders with ID. It is extremely difficult to conclude that there are any characteristics which might be considered unique to the client group. Poorly controlled studies have suggested a number of characteristics such as poor daily living and social skills, behavioural problems such as anger and aggression, psychiatric problems and mental illness, childhood abuse, school and family problems and peer influences. However, studies which have compared sexual offenders with ID to other types of offenders and non-offenders have not found these difficulties to be exclusive or, occasionally, even prominent in this client group. For example, Lindsay, Steele, Smith, Quinn and Allan (2006) found that anger and aggression, anxiety and alcohol abuse were significantly higher in other types of male offender than in sexual offenders. However, problems with daily living and some features of more impoverished relationships do appear more common in sexual offenders with ID than in other groups. In relation to abusive experiences, sex offenders with ID report higher rates of childhood sexual abuse but lower rates of physical abuse in childhood than other groups of offenders and non-offending people with ID. In terms of offence characteristics, there is some suggestion that sex offenders with ID may be more opportunistic, more likely to offend against both male and female victims and to offend across a wider range of victims than non-ID sex offenders. There is some consistency in the literature that sex offenders with ID pose a greater risk of sexual recidivism in a shorter time period than their non-ID counterparts. However, a significant methodological difference in ID studies is that participants tend to be supervised to a greater degree and so instances of inappropriate sexual behaviour may have a greater likelihood of being reported.

REFERENCES

American Psychiatric and Association. (2000). *Diagnostic and Statistical Manual of Mental Disorders-Text Revised*, 4th edn. Washington, DC: American Psychiatric Association.

Ashman, L. & Duggan, L. (2003). Interventions for learning disabled sex offenders (Cochrane Review). In, *The Cochrane Library*, Issue 1. Oxford; Update Software.

Barbaree, H. E., Seto, M. C., Langton, C. M. & Peacock, E. J. (2001). Evaluating the predictive accuracy of six risk assessment instruments for adult sex offenders. *Criminal Justice and Behavior*, 28, 490–521.

Barron, P., Hassiotis, A. & Banes, J. (2004). Offenders with learning disability: a prospective comparative study. *Journal of Learning Disability Research*, 48, 69–76.

Bartosh, D. L., Garby, T., Lewis, D. & Gray, S. (2003). Differences in the predictive validity of actuarial risk assessments in relation to sex offender type. *International Journal of Offender Therapy and Comparative Criminology*, 47, 422–38.

Beail, N. & Warden, S. (1995). Sexual abuse of adults with learning disabilities. *Journal of Intellectual Disability Research*, 3, 382–7.

Beech, A. R., Craig, L. A. & Browne, K. D. (2009). *Assessment and treatment of sex offenders: a handbook*. Chichester. John Wiley & Son.

Bjorkly, S. (2002a). Psychotic symptoms and violence towards others – A literature review of some preliminary findings – Part 1. Delusions. *Aggressive and Violent Behaviour*, 7, 605–15.

Bjorkly, S. (2002b). Psychotic symptoms and violence towards others – A literature review of some preliminary findings – Part 2 Hallucinations. *Aggressive and Violent Behaviour*, 7, 617–31.

Blanchard, R., Kolla, N. J., Cantor, J. M., Klassen, P. E., Dicky, R., Kuban, M. E. & Blak, T. (2007). IQ, handedness, and pedophilia in adult male patients stratified by referral source. *Sexual Abuse: A Journal of Research and Treatment*, 19, 285–309.

Blanchard, R., Watson, M. S., Choy, A., Dickey, R., Klassen, P., Kuban, M. & Ferren, D. J. (1999). Paedophiles: mental retardation, maternal age and sexual orientation. *The Archives of Sexual Behaviour*, 28(2), 111–27.

Bonta, J., Law, M. & Hanson, K. (1998). The prediction of criminal and violent recidivism among mentally disordered offenders: a meta-analysis. *Psychological Bulletin*, 123(2), 123–42.

BPS Professional Affairs, Board. (2001). *ID: definitions and contexts*. Leicester. The British Psychological Society. Available from, The British Psychological Society, St Andrews House, 48 Princess Road East, Leicester, LE1 7DR.

Briggs, F. & Hawkins, R.M.F. (1996). A comparison of the childhood experiences of convicted male child molesters and men who were sexually abused in childhood and claimed to be non-offenders. *Child Abuse and Neglect*, 20, 221–33.

Cantor, J. M., Blanchard, R., Robichaud, L. K. & Christensen, B. K. (2005). Quantitative Reanalysis of Aggregate Data on IQ in Sexual Offenders. *Psychological Bulletin*, 131(4), 555–68.

Caparulo, F. (1991). Identifying the developmentally disabled sex offenders. *Sexuality and Disability*, 9(4), 311–22.

Coleman, E. M. & Haaven, J. (2001). Assessment and treatment of intellectual disabled sexual abusers. In, M. S. Carich, & S. E. Mussack,(Eds), *Handbook for sexual abuser assessment and treatment*. Vermont; Safer Society Foundation, Inc.

Craig, L. A., Browne, K. D., Stringer, I. & Hogue, T. E. (2008). Sexual reconviction rates in the United Kingdom and actuarial estimates. *Child Abuse & Neglect: The International Journal, 32*, 121–38.

Craig, L. A. & Hutchinson, R. (2005). Sexual offenders with learning disabilities: risk, recidivism and treatment. *Journal of Sexual Aggression, 11*(3), 289–304.

Craig, L. A., Stringer, I. & Moss, T. (2006). Treating sexual offenders with learning disabilities in the community: a critical review. *International Journal of Offender Therapy and Comparative Criminology, 50*, 369–90.

Crocker, A. G., Cote, G., Toupin, J. & St-Onge, B. (2007). Rate and characteristics of men with an intellectual disability in pre-trial detention. *Journal of Intellectual & Developmental Disability, 32*(2), 143–52.

Day, K. (1993). Crime and mental retardation: a review. In K. Howells & C. Hollin. (Eds), *Clinical Approaches to the Mentally Disordered Offender*. Chichester, John, Wiley & Son.

Day, K. (1994). Male mentally handicapped sex offenders. *British Journal of Psychiatry, 165*, 630–9.

Dolan, M., Holloway, J., Bailey, S. & Kroll, L. (1996). The psychosocial characteristics of juvenile sexual offenders referred to an adolescent forensic service in the UK. *Medicine Science and the Law, 36*, 343–52.

Eccleston L., Ward T. & Waterman B. (in press). Theories of sexual offending and deviancy in males with intellectual disabilities: Applying the self-regulation model to sexual offenders with intellectual disabilities. In, L. A. Craig, W. R. Lindsay & K. D. Browne (Eds), *Assessment and treatment of sexual offenders: A handbook*. Chichester, Wiley-Blackwell.

Falshaw, L., Bastes, A., Patel, V., Corbett, C. & Friendship, C. (2003). Assessing reconviction, reoffending and recidivism in a sample of UK sexual offenders. *Legal and Criminological Psychology, 8*, 207–15.

Farrington, D. P. (1995). The development of offending and antisocial behaviour from childhood: Key findings from the Cambridge study in delinquent development. *Journal of Child Psychology & Psychiatry, 36*, 929–64.

Fortune, C.-A. & Lambie, I. (2004). Demographic and abuse characteristics in adolescent male sexual offenders with 'special needs'. *Journal of Sexual Aggression, 10*, 63–84.

Galea, J., Butler, J., Iacono, T. & Leighton, D. (2004). The assessment of sexual knowledge in people with intellectual disability. *Journal of Intellectual & Developmental Disabilities, 29*, 350–65.

General Accounting Office (1996). *Cycle of sexual abuse: Research inconclusive about whether child victims become adult abusers*. Report to the Chairman, Subcommittee on Crime, Committee on the Judiciary, House of Representatives, Washington DC., United States General Accounting Office.

Gibbens, T. C. & Robertson, G. (1983). A survey of criminal careers of restriction order patients. *British Journal of Psychiatry, 143*, 370–5.

Gilby, R., Wolf, L. & Goldberg, B. (1989). Mentally retarded adolescent sex offenders: A survey and pilot study. *Canadian Journal of Psychiatry, 34*, 542–8.

Gillis, M. A., De Luca, R. V., Hume, M., Morton, M. & Rennpferd, R. (1998). Some psychological dimensions of mentally retarded sex offenders. *Journal of Offender Rehabilitation, 26*, 127–39.

Glaser, W. & Deane, K. (1999). Normalisation in an abnormal world: A study of prisoners with an intellectual disability. *International Journal of Offender Therapy and Comparative Criminology, 43* (3), 338–56.

Gray, N. S., Fitzgerald, S., Taylor, J., MacCulloch, M. J. & Snowden, R. J. (2007). Predicting future reconviction rates in offenders with intellectual disabilities: The predictive efficacy of VRAG, PCL-SV, and the HCR-20. *Psychological Assessment, 19*(4), 474–9.

Griffiths, D., Hinsburger, D. & Christian, R. (1985). Treating developmentally handicapped sexual offenders: The York behaviour management services treatment program. *Psychiatric Aspects of Mental Retardation Reviews, 4*, 49–54.

Griffiths, D. & Lunsky, Y. (2003). *Sociosexual knowledge and attitudes assessment tool* (SSKAAT-R). Wood Dale, IL: Stoelting Company.

Griffiths, D. M., Quinsey, V. L. & Hingsburger, D. (1989). *Changing inappropriate sexual behaviour: A community based approach for persons with developmental disabilities.* Baltimore: Paul Brooks Publishing.

Gross, G. (1985). Activities of a development disabilities adult offender project. Washington State Developmental Disabilities Planning Council, Olympia, WA.

Grubb-Blubaugh, V., Shire, B. J. & Bausler, M. L. (1994). Behaviour management and offenders with mental retardation: The jury system. *Mental Retardation, 32*, 213–17.

Haaven, J., Little, R. & Petre-Miller, D. (1990). *Treating Intellectually Disabled Sex Offenders.* Safer Society Series number 6. Brandon, VT: Safer Society Press.

Hanson, R. K. & Bussière, M. T. (1998). Predicting relapse: A meta-analysis of sexual offender recidivism studies. *Journal of Consulting and Clinical Psychology, 66*(2), 348–62.

Hanson, R. K., Gordon, A., Harris, A. J. R., Marques, J. K., Murphy, W., Quinsey, V. L. & Seto, M. C. (2002). First report of the collaborative outcome data project on the effectiveness of psychological treatment for sex offenders. *Sexual Abuse: A Journal of Research and Treatment, 14*(2), 169–94.

Hanson, R. K. & Thornton, D. (2000). Improving risk assessment for sex offenders: A comparison of three actuarial scales. *Law and Human Behavior, 24*(1), 119–36.

Hare, R. D. (1991). *The Hare Psychopathy Checklist – Revised.* Toronto, Ontario: Multi-Health Systems.

Harris, G. T., Rice, M. E. & Quinsey, V. L. (1993). Violent recidivism of mentally disordered offenders: The development of a statistical prediction instrument. *Criminal Justice and Behavior, 20*, 315–35.

Harris, G. T., Rice, M. E., Quinsey, V. L., Lalumiere, M. L., Boer, D. & Lang, C. (2003). A multi-site comparison of actuarial risk instruments for sex offenders. *Psychological Assessment, 15*, 413–25.

Hawk, G., Rosenfield, B. & Warren, J. (1993). Prevalence of sexual offences among mentally retarded criminal defendants. *Hospital and Community Psychiatry, 44*, 784–6.

Hayes, S. (1991). Sex offenders. *Australia & New Zealand Journal of Developmental Disabilities, 17*(2), 221–7.

Hingsburger, D., Griffiths, D. & Quinsey, V. (1991). Detecting counterfeit deviance: Differentiating sexual deviance from sexual inappropriateness. *Habilitation Mental Health Care Newsletter, 10*, 51–4.

Ho, T. (1997). Mentally retarded sex offenders: Criminality and retardation. *Journal of Contemporary Criminal Justice, 13*(3), 251–63.

Hodgins, S. (1992). Mental disorder, learning deficiency and crime: Evidence from a birth cohort. *Archives of General Psychiatry, 49*, 476–83.

Hogue, T. E., Steptoe, L., Taylor, J. L., Lindsay, W. R., Mooney, P., Pinkney, L., Johnston, S., Smith, A. H. W. & O'Brien, G. (2006). A comparison of offenders with intellectual disability across three levels of security. *Criminal Behaviour & Mental Health, 16*, 13–28.

Holland, S. & Persson, P. (in press). Intellectual disability in the Victorian prison system: Characteristics of prisoners with an intellectual disability released from prison in 2003–2006. *Psychology, Crime and Law.*

Klimecki, M. R., Jenkinson, J. & Wilson, L. (1994). A study of recidivism amongst offenders with an intellectual disability. *Australia and New Zealand Journal of Developmental Disabilities, 19*, 209–19.

Lackey, L. B. & Knopp, F. H. (1989). A summary of selected notes from the working sessions of the first National Training Conference on the assessment and treatment of intellectually disabled juveniles and adult sexual offenders. In F. H. Knopp (Ed.), *Selected readings: Sexual offenders identified as intellectually disabled*. Orwell, VT: Safer Society Press.

Lambrick, F. & Glaser, W. (2004). Sex offenders with an intellectual disability. *Sexual Abuse: A Journal of Research and Treatment, 16*(4), 381–92.

Langdon, P. E. & Talbot, T. J. (2006). Locus of control and sex offenders with an intellectual disability. *International Journal of Offender Therapy and Comparative Criminology, 50*, 4, 391–401.

Langevin, R. & Pope, S. (1993). Working with learning disabled sex offenders. *Annals of Sex Research, 6* (2), 149–60.

Lindsay, W. R. (2002). Research and literature on sex offenders with intellectual and developmental disabilities. *Journal of Intellectual Disability Research, 46*, 1, 74–85.

Lindsay, W. R. (2004). Sex offenders: Conceptualisation of the issues, services, treatment and management. In, W. R. Lindsay, J. L. Taylor, & P. Sturmey,(Eds), *Offenders with developmental disabilities*. Chichester, John Wiley & Sons Ltd.

Lindsay, W. R. (2009). *The treatment of sex offenders with developmental dsabilities: A practice workbook*. Chichester, Wiley-Blackwell.

Lindsay, W. R., Bellshaw, E., Culross, G., Staines, C. & Michie, A. (1992). Increases in knowledge following a course of sex education for people with learning disabilities. *Journal of Learning Disability Research, 36*, 531–9.

Lindsay, W. R., Elliot, S. F. & Astell, A. (2004). Predictors of sexual offence recidivism in offenders with intellectual disabilities. *Journal of Applied Research in Intellectual Disabilities, 17*, 299–305.

Lindsay, W. R., Hastings, R. P., Griffiths, D. M. & Hayes, S. C. (2007). Trends and challenges in forensic research on offenders with intellectual disability. *Journal of Intellectual and Developmental Disabilities, 32*, 55–61.

Lindsay, W. R., Hogue, T. E., Taylor, J. L., Steptoe, L., Mooney, P., O'Brien, G., Johnston, S. & Smith, A. H. W. (2008). Risk assessment in offenders with intellectual disability: A comparison across three levels of security. *International Journal of Offender Therapy and Comparative Criminology, 52*(1), 90–111.

Lindsay, W. R., Law, J., Quinn, K., Smart, N. & Smith, A. H. W. (2001). A comparison of physical and sexual abuse histories: Sexual and non-sexual offenders with intellectual disability. *Child Abuse and Neglect, 25*(7), 989–95.

Lindsay, W. R. & Macleod, F. (2001). A review of forensic learning disability research. *The British Journal of Forensic Practice, 3*, 4–10.

Lindsay W. R. Michie A. M. & Lambrick F. (in press) Community-based treatment programmes for sexual offenders with intellectual disabilities. In, L. A. Craig, W. R. Lindsay, & K. D. Browne (Eds), *Assessment and treatment of sexual offenders: A handbook*. Chichester, Wiley-Blackwell.

Lindsay, W. R., Smith, A. H. W., Law, J., Quinn, K., Anderson, A., Smith, A. & Allan, R. (2004). Sexual and nonsexual offenders with intellectual and learning disabilities: A comparison of characteristics, referral patterns, and outcome. *Journal of Interpersonal Violence, 19*(8), 875–90.

Lindsay, W. R., Smith, A. H. W., Law, J., Quinn, K., Anderson, A., Smith, A., Overend, T. & Allan, R. (2002). A treatment service for sex offenders and abusers with intellectual disability: Characteristics of referrals and evaluation. *Journal of Applied Research in Intellectual Disabilities, 15*, 166–74.

Lindsay, W. R., Steele, L., Smith, A. H. W., Quinn, K. & Allan, R. (2006). A community forensic intellectual disability service: Twelve-year follow-up of referrals, analysis of referral patterns and assessment of harm reduction. *Legal & Criminological Psychology, 11*, 113–30.

Lindsay, W. R., Whitefield, E. & Carson, D. (2007). An assessment for attitudes consistent with sexual offending for use with offenders with intellectual disabilities. *Legal and Criminological Psychology, 12*, 55–68.

Linhorst, D. M., McCutchen, T. A. & Bennett, L. (2003). Recidivism among offenders with developmental disabilities participating in a case management programme. *Research in Developmental Disabilities, 24*, 210–30.

Luiselli, J. K. (2000). Presentation of paraphilias and paraphilia related disorders in young adults with mental retardation: Two case profiles. *Mental Health Aspects of Developmental Disabilities, 3,* 42–6.

Lund, J. (1990). Mentally retarded criminal offenders in Denmark. *British Journal of Psychiatry, 156,* 726–31.

Lunsky, Y., Frijters, J., Griffiths, D. M., Watson, S. L. & Williston, S. (2007). Sexual knowledge and attitudes of men with intellectual disabilities who sexually offend. *Journal of Intellectual and Developmental Disability, 32,* 74–81.

McBrien, J. A., Hodgetts, A. & Gregory, J. (2003). Offending and risky behaviour in community services for people with intellectual disabilities. *The Journal of Forensic Psychiatry and Psychology, 14*(2), 280–97.

MacEachron, A. E. (1979). Mentally retarded offenders: Prevalence and characteristics. *American Journal of Mental Deficiency, 84,* 165–76.

McGrath, R. J., Livingston, J. A. & Falk, G. (2007). Community management of sex offenders with intellectual disabilities: Characteristics, services, and outcome of a statewide program. *Intellectual and Development Disabilities, 45*(6), 391–8.

Mackinnon, S., Bailey, B. & Pink, L. (2004). *Understanding learning disabilities: A video-based training resource for trainers and managers to use with staff.* Brighton, UK. Pavilion Publishing (Brighton) Ltd.

Marshall, W. L., Anderson, D. & Fernandez, Y. (1999). *Cognitive Behavioural Treatment of Sexual Offenders.* Chichester. John Wiley & Son.

Marshall, W. L., Fernandez, Y. M., Marshall, L. E. & Serran, G. A. (2006). *Sexual offender treatment: Controversial issues.* Chichester. J. Wiley.

Michie, A. M., Lindsay, W. R., Martin, V. & Grieve, A. (2006). A test of counterfeit deviance: A comparison of sexual knowledge in groups of sex offenders with intellectual disability and controls. *Sex Abuse: A Journal of Research and Treatment, 18,* 271–8.

Morrissey, C., Hogue, T., Mooney, P., Allen, C., Johnston, S., Hollin, C., Lindsay, W. R. & Taylor, J. L. (2007). The predictive validity of the PCL-R in offenders with ID in a high secure hospital setting: Institutional aggression. *Journal of Forensic Psychiatry and Psychology, 18*(1), 1–15.

Morrissey, C., Mooney, P., Hogue, T., Lindsay, W. R. & Taylor, J. (2007). Predictive validity of psychopathy in offenders with ID in high security: Treatment progress. *Journal of Intellectual and Developmental Disability, 32*(2), 125–33.

Murphy, G. H. (2007). Intellectual disabilities, sexual abuse and sexual offending. In A. Carr, G. O'Reilly, P. Noonan Walsh & J. McEvoy (Eds), *Handbook of intellectual disability and clinical psychology practice.* London: Routledge.

Murphy, W. D., Coleman, E. M. & Haynes, M. R. (1983). Treatment and evaluation issues with the mentally retarded sex offender. In, J. G. Greer & I. R. Stuart (Eds), *The sexual aggressor: Current prospective on treatment.* Van Nostrand: Reinholt Company.

Murrey, G. J., Briggs, D. & Davis, C. (1992). Psychopathic disordered, mentally ill, and mentally handicapped sex offenders: Comparative study. *Medicine. Science and Law, 32,* 331–6.

Parry, C. & Lindsay, W. R. (2003). Impulsiveness as a factor in sexual offending by people with mild intellectual disability. *Journal of Intellectual Disability Research, 47*(6), 483–7.

Patterson, G. R. & Yoerger, K. (1997). A developmental model for late onset delinquency. In D. W. Osgood (Ed.), *Motivation and delinquency* (pp. 119–77). Lincoln: University of Nebraska.

Phillips, H., Gray, N. S., MacCulloch, S., Taylor, J., Moore, S., Huckle, P. & MacCulloch, M. (2005). Risk assessment in offenders with mental disorders. *Journal of Interpersonal Violence, 20,* 833–47.

Quinsey, V. L., Book, A. & Skilling, T. A. (2004). A follow-up of deinstitutionalised men with intellectual disabilities and histories of antisocial behaviour. *Journal of Applied Research in Intellectual Disabilities, 17,* 243–54.

Quinsey, V. L., Harris, G. T., Rice, M. E. & Cormier, C. A. (1998). *Violent offenders, appraising and managing risk*. Washington DC: American Psychological Association.

Quinsey, V. L., Harris, G. T., Rice, M. E. & Cormier, C. A. (2006). *Violent offenders, appraising and managing risk*, 2nd edn. Washington DC: American Psychological Association.

Royal College of Psychiatrists (2001). *Diagnostic criteria for psychiatric disorders for use with adults with ID/mental retardation (DC-LD)*. Occasional paper OP 48. London, Gaskell. Available from Gaskell an imprint of the Royal College of Psychiatrists, 17 Belgrave Square, London, SW1X 8PG.

Scorzelli, J. F. & Reinke-Scorzelli, M. (1979). Mentally retarded offender: A follow-up study. *Rehabilitation Counselling Bulletin*. September, 70–3.

Sequeira, H. & Hollins, S. (2003). Clinical effects of sexual abuse on people with learning disability: Critical literature review. *British Journal of Psychiatry, 182*, 13–19.

Smith, A. H. W. & O'Brien, G. (2004). Offenders with dual diagnosis. In W. R. Lindsay, J. L. Taylor & P. Strumey (Eds), *Offenders with developmental disabilities*. Chichester. Wiley.

Smith, A. H. W., Quinn, K. & Lindsay, W. R. (2000). Influence of mental illness on the presentation and management of offenders with intellectual disability. *Journal of Intellectual and Developmental Disabilities, 44*, 360–1.

Snyder, J. J. & Patterson, G. R. (1995). Individual differences in social aggression: A test of a reinforcement model of socialisation in the natural environment. *Behaviour Therapy, 26*, 371–91.

Sparrow, S. S., Balla, D. A. & Cicchetti, D. V. (1984). *Vineland's adaptive behaviour scales; interview edition, expanded form*. American Guidance Service Inc, Circle Pines, MN.

Steptoe, L., Lindsay, W. R., Forrest, D. & Power, M. (2006). Quality of life and relationships in sex offenders with intellectual disability. *Journal of Intellectual and Developmental Disability, 31*(1), 13–19.

Swanson, J. W., Borum, R., Swartz, M. S. & Monahan, J. (1996). Psychotic symptoms and disorders and the risk of violent behaviour in the community. *Criminal Behavior & Mental Health, 6*, 317–38.

Swartz, M. & Masters, W. (1983). Conceptual factors in the treatment of paraphilias: A preliminary report. *Journal of Sex and Marital Therapy, 9*, 3–18.

Talbot, T. J. & Langdon, P. E. (2006). A revised sexual knowledge assessment tool for people with intellectual disabilities: Is sexual knowledge related to sexual offending behaviour? *Journal of Intellectual Disability Research, 50*(7), 523–31.

Thomas, D. H. & Singh, T. H. (1995). Offenders referred to a learning disability service: A retrospective study from one county. *Mental Handicap, 23*, 24–7.

Thompson, D. & Brown, H. (1997). Men with intellectual disabilities who sexually abuse: A review of the literature. *Journal of Applied Research in Intellectual Disabilities, 10*(2), 125–39.

Thornton, D. (2002). Constructing and testing a framework for dynamic risk assessment. *Sexual Abuse: A Journal of Research and Treatment, 14*(2), 139–53.

Timms, S. & Goreczny, A. J. (2002). Adolescent sex offenders with mental retardation: Literature review and assessment considerations. *Aggression and Violent Behavior, 7*(1), 1–19.

Walker, N. & McCabe, S. (1973). *Crime and Insanity in England*. Edinburgh University Press, Edinburgh.

Ward, T. & Hudson, S. M. (1998). A model of the relapse process in sexual offenders. *Journal of Interpersonal Violence, 13*, 700–25.

Webster, C. D., Eaves, D., Douglas, K. S. & Wintrup, A. (1995). *The HCR-20: The assessment of dangerousness and risk*. Vancouver, Canada: Simon Fraser University and British Colombia Forensic Psychiatric Services Commission.

Webster, C. D., Douglas, K. S., Eaves, D. & Hart, S. D. (1997). *HCR-20: Assessing risk for violence, version 2*. Burnaby, British Columbia, Canada: The Mental Health, Law, and Policy Institute of Simon Fraser University.

Wechsler, D. (1999). *Wechsler adult intelligence scale*, 3rd edn. London: Psychological Corporation.

Wildenskov, H. O. T. (1962). A long-term follow up of subnormals originally exhibiting severe behaviour disorders or criminality. *Proceedings of the London Conference on the Scientific Study of Mental Deficiency*. London: May & Baker.

Wilson, M. (2004). The community and family context in understanding juvenile crime. In A. Needs & G. Towl (Eds), *Applying Psychology, to Forensic Practice*. Oxford: BPS Blackwell.

World Health Organization. (1992). *ICD-10 Classification of Mental and Behavioural Disorders – Clinical Descriptions and Diagnostic Guidelines ICD-10-CDDG*. Geneva: WHO.

3

Developmental Pathways in Intellectually Disabled Sexual Offenders

SUSAN C. HAYES

INTRODUCTION

This chapter reviews the developmental pathways from adverse childhood experiences to juvenile sex offending and adult sex crimes. The influence of a person having an intellectual disability (ID) in relation to these developmental pathways is specifically considered and this is compared to individuals with neurodevelopmental deficits (such as attention deficit hyperactivity disorder (ADHD)) and young people without deficits or disabilities.

DEVELOPMENTAL PATHWAYS

Developmental pathways are characterised by a series of stages that unfold over time, usually in a predictable manner. The developmental pathway behaviour that leads to offending is distinct from the pathways that are followed by other individuals. Single or multiple factors may influence the pathways towards offending behaviour; an understanding of the genesis of these factors, and their influence on the developmental pathway may assist in the process of understanding problem behaviours and intervening in an effective and timely fashion to prevent the development of more serious behaviours (Kelley, Loeber, Keenan & DeLamatre, 1997).

The development of problem behaviour is more than just an erratic sequence of behaviours that are unpredictable and independent of each other. Service providers need to be aware that developmental sequences in problem behaviour may represent systematic changes in

Assessment and Treatment of Sexual Offenders with Intellectual Disabilities: A Handbook
Edited by Leam A. Craig, William R. Lindsay and Kevin D. Browne
© 2010 John Wiley & Sons, Ltd.

behaviour of individuals over time. Developmental pathways that contribute to offending behaviour have the following features:

- Most individuals who advance to behaviours along a pathway will have displayed behaviours characteristic of the earlier stages in the temporal sequence, which may not have been consistently noted or responded to.
- Not all individuals progress to the most serious outcome(s); typically, increasingly smaller numbers of individuals reach more serious levels within a pathway because as the severity of the behaviours escalates so too does the likelihood of intervention or increased supervision.
- Individuals who reach a more serious level in a pathway tend to continue to display behaviours typical of earlier levels rather than to replace them with the more serious acts, that is, they add to and diversify their actions (Loeber, Stouthamer-Loeber, Van Kammen & Farrington, 1991).
- The severity of their behaviour tends to be an outcome of repetition of the acts, the increasing age of the offender (especially as they move from adolescence to young adulthood) and the increasing range of their antisocial acts.

The body of work by Rolf Loeber and colleagues, especially in the Pittsburgh Youth Study (Kelley, Loeber, Keenan & DeLamatre, 1997) summarises the approximate ordering of the different manifestations of disruptive and antisocial behaviours in childhood and adolescence, commencing soon after birth and progressing along the age spectrum, in the following manner:

- difficult temperament
- hyperactivity
- overt conduct problems or aggression
- withdrawal
- poor peer relationships
- academic problems
- covert or concealing conduct problems such as lying or stealing
- association with deviant peers
- delinquency, coming to the attention of police
- recidivism

The person with ID may express some of these behaviours as a concomitant of their condition (such as academic problems or hyperactivity), thereby possibly rendering them more prone to the development of disruptive or offending behaviour, but also making it more difficult to identify the early markers which might indicate later offending. Furthermore, the development of verbal skills enables non-disabled individuals to learn to solve problems without physical aggression, an area which may challenge the person with ID.

The age trajectory of offending behaviour has been identified as commencing as oppositional and conduct problems in early to middle childhood, with an offending peak in adolescence or early adulthood, followed by a decline (Tremblay, 2000; Elliot, 1994), although involvement in violent crime may continue until the offender is in their 30s–40s (Tolan and Gorman-Smith, 1998). However, with sexual offences the age distribution appears to be bi-modal, with a peak in early adolescence and another in mid to late 30s

(Smallbone and Wortley, 2004). In contrast with non-sexual offenders, the ages of convicted sex offenders tend be distributed across the lifespan (ibid.).

The focus of this chapter is on the specific development of sexual offending behaviour, which may differ from the development of other antisocial behaviours which lead on to property violations, aggression or assault and offences involving deception, such as stealing or credit card fraud. Much of the research and clinical endeavour in the area of sexual offending concentrates on the non-disabled group, and there is speculation about the degree to which sexual offenders with ID are similar to their non-disabled counterparts. (Discussion of theories of sexual offending and deviancy in males with ID can be found in Chapters 2 and 4 of this volume; the issue of family violence and abuse is the topic of Chapter 5.) The dearth of research and the limitations of existing research on developmental characteristics of sexual offenders with ID mean that it is necessary to draw upon studies of non-disabled populations of offenders, although doing so raises the issue of whether the developmental pathways are identical for the two groups. This chapter utilises much of the research on non-disabled offending groups and attempts to indicate where the experience of their disabled counterparts may differ.

Research on non-disabled sexual offenders indicates that it is not necessarily the case that sexual offending behaviour targeting child victims has early onset; the researchers postulate that studies establishing early onset tend to focus on deviant sexual interests or fantasies rather than the emergence of the sexual offending behaviour (Smallbone and Wortley, 2004). First sexual contact with a child in Smallbone and Wortley's study was on average at the age of 32, and as they comment, this is an age when adults may have opportunities for increased contact with children through family links or through their work or recreational activities. Most adult child molesters who participated in their study reported a history of non-sexual offences, consistent with Loeber, Stouthamer-Loeber, Van Kammen and Farrington's (1991) findings concerning increasing diversity of antisocial acts. Smallbone and Wortley (2004) comment that 'men who have already some experience of serious rule-breaking, dishonesty, exploitation, and/or aggression may be more likely to *take* the opportunities to sexually abuse a child' (p. 295). Therefore, the developmental pathway for sexual offending may commence with non-sexual offending, which needs to be borne in mind when assessing and intervening with non-sexual offenders.

PATHWAY MODELS

The findings of Smallbone and Wortley (2004) concerning the link between rule-breaking behaviour generally and sexual offending accord with Ward and Siegert's Pathways Model of sexual offending (Ward and Siegert, 2002), an approach which knits together the most salient features of previous theories of child sexual offending and which also incorporates the developmental disruptions which occur in the background of many sexual offenders. As indicated by the body of work by Loeber and associates (Kelley, Loeber, Keenan & DeLamatre, 1997; Loeber, Stouthamer-Loeber, Van Kammen & Farrington, 1991), the Pathway Model allows for multiple developmental trajectories that lead towards sexual offending. The Pathway Model suggests four core mechanisms – intimacy and social skills deficits, distorted sexual scripts, emotional dysregulation and antisocial cognitions, as well as a fifth pathway that involves multiple dysfunctional mechanisms.

An alternative aetiological model has been developed (Knight and Sims-Knight, 2003, 2004); these authors stress the lack of information about the appropriateness of applying adult models to juvenile sexual offenders. A similar issue could be raised in relation to applying models developed for non-disabled offenders to sexual offenders with ID.

The Knight and Sims-Knight model of the origins of sexual aggression proposes that early abuse experiences (including physical, verbal and sexual abuse) combine with personality predispositions to produce three latent traits that predict sexual aggression. These three traits are (i) arrogant, deceitful personality/emotional detachment, (ii) impulsivity/antisocial behaviours and (iii) sexual pre-occupation/hyper-sexuality.

These authors comment that physical and verbal abuse first of all increase the likelihood of development of arrogant, deceitful personality/emotional detachment and, secondly, serve as a model for aggression, thus increasing the likelihood of aggressive and acting-out behaviour; both of these factors are similar to factors in Hare's Psychopathy Checklist (Hare, Harpur, Hakstian, Forth, Hart & Newman, 1990). Sexual abuse, on the other hand, leads to sexual preoccupation and compulsivity which in turn increases the possibility of aggressive sexual fantasies. Knight and Sims-Knight (2003) found that arrogant and deceitful personality/emotional detachment predicted sexual fantasy and antisocial behaviour/aggression, which is a significant predictor of sexual offending. Impulsivity/antisocial behaviours predicted sexual coercion directly and also through sexual fantasy; those offenders who commenced their sexually coercive behaviour in adolescence showed significantly more antisocial behaviour as juveniles than those offenders who began offending as adults. Lastly, sexual drive and promiscuity were found to be higher among sexually coercive participants. These authors discuss the role of sexual drive, postulating that sexual deviance plus sexual drive are important predictors of recidivism and that these factors are associated with use of pornography, aggression towards women, sadism, anger and pre-planning of offences (Knight and Sims-Knight, 2004). The three traits that define the three paths in the model were found to predict sexual coercion against women in both adolescents and adults and relate to the concept of psychopathology. It is also suggested that the three traits are important targets for treatment.

CHILDHOOD ABUSE OR NEGLECT

There are more similarities between sex offenders with ID and non-sex offenders with ID, as well as non-disabled offenders, than there are differences (Hayes, 2002). One area of similarity between the two groups is the high level of prior sexual and physical abuse of all offender groups (ibid.; McElroy et al., 1999).

While having been the victim of abuse or neglect as a child is seen as an important factor related to later sexual offending there are differing views as to the way in which abuse and neglect contribute to later offending. It is widely accepted that childhood abuse can interfere with attachment, that is, the degree to which a young child can rely on his or her caregiver as a source of security or protection; the capacity to establish secure affectional bonds with others is seen as a principal feature of effective personality functioning and mental health. A study of over 800 non-disabled young adults showed that over one-quarter reported some kind of prior verbal, physical or sexual abuse, with considerable overlap between the three categories of abuse (Styron and Janoff-Bulman, 1997). The abused participants reported their childhood and adult relationships to be less secure than their non-abused counterparts. They tended to be less securely attached as children to their mother and father and less securely attached as adults to their romantic partner. They were also more depressed and more likely to use destructive behaviours in conflict situations, including verbal aggression and more importantly, physical aggression towards their partners.

It has been postulated that youths growing up in high crime/high violence environments dominated by males who show antisocial behaviours may conclude that aggression and threat are adaptive mechanisms in such a situation. On the other hand, they may perceive that behaviours which are considered adaptive in the mainstream of society, such as trust, cooperation, tolerance and empathy, create vulnerability and are non-adaptive (Hunter, Figueredo, Malamuth & Becker, 2004). Boys and young men with ID may often grow up in environments marked by interpersonal violence and aggression, in families, group homes (Brown and Stein, 1997), larger residential institutions and, later, young offender institutions. The lack of appropriate non-violent role models can result in the development of harmful attitudes regarding sexual partners and can inhibit the acquisition of pro-social relationship skills. In turn, such youths are at a disadvantage because they have not developed the social skills that are valued, especially in sexual relationships, and their psychosocial deficits are likely to increase the reliance on violence and aggression in both sexual and non-sexual interactions (Hunter, Figueredo, Malamuth & Becker, 2004). Psychosocial deficits and egotistical–antagonistic masculinity have been shown to play mediating roles in young men who have been exposed as children to violence against women, and male-modelled antisocial behaviour, in the development of both sexual and non-sexual aggression (ibid.).

By extrapolation, this picture suggests that people with ID who have experienced childhood abuse will tend to have difficulty maintaining adult relationships, may employ abuse and physical violence in their relationships and probably lack skills of conflict resolution. Furthermore, they will probably have a higher propensity towards depression (Hayes, 2004).

In a study comparing non-disabled women with histories of child abuse and neglect with non-abused women, the abused group had significantly greater levels of impairments in physical, social, occupational and emotional role functioning, more physical symptoms, more health-risk behaviours and greater numbers of medical diagnoses (Walker *et al.*, 1999). Many women reported more than one category of abuse, and a higher number of abuse categories was associated with an increased risk of adverse health outcomes. In some women, maladaptive coping mechanisms, including somatisation, smoking, alcohol abuse, unsafe sex practices and obesity were related to the maltreatment experience.

It is reasonable to assume that people with ID who have been the victim of abuse will develop a similar range of impairments and symptoms, and this was borne out in a study examining psychological disturbance associated with sexual abuse of people with ID in comparison to a non-abused group; this study found that those who had been abused presented with more severe behaviour problems, especially aggressive and agitated behaviours, self-harm, temper outbursts and mood swings, as well as social withdrawal and stereotypical behaviours (Sequeira, Howlin & Hollins, 2003). There was a higher incidence of psychiatric diagnoses in the abused group and more severe depression and anxiety. As the severity of abuse increased so too did the severity of the symptoms. In particular, inadequate daily living skills, a chronic physical condition, social incompetence and negative life events were predictive of *DSM-IV* disorder in children with ID. Of special note were the findings that disruptive behaviour (as defined by the *Diagnostic Interview Schedule for Children – Parent Version: DISC-IV-PV*) was specifically predicted by inadequate daily living skills, family dysfunction and low parental education, while mood disorder was uniquely predicted by negative life events (Dekker and Koot, 2003). These results indicate the links between abuse or neglect and subsequent behavioural, psychological and psychiatric disorders in people with ID, which in turn might be related to subsequent offending behaviour.

This leads to the important issue, therefore, of whether sexual offenders with ID have experienced abuse, and whether the abuse appears to be linked with adverse health and mental health outcomes.

Among sexual offenders with ID, high rates of physical and sexual abuse have been found, and the history of abuse may correlate with depression, suicidal ideation and suicide attempts (Hayes, 2004), although depression has not been consistently noted in all research with this group compared with non-sexual offenders (Lindsay, Law, Quinn, Smart & Smith, 2001). Those sex offenders with ID who have symptoms of depression may be more likely to use violence or to have threatened violence in the commission of the offence, which is consistent with the findings of the research reporting deficits in conflict resolution skills (Styron and Janoff-Bulman, 1997).

These results are consistent with other studies of physical and sexual abuse histories for offenders with ID (Lindsay, Law, Quinn, Smart & Smith, 2001). These researchers concluded that sexual abuse in childhood may be a significant variable in the development of sexual offending in adulthood, whereas physical abuse in childhood was significantly more prevalent among non-sexual offenders. More women than men offenders with ID have been sexually abused, whereas rates of physical abuse were comparable for both men and women offenders with ID (Lindsay et al., 2004).

There are, however, significant numbers of individuals who have been the victims of childhood physical or asexual abuse who do not become sexual offenders, and on the other hand, significant numbers of sexual aggressors who have not been subjected to childhood abuse. A study of sexually aggressive children and adolescents found that nearly three-quarters had not experienced childhood abuse (Fago, 2003). An examination of other developmental characteristics that may have related to the sexually aggressive behaviour identified a high prevalence (82 per cent) of ADHD and other neuro-developmental disorders. Deficits in executive functioning had a prevalence rate that was 20 times greater than the figure for the general population. Fago (2003) theorised that children with ADHD tended to have many of the characteristics of sexual offenders, including lack of interpersonal sensitivity and empathy; attraction to dangerous, stimulating and high-risk behaviours; tendency towards hypersexuality; and difficulty imposing limits and structure on their own behaviour. These characteristics may be also found in some sexual offenders with ID.

In comparison with non-offenders, sex offenders with ID are more likely to have suffered attachment disruption in early childhood, to have experienced childhood abuse, to be aggressive and to have few conflict resolution skills, to have deficits in executive functioning and to have developed psychiatric, behavioural and emotional problems related to these negative early experiences. Their manner of relating to the world has been seriously affected by these early experiences, and the reversal of these effects will not occur overnight.

EARLY ONSET OF SEXUAL OFFENDING

It is only relatively recently that child and adolescent sexual offending has been regarded as a serious indicator of subsequent and ongoing offending behaviour. There was a tendency to adopt a 'they will grow out of it' perspective, viewing the behaviour as a form of inappropriate sexual experimentation (Bullens, van Wijk & Mali, 2006). Subsequent research found that adolescent inappropriate sexual behaviour often endured into adulthood, with recidivism rates for sexual offences varying from 2 per cent to over 40 per cent, depending upon the type, size and source of the sample (Parks and Bard, 2006), and public attitudes became more intolerant of lenient treatment of adolescent sexual offenders.

Developmental factors have been shown to be related to deviant sexual preferences in adult rapists (Beauregard, Lussier & Proulx, 2004), specifically a background characterised by a sexually inappropriate family environment, use of pornography during childhood and adolescence and deviant sexual fantasies during childhood and adolescence.

The criminal careers of adolescent sexual and non-sexual offenders differ, in that the former commence their offences at an earlier age (except for exhibitionists), and tend to have shorter criminal career (Bullens, van Wijk & Mali, 2006). Many started their offending with a sexual offence and subsequently branched into property offences. Possible explanations for this trend are that the sexual offenders discover that juvenile sex offenders are fairly low in the pecking order of juvenile offenders generally and so they replace this type of offence with other more 'acceptable' offences, and also learn to commit property offences in order to purchase sex (ibid.). These are complex realisations and decisions which may not readily arrived at by sexual offenders with ID, who may therefore persist with sexual offending.

Researchers warn against regarding all sexual offenders as having the same characteristics, because different patterns of offending and violence have been noted between child molesters, peer/adult rapists, exhibitionists and those who commit mixed offences (Bullens, van Wijk & Mali, 2006; Parks and Bard, 2006). General delinquent behaviour is associated with both sexual and non-sexual recidivism and therefore is a risk factor which cannot be ignored. Some of the other factors that need to be taken into consideration include motivational patterns (sexual motivation as compared with impulsivity or anger), age of onset and persistence of sexual offending, lower social competency and clusters of background variables, including demographic characteristics, histories of abuse, psychiatric diagnoses and offence type (Andrade, Vincent & Saleh, 2006). It is unclear whether the factors that differentiate between various types of sexual offenders would be similar for offenders with ID.

Knight and Sims-Knight (2004) draw attention to the differences between adult and adolescent sexual offenders, citing three issues relating to the different developmental stages of the two groups and the difficulties of predicting the developmental pathway of adolescent sexual offenders. These three issues are

1. the developmental timeline for coalescence of particular attitudes and behavioural traits;
2. the problem with adolescent samples of differentiating between those for whom problematic sexual acts will be limited to adolescence and those for whom sexually coercive behaviour will be evident throughout their lifetime;
3. the increased difficulty within adolescent samples of determining those who choose age-appropriate victims and those who fixate on children as sexual objects.

These differentiations become even more problematic within the population of offenders with ID, with their different developmental timelines and the possibility that age appropriate peers may be those with an appropriate mental rather than chronological age.

Major mental illness, including paraphilic disorders, substance abuse, impulse control, anxiety, mood disorders and eating disorders have been noted in adult male sexual offenders (McElroy *et al.*, 1999). Among juvenile sexual offenders, the major disorders that have been noted include paraphilia, conduct disorder, ADHD, depressive disorder, bipolar disorder and substance abuse (Galli, McElroy, Soutullo, Kizer, Raute & Keck, 1999). These findings, when extrapolated to the group with ID, indicate the significance of thorough assessment of major mental illnesses using criteria appropriate for the ID group, to plan for better treatment and to understand the motivational aspects of the crime and its relationship to the presence of mental illness (Andrade, Vincent & Saleh, 2006).

Following on from the conclusions of Andrade Vincent and Saleh (2006), difficulties with assessing sexual offenders with ID include the fact that many such individuals display behavioural or emotional symptoms characteristic of a form of psychopathology at some point, and yet the expected developmental trajectory of an individual with ID is difficult to define, while tools and strategies for classifying major mental disorder in this group continue to experience reliability and validity difficulties.

The differences between adult and adolescent non-disabled sexual offenders highlights the fact that there may also be significant differences between sexual offenders with ID and their non-disabled counterparts, as well as between adult and adolescent sex offenders with ID. The developmental trajectories of the two latter groups have not been the subject of comprehensive research which could inform evidence-based clinical practice and intervention.

CONCLUSIONS

As many of the research studies indicate, the developmental pathways of sexual offenders are of interest not solely because of their aetiological significance but more importantly as signposts for early intervention prior to the commission of an offence and in order to the target areas for treatment (see Part III). There has been insufficient research and clinical evidence-based practice concerning the developmental pathways of sexual offenders with ID, however. While it is clear that sexual offenders with ID are not a homogeneous group any more than their non-disabled adult and juvenile counterparts, there is a need for further work to establish and evaluate useful developmental pathway models for this group.

While early identification of the characteristics that may set a young person on the pathway to subsequent offending behaviour and the implementation of early intervention are ideals, there are especial difficulties and barriers within the population of youngsters with ID. It is difficult enough for parents of non-disabled children to perceive a pattern of behaviour that may lead to later offending; parents tend to have limited knowledge of typical child and adolescent development, they may not know how to respond to the behaviour and may not know how to access resources to assist them to handle their problem children (Kelley, Loeber, Keenan & DeLamatre, 1997). It is even more difficult for parents of children with ID, who are attempting to cope with new difficulties and unexpected behaviours, frequently with little assistance from family or professionals. Teachers and other service providers may be of little assistance because they might not have previously encountered challenging sexual or disruptive behaviour, and they may not be familiar with the field of ID generally. Furthermore, the child may not be consistently monitored by one professional or a team of professionals who can perceive the progression of behaviour into more serious and disruptive realms. Children with

ID frequently change schools, and professionals come and go in the services and in the lives of the family or carers. The troublesome young people may not be referred to mental health or young offender services until the behaviour becomes manifestly unacceptable and possibly dangerous to the young person or to others. The service providers and parents may not know which behaviours are serious enough to warrant intervention, or when a cluster of behaviours become significant (Kelley, Loeber, Keenan & DeLamatre, 1997). The frequency, duration, intensity, provocation and age of onset of the index behaviours may not be clearly identified and documented (ibid.), even though these are important dimensions in determining how significant the antisocial behaviour may be. There may be no clear indicators as to whether the child is likely to 'grow out of' the problematic behaviour, or whether the apparent discontinuation of the behaviour is a latency period or a manifestation that the individual is becoming more adept at concealing the behaviour. Changing the trajectory of a developmental pathway in a young person is a lengthy and difficult project, necessitating multi-agency and family involvement and long-term consistent commitment, policy support and funding. The earlier the investment in young people's lives, the more cost-effective the intervention to prevent sex offending.

REFERENCES

Andrade, J. T., Vincent, G. M. & Saleh, F. M. (2006) Juvenile sex offenders: A complex population, *Journal of Forensic Sciences, 51*, 163–7.

Beauregard, E., Lussier, P. & Proulx, J. (2004) An exploration of developmental factors related to deviant sexual preferences among adult rapists, *Sexual Abuse: A Journal of Research and Treatment, 16*, 151–61.

Brown, H. & Stein, J. (1997) Sexual abuse perpetrated by men with intellectual disabilities: A comparative study, *Journal of Intellectual Disability Research, 41*, 215–24.

Bullens, R., van Wijk, A. & Mali, B. (2006) Similarities and differences between the criminal careers of Dutch juvenile sex offenders and non-sex offenders, *Journal of Sexual Aggression, 12*, 155–64.

Dekker, M. C. & Koot, H. M. (2003) *DSM-IV* disorders in children with borderline to moderate intellectual disability. II: Child and family predictors, *American Academy of Child and Adolescent Psychiatry, 42*, 923–31.

Elliot, D. (1994) Serious violent offenders: onset, developmental course, and termination - The American Society of Criminology 1993 Presidential Address, *Criminology, 32*, 1–21.

Fago, D. (2003) Evaluation and treatment of neurodevelopmental deficits in sexually aggressive children and adolescents, *Professional Psychology: Research and Practice, 34*, 248–57.

Galli, V., McElroy, S. L., Soutullo, C. A., Kizer, D., Raute, N. & Keck, P. E. (1999) The psychiatric diagnoses of twenty-two adolescents who have sexually molested other children, *Comprehensive Psychiatry, 40*, 85–8.

Hare, R., Harpur, T., Hakstian, A., Forth, A., Hart, S. & Newman, J. (1990) The revised psychopathy checklist: Reliability and factor structure, *Psychological Assessment, 56*, 741–7.

Hayes, S. (2002) Adaptive behaviour and background characteristics of sex offenders with intellectual disabilities. International Association for the Scientific Study of Intellectual Disability Conference Dublin. Unpublished paper.

Hayes, S. (2004) The relationship between childhood abuse and subsequent sex offending (Abstract), *Journal of Intellectual Disability Research, 48*, 464.

Hunter, J. A., Figueredo, A. J., Malamuth, N. M. & Becker, J. V. (2004) Developmental pathways in youth sexual aggression and delinquency: Risk factors and mediators, *Journal of Family Violence, 19*, 233–42.

Kelley, B. T., Loeber, R., Keenan, K. & DeLamatre, M. (1997) Developmental pathways in boys' disruptive and delinquent behavior, In *Juvenile Justice Bulletin* US Department of Justice, Office of Justice Programs, Washington.

Knight, R. A. & Sims-Knight, J. E. (2003) The developmental antecedents of sexual coercion against women: Testing alternative hypotheses with structural equation modeling, *Annals of the New York Academy of Sciences, 989*, 72–85.

Knight, R. A. & Sims-Knight, J. E. (2004) Testing an etiological model for male juvenile sexual offending against females, *Journal of Child Sexual Abuse, 13*, 33–55.

Lindsay, W., Law, J., Quinn, K., Smart, N. & Smith, A. (2001) A comparison of physical and sexual abuse: Histories of sexual and non-sexual offenders with intellectual disability, *Child Abuse and Neglect, 25*, 989–95.

Lindsay, W., Smith, A., Quinn, K., Anderson, A., Smith, A., Allan, R. & Law, J. (2004) Women with intellectual disability who have offended: Characteristics and outcome, *Journal of Intellectual Disability Research, 48*, 580–90.

Loeber, R., Stouthamer-Loeber, M., Van Kammen, W. & Farrington, D. (1991) Initiation, escalation and desistance in juvenile offending and their correlates, *Journal of Criminal Law and Criminology, 82*, 36–82.

McElroy, S. L., Soutullo, C. A., Taylor, P., Nelson, E. B., Beckman, D. A., Brusman, L. A., Ombaba, J., M, Strakowski, S. M. & Keck, P. E. (1999) Psychiatric features of 36 men convicted of sexual offences, *Journal of Clinical Psychiatry, 60*, 414–20.

Parks, G. A. & Bard, D. E. (2006) Risk factors for adolescent sex offender recidivism: Evaluation of predictive factors and comparison of three groups based upon victim type, *Sex Abuse, 18*, 319–42.

Sequeira, H., Howlin, P. & Hollins, S. (2003) Psychological disturbance associated with sexual abuse in people with learning disabilities: Case-control study, *British Journal of Psychiatry, 183*, 451–56.

Smallbone, S. W. & Wortley, R. K. (2004) Onset, persistence, and versatility of offending among adult males convicted of sexual offenses against children, *Sexual Abuse: A Journal of Research and Treatment, 16*, 285–98.

Styron, T. & Janoff-Bulman, R. (1997) Childhood attachment and abuse: Long-term effects on adult attachment, depression and conflict resolution, *Child Abuse & Neglect, 21*, 1015–23.

Tolan, P. & Gorman-Smith, D. (1998) Development of serious and violent offending careers, In R. Loeber & D. Farrington (Eds), *Serious and violent juvenile offenders: Risk factors and successful interventions* (pp. 68–85). Sage, Thousand Oaks, CA

Tremblay, R. (2000) The origins of youth violence, *Canadian Journal of Policy Research 1*, 19–24.

Walker, E. A., Gelfand, A., Katon, W. J., Koss, M. P., Von Korff, M., Bernstein, D. & Russo, J. (1999) Adult health status of women with histories of childhood abuse and neglect, *American Journal of Medicine, 107*, 332–9.

Ward, T. & Siegert, R. (2002) Toward a comprehensive theory of child sexual abuse: a theory knitting perspective, *Crime and Law, 8*, 319–51.

4

Adolescents with Intellectual Disability and Family Sexual Abuse

KEVIN D. BROWNE AND MICHELLE MCMANUS

INTRODUCTION

In 2006, the police in England and Wales recorded 1,344 incest or familial sexual offences compared to 966 the year before. The 39 per cent increase was thought to have been influenced by the Sex Offences Act 2003 (Nicholas, Kershaw & Walker, 2007). The Sex Offences Act 2003 revised the crime of incest and replaced it with the offence *familial sexual abuse* which also covered sexual offences by a cohabitee/carer in the family who may not be a blood relative to the child. The offence encompasses sex abuse by step, foster and adoptive siblings, parents and grandparents and friends and relatives living in the family as well as blood relatives. Furthermore, the 2003 Act covers sexual abuse by acquaintances and extended family members with the new offence of *abuse of position of trust*.

It has been recognised that at least a third of adult sex offenders are known to have committed sexual assaults on children during their own teenage years (Elliott, Browne & Kilcoyne, 1995; Masson & Erooga, 1999; Erooga & Masson, 2006) and between 50 per cent and 80 per cent of adult sex offenders acknowledge a sexual interest in children during adolescence (Abel, Osborn & Twigg, 1993; Hoghughi, Bhate & Graham, 1997). Indeed, teenage male perpetrators aged 20 and younger account for about one-third of all allegations of sexual abuse (Davis & Leitenberg, 1987; Glasgow, Horne, Calam, & Cox, 1994; Watkins & Bentovim, 1992), two-thirds of all cautions and reprimands and approximately one-fifth of those convicted of a sexual offence in the UK (Erooga & Masson, 2006). This was confirmed by the Irish prevalence study which found that victims of sexual abuse claimed the perpetrator was a child (under 17 years) in one out of four cases (McGee, Garavan, De Barra, Byrne & Conroy, 2002).

Assessment and Treatment of Sexual Offenders with Intellectual Disabilities: A Handbook
Edited by Leam A. Craig, William R. Lindsay and Kevin D. Browne
© 2010 John Wiley & Sons, Ltd.

Since the mid 1990s, much attention has been given to the apparent over-representation of intellectual disability (ID) in services for sexual offenders (Day, 1994; Murphy, Harnett & Holland, 1995; O'Callaghan, 1998; Langevin & Curnoe, 2008). Much of the research about people who commit sex offences take samples from hospitals, secure units, treatment programmes and prisons. This may lead to an over-representation of sex offenders with ID within the literature and the assumption that individuals with ID are disproportionately more likely to be involved in sex offences compared to the general population (O'Callaghan, 1999).

However, little is known about the psychological development of sex offenders with ID, and the influence of family experiences on them, prior to their involvement with the health social and police services. The exception is the established fact that a higher proportion of this group have been victims of physical and sexual abuse during their childhood compared to other offenders and the population as a whole (See Hayes, Chapter 3). In fact, infants and children with intellectual and/or physical disabilities are at least twice as likely to be maltreated compared to children without disabilities (Browne & Herbert, 1997; Browne, Douglas, Hamilton-Giachritsis & Hegarty, 2006; Crosse, Kaye & Ratnofsky, 1993).

This chapter seeks to identify the extent and characteristics of family sexual abuse and considers the part played adolescents with ID in relation to sibling abuse and incest. Previous victimisation, the role of parents/carers and the potential impact on the family are discussed with the aim of identifying opportunities for prevention of sex offences in the family by adolescents and young adults with ID.

THE EXTENT OF SEXUAL ABUSE OF CHILDREN

The World Health Organization defines the sexual abuse of children as 'the involvement of a child in sexual activity, by either adults or other children who are in a position of responsibility, trust or power over that child, that he or she does not fully comprehend, is unable to give informed consent to, or for which the child is not developmentally prepared, or else that violates the laws or social taboos of society' (Butchart, Harvey, Mian & Furniss, 2006, p. 10).

Incidence

Evidence from victim surveys and prevalence studies in the UK consistently indicates that the number of people who anonymously report abuse in childhood is much more than the detected incidence rate of 2 children in every 10,000 identified as victims of sexual abuse, 60 per cent of these are girls and 40 per cent are boys (Creighton, 2002). In England on the day of 31 March 2008, 27 children per 10,000 (0–17 years) were the subject of a child protection plan for actual or highly suspected abuse and/or neglect. Of these 29,200 children on the register, 2,044 were registered for sexual abuse, which represents 7 per cent of cases. A further 2,336 (8 per cent) children were registered under mixed abuse, some of which included sexual abuse (Department for Children, Schools and Families, 2008). These incidence figures, when compared to prevalence rates, indicate that there is a significant 'dark figure' of unreported sexual crime on children as they represent less than one-tenth of anonymous reports of sexual abuse in childhood (Gilbert, Spatz-Widom,Browne, Fergusson, Webb & Janson, 2009). One reason for this discrepancy is that only a quarter of English adults who had unwanted sexual experiences or sex with someone five years older or more as a child chose to disclose the event, usually at a later date. This disclosure was usually to a friend, less often to a family member and rarely to the police (Cawson, Wattam, Brooker & Kelly, 2000).

According to the American Humane Association (McDonald *et al.*, 2005), the incidence of sexual abuse cases also represents 7 per cent of all child maltreatment referrals and 44 per cent of the cases were perpetrated in the family. Biological parents were alleged perpetrators in only 3 per cent of these cases. The male parent/caregiver (biological or non-biological) was thought to be responsible in 11 per cent of cases, other relatives (grandparent, siblings, cousins, uncles) accounted for 30 per cent of cases.

Prevalence

An early prevalence study of sexual abuse as a child, retrospectively reported by British adults (Baker & Duncan, 1985), found that 12 per cent of women and 8 per cent of men recall sexually abusive experiences in their childhood. More recent prevalence studies of over 3,000 adults who also gave retrospective self-reports about their childhood in England (Cawson, Wattam, Brooker, & Kelly, 2000) and Ireland (McGee, Garavan, De Barra, Byrne & Conroy, 2002) showed that contact sexual abuse had been experienced by 11 per cent of English children and 18.3 per cent of Irish children.

Similarly, the prevalence of sexual abuse of children has been estimated in the USA by David Finkelhor and his colleagues (Finkelhor, Hotaling, Lewis & Smith 1990). They interviewed 1,481 women and 1,145 men by telephone and found that 15 per cent of women and 9.5 per cent of men were found to have been victims of sexual intercourse during childhood. In addition, 20 per cent of women and 5 per cent of men admitted to being touched, grabbed or kissed as a child. An international comparison of 21 countries, around the same time, showed that the prevalence of sexual abuse of children ranged from 7 per cent to 36 per cent for women and 3 per cent to 29 per cent for men (Finkelhor, 1994). According to these studies, girls were between 1.5 and 3 times more likely to be sexually abused than boys. Up to 56 per cent of the girls and 25 per cent of the boys were sexually abused within the family environment, the abuse perpetrated by blood relatives, step-parents, foster carers and adoptive parents. In Ireland, 24 per cent of women and 14 per cent of men reported being sexually abused as children by a member of their family (McGee, Garavan, De Barra, Byrne & Conroy, 2002). In Romania, when young teenagers (aged from 13 to 14 years) were surveyed about maltreatment in the family home (Browne, Cartana, Momeu, Paunescu, Petre, & Tokay, 2002), 9 per cent claimed to have been sexually abused by a family member.

Relationship to Perpetrator, Duration and Disclosure

In a survey of 930 randomly selected women in San Francisco, Russell (1986) found that 150 (16 per cent) of the women reported they had been victims of sexual abuse by a relative before the age of 18 years (as a child). Furthermore, fewer than 20 described the experience in a positive or neutral way. Nevertheless, they suffered as much or even greater trauma than those women who described the experience as negative. For all women father/stepfather–daughter incest was found to be the most traumatic, which was reported in 24 per cent of cases. Uncles were responsible for 25 per cent of cases, 18 per cent were first cousins (2 per cent of whom were female), 17 per cent were brothers/stepbrothers, 10 per cent were other relatives (2 per cent of whom were female), 6 per cent were grandfathers and 1 per cent were mothers.

Early clinical sample studies of the extent of sexual abuse within English families (Bentovim & Boston, 1988; Mrazek, Lynch & Bentovim, 1981) did not distinguish sibling perpetrators and included offences from brothers and sisters in a category of 'other relatives'. For example, Mrazek, Lynch and Bentovim's (1981) review of 202 sexual abuse victims in England found that biological parents were responsible in 22 per cent of cases (2 per cent of whom were mothers), stepfathers 12 per cent, other relatives 9 per cent, acquaintances 31 per cent and strangers 26 per cent. Similarly, a survey of adult male sex offenders by Elliott, Browne and Kilcoyne (1995) found that approximately one-third of convicted offenders were intrafamilial offenders, one-third were extrafamilial acquaintances known to the child and one-third were strangers.

Finkelhor (1986) observed that most USA sexual abuse victims outside the family (60 per cent) described a single unpleasant experience. Consequently, they avoided the perpetrator or told a parent/guardian, who helped them to prevent it happening again. However, victims of sexual abuse by family members or friends of the family (40 per cent) described sexual assaults on an episodic or regular basis. The average duration for female victims of sexual abuse within the family was 31 weeks. Similarly, in Ireland 60 per cent of cases experienced a single abusive event, for those 40 per cent of cases who experienced ongoing sexual abuse (58 per cent of girl victims and 42 per cent of boy victims) the duration was over one year and was more likely to be perpetrated by a family member or friend of the family. Four out of five victims reported that they knew their offender prior to the sexual assault and 67 per cent of girl victims and 62 per cent of boy victims reported that the sexual abuse took place before they reached 12 years of age. Over a third (36 per cent) of those who had experienced sexual abuse as a child believed that their abuser was also sexually assaulting other children at the same time (McGee, Garavan, De Barra, Byrne & Conroy, 2002).

In cases of sexual abuse of children, only 5 per cent are disclosed and 2 per cent reported to the police at the time of the event or shortly after, half of which (1 per cent) are prosecuted (Kelly, Regan & Burton, 1991). The same small proportion (2 per cent) of cases reported to the police has also been found in the USA (Russell, 1983, 1986). Generally, studies (e.g., Davenport, Browne & Palmer, 1994) show that proximity in the relationship between victim and offender influences the disclosure of sexual abuse such that abuses by a close relation within the immediate family are even less likely to be disclosed than those perpetrated by those more distant in the circle of extended family/friends or those involving a stranger. Furthermore, male victims are less likely to disclose than female victims as the experience is more likely to be homosexual and there is a cultural reluctance to see males as victims of sexual assaults (Rogers & Terry, 1984).

The Risk to Children with Disabilities

The relative risk of child maltreatment for children with disabilities compared to children without a disability has been determined from a large US epidemiological study of 50,278 children (Sullivan & Knutson, 2000). The study identified 4,503 maltreated children from this population, 1,012 of whom also had a disability. As only 8 per cent of US children have some form of disability, it was found that they were 3.4 times more likely to be abused and/or neglected. Overall, 31 per cent of children with a disability were maltreated compared to 11 per cent of children without a disability. Table 4.1 presents the relative risk (as a multiplication factor) of child maltreatment for children with different types of disabilities compared to children without a disability (x 1) as reported by Kendall-Tackett, Lyon, Taliaferro and Little (2005) based on the above study.

Table 4.1 Relative risk of child maltreatment for children with disabilities compared to children without a disability (X 1) (Adapted from Kendall-Tackett, Lyon, Taliaferro & Little, 2005 and based on data on 50,278 US children from Sullivan & Knutson 2000)

Child's Disability	Neglect	Physical Abuse	Sexual Abuse	Psychological/ Emotional Abuse
Hearing Difficulties	X 2	X 4	X 1	X 2
Speech/Language Difficulties	X 5	X 5	X 3	X 1
Developmental Delay	X 4	X 4	X 4	X 4
Learning Disabilities	X 2	X 2	X 2	X 2
Behavioural Disorders	X 7	X 7	X 5.5	X 7
No Disability	X 1	X 1	X 1	X 1

Children with disabilities are especially vulnerable to maltreatment because of their need for personal care and powerlessness which results in compliance and caregivers making choices for them (Westcott & Jones, 1999). Difficulties in language, speech or vocabulary and impaired or limited cognitive abilities may result in social and emotional isolation, enhancing the risk of abuse and inhibiting disclosure and detection. Sex education and information about abuse prevention reduces this risk, but children with disabilities are often left out of these initiatives as they are perceived as unable to benefit. A lack of support for families caring for a disabled child, and a failure to screen the care staff and the professionals who work with them, creates a further risk of abuse and neglect, especially if the child is placed in institutional care. All children lack the ability to protect themselves from abusive older children, teenagers and adults and find it difficult to communicate their feelings about being bullied and maltreated. However, this is especially a problem for children with disabilities (Morris, 1999).

Depending on the form the ID takes, the chances of being sexually abused as a child increase dramatically (see Table 4.1). However, any form of abuse and/or neglect experienced by a child increases the probability of antisocial behaviour disorders and sex offences as a teenager and adult (Browne, Hamilton-Giachritsis & Vettor, 2007). A retrospective case note review of 300 English 'psychiatric in-patients' admissions with ID (Balogh *et al.*, 2001), aged between 9 and 21 years, found information on sexual maltreatment for 23 boys and 20 girls (14 per cent of cases). There was evidence of victimisation alone for 21 cases (7 per cent), both victimisation and perpetration in 16 cases (5 per cent) and perpetration alone in 6 male cases (2 per cent). In total, there were 22 sex offenders; 17 boys and 5 girls aged between 9 and 18 years, of whom 73 per cent had also been victims of sexual abuse earlier in childhood. Of the 37 victims, the relationship to their childhood abuser was known in 34 of the cases: 20 (61 per cent) had been sexually abused by a family member, 10 (30 per cent) by an acquaintance and 3 (9 per cent) by a stranger. Hence, it appears that children with intellectual disabilities are more likely to be sexually abused by a family member and less likely by a stranger than are non-disabled children.

SIBLING SEXUAL ABUSE AND INCEST

With regard to the family context, the sexual maltreatment of brothers and sisters by their siblings is much more common than was once thought. Even though there is more written about father–daughter incest and sexual abuse, sibling incest and sexual abuse by half, step- and surrogate brothers and sisters is widely accepted as the most prevalent type of intrafamilial sexual assault (Adler & Schutz, 1995; Carlson, Maciol & Schneider, 2006; O'Brian, 1991). To a certain extent this has been the result of a reappraisal of what was once considered sexual exploration between brothers and sisters, which occurs for approximately 15 per cent of girls and 10 per cent of boys (Finkelhor, 1980). This has been more appropriately described as exploitation where the age difference between the siblings is greater than five years (De Long, 1989; Finkelhor, 1980), although it has been observed that adolescent incest offenders were less likely to be court ordered for treatment than non-incestuous adolescent offenders (O'Brian, 1991).

Various factors that are bound up in the context of the family result in the extent of sibling incest and sexual abuse being relatively unknown. However, in a study of family conflict, 2 per cent of English undergraduate students reported being sexually maltreated by a sibling on at least one occasion (Browne & Hamilton, 1998). Often this sexual maltreatment was associated with physical abuse and bullying, a fact that has been confirmed by a number of American studies for both boys and girls (De Long, 1989; Johnson, 1988, 1989). These studies also demonstrated that sibling maltreatment of both a physical and sexual nature is not restricted to older teenagers and young adults in the family and has been observed in young children (Cantwell, 1988). For example, Johnson (1988) noted that 46 per cent of a sample of 47 sexually abusive adolescent boys were involved in the abuse of their siblings. Similarly, Pierce and Pierce (1987) reported in their study that of the 59 sex offences committed by 37 juvenile offenders, 40 per cent were against sisters and 20 per cent were against brothers. Similarly, 43 per cent of young sex offenders referred to a 'Sexual Abuse Counselling and Prevention Program' in Melbourne, Australia had sexually abused a sibling; 'the majority of their victims were less than 10 years of age'. Two-thirds of victims had suffered penetration sexual offences and the use of force and for one-third the abuse had been occurring for more than one year (Flanagan & Hayman-White, 1999).

Adler and Schutz's (1995) study of male adolescent sibling incest offenders (n = 12) who had been referred to a clinical service, found 58 per cent (n = 7) were recorded as having learning problems or behavioural problems in school; however, only 4 (33 per cent) had a diagnosis for a specific 'learning disorder'.

The availability of younger victims in the household and parents not providing adequate supervision are risk factors associated with inappropriate sexual behaviour from adolescents in the family. Intervention with such families often involves adult members of the family being questioned on where the sexual behaviours shown by their children were learnt and how they developed to become abusive and problematic (e.g., being exposed to inappropriate sexual behaviours such as observing the sexual intercourse of parents, access to pornography etc. (Worling, 1995)). Often there is a blurring of boundaries surrounding the identification of inappropriate sexual behaviour, with much being referred to as exploratory – for example, the parents would say 'boys will be boys'. Likewise, the parents see it as mutually consenting sex play acting out 'doctors and nurses' or 'mothers and fathers'. Consequently, the perpetrator is not held responsible for his/her actions and has license to continue (O'Brian, 1991; Wiehe, 1997; Worling, 1995). This minimisation and ignorance of wrongdoing is liable to have long-term consequences for the victim.

Victims of sibling sexual abuse, in the context of denial and minimisation, may see themselves as cooperative and willing participants and able to stop the perpetrator if they wish. Hence, they may blame themselves for the abuse and take responsibility for the family distress, unwanted intervention and scrutiny (Caffaro & Conn-Caffaro, 2005). This turmoil may result in the victim repressing their emotions, denying or retracting allegations and, later, in mental health problems.

Sibling relationships are seen as a one of the most important, enduring relationships in human life (Caffaro & Conn-Caffaro, 2005). Siblings share family histories and, particularly in adverse, neglectful or abusive environments, they may seek each other's company to achieve their required levels of affection and support, previously termed 'secret coalition' (Carlson, Maciol & Schneider, 2006). In turning to each other, the advent of puberty increases the likelihood of this rapport being sexualised. Indeed, research has reported a link between family dysfunction and sibling incest which is sometimes mediated through physical and/or sexual abuse of the children (Wiehe, 1997; Worling, 1995). Hence, a lack of parental supervision is a common characteristic seen in cases of sibling incest and sexual abuse that often represents a deeper individual and family pathology (O'Brian, 1991).

From an attachment perspective, children from 'average' families usually experience sensitive and consistent parenting and learn to perceive their social environment in a positive way. As a consequence, they develop a positive sense of self and a positive view of others. By contrast, children from abusive, neglectful or disorganised families are highly likely to have an insecure attachment to their primary caregiver and other members of the family as a result of harsh or inconsistent parenting (Morton & Browne, 1998). This hinders the development of a positive self-image and these children are more likely to have a negative view of self and a negative view of others, which in turn lessens the development of empathy towards the others, making it emotionally easier to offend and harm others (Browne & Herbert, 1997).

A concern is that sibling incest and abuse tends to endure over long periods, resulting in more serious offences being committed over time (Cyr, Wright, McDuff & Perron, 2002). It is likely to continue until someone reports the sexualised sibling relationship, which is not usually the victim or the offender (Adler & Schutz, 1995). Once 'discovered', it is common for victims to report the sexual abuse lasting up to five years (Bass, Taylor, Knudson-Martin & Huenergardt, 2006), with some reporting much longer periods (Carlson, Maciol & Schneider, 2006; Rudd & Herzberger, 1999). Hence, the consequences for the victims are profound because of the serious nature of the abuse, the duration of the abuse, the betrayal of trust in such a close relationship and the feelings of vulnerability and lack of parental care and protection (Davenport, Browne & Palmer, 1994).

Disclosure by victims is problematic in sibling abuse and incest (45 per cent in Caffaro and Conn-Caffaro (2005) had not disclosed before interview). In families where there is a lack of appropriate supervision/power or a hierarchal structure within the family the victim may feel reluctant to report such behaviour through fear of not being believed, being blamed for the behaviour, or being responsible for the break-up of the family (Bass, Taylor, Knudson-Martin & Huenergardt, 2006; Carlson, Maciol & Schneider, 2006). Similarly, these same reasons can be applied to parents who are aware of sibling abuse but are reluctant to report because they fear the consequences of having the victim and offender removed and the rest of the family being scrutinised (Deisher, Wenet, Paperny, Clark & Fehrenbach, 1982; DiGiorgio-Miller, 1998). The unfortunate dilemma of a mother is expressed effectively by Burnham, Moss, deBelle and Jamieson: *'she was scared to blame her son, in case he felt abandoned, yet if she did not blame him she felt her daughter would think she was condoning what he did and feel betrayed'* (1999, p. 161; emphasis added).

Therefore, it is not surprising that sibling incest rarely comes to the attention of services at the time the offence occurs. Much of what is known has been gathered from adult offenders retrospectively reporting their experiences in their family of origin. This ultimately limits our knowledge and exploration of sexual abuse and incest in the family, especially in relation to the role of ID.

ADOLESCENT SEX OFFENDERS

Adolescent and teenage sex offenders, sometimes referred to as juvenile sex offenders, are not a homogeneous group and may be categorised into a number of subgroups based on their personal characteristics and the nature of their offences (Barbaree & Marshall, 2006; Gerhold, Browne & Beckett, 2007). Interestingly, O'Brian (1991) categorised his adolescent male sex offenders (n = 170) into one of 4 groups: (i) sibling incest (n = 50); (ii) child molester, non-family (n = 57); (iii) non-child offender (n = 38); (iv) mixed offender (n = 25) residual category, which included those who had multiple victims who were siblings/non-familial/peers/adults. This may be the situation with some of the offenders who are less discriminatory in their choice of victim and are more influenced by access and opportunity offenders with ID. From his group as whole he found 60 per cent had a below average school performance, with sibling incest offenders more likely (60 per cent) than the other three categories to have had previous referrals to therapy.

Most adult sexual offenders admit to taking advantage of younger children during their teenage years, and the majority confess to being physically and/or sexually assaulted themselves by other teenagers and adults (Elliott, Browne & Kilcoyne, 1995). Indeed, retrospective self-report studies have revealed that 60 per cent to 80 per cent of sex offenders with a history of childhood victimisation began molesting children as adolescents (Groth, Hobson & Garry, 1982), and it has been estimated that these individuals perpetrate 50 per cent of the sex crimes against boys and up to 20 per cent of offences against girls (Rogers & Terry, 1984). Indeed, it has been estimated that the probability of committing sex offences against children is 5.4 times greater for male victims of sexual maltreatment than for males with no such history (Lee, Jackson, Pattison & Ward, 2002).

Skuse and colleagues (Skuse et al. 1998) carried out a retrospective case control study to investigate the risk factors for abused adolescent boys becoming abusers themselves. It was found that experiencing and/or witnessing intrafamilial violence in general and discontinuity of care were significant factors that distinguished those who became abusers and those who did not. Therefore, sexually abusive behaviour towards other children may not be directly related to the sexual abuse suffered as a child as a variety of severe family problems and all forms of abuse and neglect are implicated (Veneziano & Veneziano, 2002).

It has been suggested that males pose greater risk than females of becoming an abuser (Summit, 1983) and that this risk also depends on the onset, type, frequency, duration and severity of maltreatment suffered as a child. People's responses to disclosure by the victim also have a strong influence on their risk of offending behaviour. The relationship to the perpetrator (s) and the number of perpetrators are also significant especially when the person has experienced recurrent victimisation (Hamilton, Falshaw & Browne, 2002). The risk may be further exacerbated by the victim's temperamental personality (Finkelhor, 2008).

In a study of 139 adolescent sex offenders attending a clinic in the USA, Becker (1988) found that 27 (19 per cent) disclosed in an initial interview that they had been victims of sexual abuse earlier in their childhood. It was reported that 15 per cent of non-disabled juvenile sex offenders had previously been sexually abused by a family member or relative (4 per cent of which were siblings), 59 per cent were victims of an adult outside the family and 26 per cent of a peer or older child outside the family (4 per cent female perpetrator). Thus, approximately a third had been sexually abused by another child and nearly nine out of ten (89 per cent) knew the adult or child perpetrator. The finding that most non-disabled juvenile sex offenders were abused by a known acquaintance outside the family is consistent with an earlier study (Rogers & Terry, 1984) but differs from the findings of later studies on juvenile sex offenders with ID (Balogh *et al.*, 2001; Fyson, 2007a; Lindsay *et al.*, 2001) both in terms of the prevalence of earlier sexual victimisation (38 to 87 per cent) and the proportion of perpetrators outside the family (39 to 50 per cent). The English prevalence (12.7 per cent) of earlier sexual victimisation of people with ID who do not commit sex offences (Lindsay, Law, Quinn, Smart & Smith, 2001) is approximately the same as that found in the general population (11 per cent) (Cawson, Wattam, Brooker & Kelly, 2000).

ADOLESCENT SEX OFFENDERS WITH INTELLECTUAL DISABILITY

Studies frequently report that ID and educational problems are over-represented among samples of adolescent sexual abusers (Fyson, 2007a; Lindsay *et al.* 2002). O'Callaghan (1998), the former Programme Director at G-MAP (an independent organisation which seeks to work with young people identified as displaying inappropriate sexual behaviours) reported that around half of the young people referred were assessed as having some level of ID. However, the prevalence quoted in other studies ranges between 44 and 80 per cent. For example,

- 46 per cent of 121 young sexual offenders investigated were categorised as ID (Dolan, Holloway, Bailey and Kroll (1996);
- 44 per cent of adolescent sex offenders in a secure setting had learning difficulties (Epps, 1991);
- 53 per cent of young people referred to the London-based Young Abusers Project were deemed to be ID (Hawkes, Jenkins & Vizard, 1997); and
- 80 per cent of adolescents in a residential programme for sex offending were assessed as ID (Boswell & Wedge, 2002).

Many authors seek to explain this imbalance by focusing on the key characteristics that seem to differentiate adolescent sex offenders with ID from their non-disabled counterparts. For example, Thompson and Brown (1997) identified a number of factors associated with a lack of privacy: individuals with ID are likely to encounter increased supervision and naivety about admitting their sexual activities; often the sex offending takes place in public settings because of their lack of sex education and opportunistic style; they are seen as less adept at disguising or hiding their sexual activities and offences and are often unaware that what they have done is wrong.

Other authors have observed that adolescent sex offenders with ID tend to be less discriminating in their choice of victim and are less likely to involve planning in their sex offences, sexually assaulting those who are accessible in terms of proximity and/or vulnerability (O'Callaghan, 1999; Langevin & Curnoe, 2008). They have also been reported as having a greater external locus of control and being less able to maintain self-control of their sexual urges in comparison to adolescents without ID (Rose, Jenkins, O'Connor, Jones & Felce, 2002). Hence, they tend to be less preferential in the sex and age of their victims (Tudiver, Broekstra, Josselyn & Barbaree, 1998), which implies that the offences are more impulsive and opportunistic (Thomson & Brown, 1997).

Nevertheless, victims of adolescent sex offenders with ID tend to be younger than them rather than a member of their peer group (Fyson, 2007b). This is linked to deficits in their social skills that limit their ability to interact with others within their own age range. Rather, this group of individuals with ID have a psychosocial pairing with children who are of a similar developmental age to themselves (Craig, in press; Murrey, Briggs & Davies, 1992).

Furey (1994) found that 42 per cent of cases of sexual abuse involving adult victims with ID were committed by an individual who also had ID. The risk of sibling abuse within group or family containing individuals with ID is significant as individuals with ID who commit sex offences have a propensity to victimise those in close proximity.

There seems to be a tendency to deny adolescents categorised with ID the possibility of appropriate sex education and opportunities to discuss and express their sexual identity. This may have an adverse impact, in the short- and long-term, with regard to their knowledge of sex and intimacy or what constitutes appropriate personal boundaries and acceptable sexual behaviour (Fyson, 2007b; O'Callaghan, 1998, 1999). Indeed, Murphy (2003) found that only 55 per cent of young people with ID completed school sex education compared to 98 per cent of young people without ID. Therefore, individuals with ID are at a higher risk of committing sex offences unwittingly and unknowingly.

Tudiver, Broekstra, Josselyn and Barbaree (1998), in their guidance on individuals with developmental delay, state there is a myth that these individuals are 'asexual' and are often seen as childlike, which has a negative impact on their development. This reinforces the minimisation by those around the individual of any inappropriate behaviour, believing it to be child-play, and removes the opportunity for the unwanted behaviour to be challenged and changed. Without appropriate intervention, the risk of later sexual offences is increased.

A similarity between adolescent sex offenders with and without ID is the increased likelihood of family dysfunction and evidence of the intergenerational transmission of abuse (Browne, Hamilton-Giachritsis & Vettor, 2007; Lindsay et al., 2002; Tudiver, Broekstra, Josselyn & Barbaree, 1998). However, the prevalence of prior victimisation and risk factors that facilitate the 'cycle of violence' may be greater in those offenders with ID.

SIBLING ABUSE AND INCEST INVOLVING ADOLESCENT SEX OFFENDERS WITH INTELLECTUAL DISABILITY

The amalgamation of research on adolescent sex offenders with ID and research on adolescents who sexually abuse siblings in the family has barely been touched upon in academic literature. It is evident from the research presented above that within both of these two areas of research there are the problems with identification, assessment and intervention. Thus, together they present a 'double-barrier' to knowledge and exploration of sexual abuse and incest in the family. However, these two separate areas of research seem to share a number of common factors. Table 4.2 presents the common factors associated with adolescent sex offenders with ID and adolescents who sexually abuse siblings in the family.

Kelly, Richardson, Hunter and Knapp (2002) reported 50 per cent of adolescent male sex offenders had special educational needs, with around 12 per cent classified as intrafamilial. Tudiver, Broekstra, Josselyn and Barbaree (1998) developed guidance addressing the needs of what they termed 'developmentally delayed' sex offenders. They found that in the majority (75 per cent) of serious sexual incidents (hands on offence/oral offence/penetrative offence) the victim was known to the offender, with 5 per cent reported as being a sibling. Similarly, Fyson (2007b) investigated 15 young people with ID who had committed sex offences and found that two individuals (13.3 per cent) in her sample had sexually abused their siblings. Three cases were offences against victims who themselves had some sort of disability.

Although research on adolescent sex offenders with ID describes their offending as likely to be of a serious or violent nature (Lindsay, 2002), the duration and easy access shown in sibling incest research highlights the risk of individuals with ID developing sexually abusive behaviours over time. Severe consequences can occur when early warning signs are minimised or ignored and as a result the behaviour is not dealt with. This may gradually escalate into more serious offending causing increased victim trauma and the likelihood that the offender will be put on the sex offender register (Lindsay, 2002). Fyson (2007b) found a typical reluctance to report sibling incest and suggested that the phenomenon is under reported and the prevalence among young people with ID is higher than she observed in this investigation. A retrospective study of 'survivors' of sibling incest supports this observation (Carlson, Maciol & Schneider, 2006).

A common problem with sibling abuse and adolescent sex offences is the inability of key carers to distinguish between inappropriate and normal sexual behaviour. Hinsberger, Griffiths and Quinsey (1991) use the term 'counterfeit deviance' to describe the behaviour of adolescents with ID as deviant yet influenced by factors such as lack of sexual knowledge accompanied by sexual naivety, poor social skills and opportunities to explore and express sexual relationships (see Chapter 2 in this volume).

Knowing the possible consequence of identifying sexually inappropriate behaviour carries with it the potential for unwarranted intervention (DiGiorgio-Miller, 1998), reporting such behaviour is a complex decision for parents, who do not want to see their child further labelled as a 'sex offender'. Admitting there is a problem may also bring guilt on parents with regard to their parental abilities, as it may involve admitting to a failure in their parental skills. This carries the additional fear of the victim as well as the perpetrator being removed from the family and the home environment while under investigation and assessment (ibid.).

Therefore, research suggests that parents are unlikely to report sibling abuse (Bass, Taylor, Knudson-Martin & Huenergardt, 2006) and carers of individuals with ID in school adopt the same behaviour (Fyson, 2007a; 2007b). However, an individual with ID left unchallenged and untreated with regard to their sexually abusive behaviours is at risk of increased frequency, intensity and duration of their sexual offending. This escalation, in turn, will exacerbate the trauma experienced by the victim(s) both in the short and long term, which is common to all sibling incest victims (Wiehe, 1997). In both contexts there is a reluctance of carers and parents to identify and report inappropriate sexual behaviour. They interpret the sexualised behaviour as play or exploration and are unsure how to tackle the problem. A reluctance to report sexual abuse in the family ensues, which seeks to maintain the family homeostasis. Parents face a

Table 4.2 Common factors associated with adolescent sex offenders with intellectual disabilities and sibling abuse/incest in the family

Common Factors in Adolescent Sex Offenders	Intellectual Disability Research	Sibling Abuse/Incest Research
Dysfunctional Family	Day (1993); Firth *et al*. (2001); Hayes, 1991; Lindsay *et al*. (2002); O'Callaghan, 1999; Fyson (2007a, b)	O'Brian (1991); Adler & Schutz (1995); Worling (1995); Rudd & Herzberger (1999); Smith & Israel (1987); Caffaro & Conn-Caffaro (2005): Worling (1995); Carlson et al. (2006); Bass *et al*. (2006)
Prior Victimisation (Physical)	Day (1993); Lindsay *et al*. (2001); Fyson (2007a, b)	Adler & Schutz (1995); O'Brien (1991); Rudd and Herzberger (1999); Cyr *et al*. (2002); Caffaro & Conn-Caffaro, (2005)
Prior Victimisation (Sexual)	Thompson & Brown (1997); Lindsay *et al*. (2001); Firth *et al*. (2001); Fyson (2007a, b)	O'Brian (1991); Smith & Israel (1987); Worling (1995); Cyr *et al*. (2002); Rudd & Herzberger (1999); Carlson *et al*. (2006)
Lack Parental/Carer Supervision	Fyson (2007a, b); O'Callaghan (1998); Firth *et al*. (2001); Tudiver *et al*. (1998);	O'Brian (1991); Rudd & Herzberger (1999); Worling (1995); Caffaro & Conn-Caffaro (2005)
School/Behavioural Problems	Day (1993); Hayes, 1991; Lindsay *et al*. (2002); Tudiver *et al*. (1998); Langevin & Cunroe (2007)	Wiehe (1997): Bass *et al*. (2006); Caffaro & Conn-Caffaro (2005); Adler & Schutz (1995); Bass *et al*. (2006)
Parents/Carers Discourage Sexual Expression	Murphy (2003); O'Callaghan, 1998, 1999; Tudiver *et al*. (1998); Murphy (2003)	Smith & Israel (1987); Meiselman (1987); Adler & Schtuz (1995)
Exposed to inappropriate age sexual behaviours	Firth *et al*. (2001); Craft (1994)	Worling (1995); Caffaro & Conn-Caffaro (2005)
Confusion Regarding What is Inappropriate/Appropriate Behaviour	O'Callaghan, (1999); Fyson (2007a, b); Tudiver *et al*. (1998)	DiGiorgio-Miller (1998); Wiehe (1997); Caffaro & Conn-Caffaro (2005); Carslon *et al*. (2006)

Table 4.2 (*Continued*)

Common Factors in Adolescent Sex Offenders	Intellectual Disability Research	Sibling Abuse/Incest Research
Easy access to Victims/Less Discriminatory in Victim/ Impulsive	Lindsay (2002); Firth *et al.* (2001); O'Callaghan, (1999); Tudiver *et al.* (1998)	O'Brian (1991); Worling (1995); Rudd & Herzberger (1999); Caffaro & Conn-Caffaro (2005); Bass *et al.* (2006)
Variety of Sexual Offences Committed	Lindsay (2002); Firth *et al.* (2001); Lindsay *et al.* (2002); O'Callaghan (1998); Langevin & Cunroe (2007); Rose *et al.* (2002)	O'Brian (1991); Adler & Schutz (1995); Caffaro & Conn-Caffaro (2005); Carlson et al. (2006); Bass *et al.* (2006)
Parental or Carer Denial/ Minimisation	Swanson & Garwick (1990 in Lindsay *et al.* 2002); O'Callaghan (1999); Tudiver *et al.* (1998)	Adler & Schutz (1995); O'Brian (1991); Rudd & Herzberger (1999); Caffaro & Conn-Caffaro (2005)
Reluctance of Parents/ Carers to Report	Rose *et al.* (2002); Fyson (2007a, b; Lindsay (2002); Tudiver *et al.* (1998)	Rudd & Herzberger (1999); DiGiorgio-Miller (1998); Caffaro & Conn-Caffaro (2005); Carlson *et al.* (2006); Bass *et al.* (2006)

dilemma when their child with ID is sexually abusing a sibling. Parents will want to protect the bother and/or sister by reporting the sexual abuse in the family, but will also want to protect their child with ID, who is vulnerable. The parent will fear blame, family breakdown, inadequate intervention and the further labelling of their child as a sex offender (Burnham, Moss, deBelle & Jamieson, 1999). Research in general on sibling abuse often highlights the responsibility of the parents who tend to minimise the inappropriateness of such acts, believing this to be mutual, exploratory 'sex play' (O'Brian, 1991; Rudd and Herzberger (1999).

Not surprisingly therefore, the abuse of brothers and sisters in the family (full, half, step- and surrogate siblings) by offenders who have ID, has rarely been discussed within literature, regardless of the potential risk to siblings. A growth of research has recently developed on sibling abuse which is now recognising sibling incest as the most prevalent form of incestuous behaviour, but again the presence of ID has largely been neglected. In addition to parents, there is reluctance on the part of schools and institutions to report sexually inappropriate behaviours. Fyson (2007a, b) has conducted some analysis of this problem using surveys distributed to special schools. She highlighted problems with the identification of inappropriate sexual behaviour and also the lack of guidance on appropriate interventions to support the decisions of teachers or parents/carers to report. However, she found that 88 per cent of special schools reported the occurrence of sexually inappropriate behaviours. The behaviours ranged from

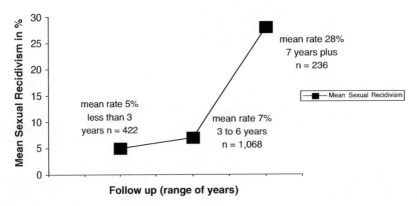

Figure 4.1   Mean rates for sexual recidivism for juvenile sex offenders (n = 1,315) across 12 studies dependent on length of follow-up (from Gerhold, Browne & Becket, 2007)

public masturbation (58 per cent) to attempted or actual penetration (15 per cent). This indicates that even within closely monitored, regulated environments, serious acts of abuse occur.

INTERVENTION

Until relatively recently, most juvenile sexual offending was considered 'exploratory' behaviour and something that would cease with age in a similar way to non-violent delinquent behaviour (Ryan & Lane, 1997). However, research indicates that juvenile sex offending does not decline over time without appropriate intervention. Gerhold, Browne and Beckett (2007) reviewed 12 studies of sexual recidivism in adolescent sex offenders with an overall sample of 1,315 juvenile sex abusers with an average age of 15. The overall average for recidivism in these studies was 14 per cent for sexual offending and 44 per cent for non-sexual offending. However, it was discovered that those studies with longer follow-up periods had a higher percentage of young people sexually re-offending (see Figure 4.1). Indeed, 28 per cent had re-offended within seven years. These studies suggest that without appropriate intervention and referral to youth services for inappropriate sexual behaviour, these teenagers may go on to commit sexual offences as adults.

Case study
Rose, Jenkins, O'Connor, Jones and Felce (2002) highlighted the case of a sex offender with ID aged 17 living with his father and stepmother, who had two young children. When assessed using the WAIS-R (Wechsler, 1984) he scored in the mild ID (66) range. He had a previous conviction for sexually assaulting an 8-year-old boy which led to prosecution and a two-year probation order with a requirement to attend group work. One of the main concerns was the risk of him abusing the young children at home because of the ease of access. The authors describe a gradual improvement of behaviour following intervention as the teenager responded to treatment over the next few months. Nevertheless, he became involved in another incident of sexual assault on a child and he was removed from his family and institutionalised to protect his siblings. This very briefly emphasises the potential risks to families.

Therefore, interventions must be focused on comprehensive assessment (to identify criminogenic need) and appropriate treatment to prevent further offending behaviour and victimisation. This involves a combination of individual, group and family therapy carried out by professionals trained specifically to work with young people with ID and their families on sexual victimisation and offending. Some intervention approaches applied to non-disabled juveniles with antisocial behaviour problems may be applicable; such as basic sex education, impulse control skills, anger management, challenging distorted thinking patterns, relapse prevention techniques, life skills and self-esteem. However, these approaches must be first adapted to the needs of people with ID and evaluated.

Assessment obviously includes an evaluation of the individuals intellectual functioning (even if one has been carried out before). In a Canadian sample of 71 male and 14 female 'developmentally delayed' sex offenders (aged from 13 to 78 with a mean of 33.5 years) Tudiver, Broekstra, Josselyn and Barbaree (1998) found the following intellectual functioning:

- 6 per cent low to average
- 19 per cent borderline
- 34 per cent mild
- 33 per cent moderate
- 6 per cent severe/profound

A third were living with their families, 47 per cent in group or foster homes and 20 per cent within institutions (not living in the community). Half were unemployed, 24 per cent in the workforce and 26 per cent in school. Three-quarters of their victims were known to them (5 per cent siblings) and half were also 'developmentally delayed'. In relation to this an assessment of their sexual knowledge revealed that

- 10 per cent were well-informed;
- 44 per cent had a moderate level of information;
- 19 per cent possessed little correct information;
- 27 per cent were not well informed.

In terms of assessing appropriate sexual curiosity and exploration by children and young people; normal sexual interest involves mutual interest and consent between individuals of a similar age, size and development. It is playful and limited in type and frequency at any one particular stage. Adult sexual knowledge and activity is acquired over a number of years, slowly and in strict sequence from kissing, touching over clothes, touching under clothes, manipulation of genitals, masturbation and penetration through exploration with consenting peers. It is expected that 40–75 per cent of children will engage in some exploratory gender role play and sexual behaviour before the age of 13 (Johnson & Friend, 1995).

Family Work

Bentovim (2007), summarises the main approaches to working with families were sexual abuse has occurred. This is done within a legal framework of child care and protection. The steps are as follows:

- assigning responsibility for the abuse;
- treatment focused on parenting;
- treatment focused on family relationships;
- treatment focused on acknowledging the origins and effects of abuse;
- treatment to help the perpetrator within a context of safety (which may require the perpetrator to be separated from the family in the short term and sometimes long term);
- abuse-focused therapy for the victim.

Family work is important, especially when the sexual abuse victim and/or perpetrator in the family is being blamed or scapegoated for the family problems. All family members should evaluate their family organisation, behaviour, boundaries, availability and supervision with regard to children and young people in the home. Work between the child victim or perpetrator and the non-abusive family members should not be ignored, and indeed is essential to their rehabilitation.

CONCLUSIONS

The limitations of this chapter have necessitated reliance on previous literature, which has been amalgamated from studies that often (especially within sibling incest) have small sample sizes. The difficulties in conceptualising, identifying and assessing child and adolescent sex offenders often leaves researchers with no choice but to source their samples from clinical/therapeutic services. These tend to be young adults who are being treated for other problems such as anger (Lindsay *et al.*, 2002), often in addition to their abusive behaviour. This suggests we are only capturing the most visible and problematic offenders. Subsequently, many authors admit their research findings are probably a gross underestimation of the actual problem. There is growing recognition of female perpetrators within sibling incest and adolescent sex offences, with figures reported to be as high as one in five cases (Vizard, Monck & Misch, 1995). This is an area that warrants further investigation.

REFERENCES

Abel, G., Osborn, C. & Twigg, D. (1993). Sexual assault through the life span: Adult offenders with juvenile histories. In H.E. Barbaree, W.L. Marshall, and S.M. Hudson (eds), *The juvenile sex offender* (pp. 104–17). New York: Guildford.

Adler, N.A. & Schutz, J. (1995). Sibling incest offenders. *Child Abuse and Neglect*, 19 (7), 811–19.

Baker, A.W. & Duncan, S.P. (1985). Child sexual abuse: A study of prevalence in Britain. *Child Abuse and Neglect*, 8, 457–467.

Balogh, R., Bretherton, K., Whibley, S., Berney, T., Graham, S., Richold, P., Worsley, C. & Firth, H. (2001). Sexual abuse in children and adolescents with intellectual disability. *Journal of Intellectual Disability Research*, 45 (3), 194–201.

Barbaree, H. & Marshall, W. (2006). An introduction to the juvenile sex offender: Terms, concepts and definitions. In H. Barbaree and W. Marshall (eds), *The Juvenile Sex Offender*. New York: Guildford Press.

Bass, L.B., Taylor, B.A., Knudson-Martin, C. & Huenergardt, D. (2006). Making sense of abuse: Case studies in sibling incest. *Contemporary Family Therapy, 28* (1), 87–109.

Becker, J.V. (1988). The effects of sexual abuse on adolescent offenders. In G. Wyatt & G. Powell (eds), *Lasting effects of child sexual abuse* (pp. 193–208). Beverly Hills CA: Sage Publ.

Bentovim, A. (2007). Working with abusing families. In K. Wilson and A. James (eds), *The Child Protection Handbook*, 3rd edn. (pp. 451–78). London: Bailliere-Tindall/Elsevier.

Bentovim, A. & Boston, P. (1988). Sexual abuse basic issues: Characteristics of Children and Families. In A. Bentovim, A. Elton, J. Hildebrand, M. Tranter; & E. Vizard (eds), *Child sexual abuse within the family: Assessment and treatment* (pp. 16–39). London: Wright Publ.

Boswell, G. & Wedge, P. (2002). Sexually abusive adolescent males: An evaluation of a residential therapeutic facility *Community and Criminal Justice. Monograph 3.* Leicester: DeMontfort University.

Browne, K.D., Cartana, C., Momeu, L., Paunescu, G., Petre, N. & Tokay, R. (2002). *Child abuse and neglect in Romanian families: A national prevalence study.* WHO Regional Office for Europe, Copenhagen, Denmark.

Browne, K.D., Douglas, J., Hamilton-Giachritsis, C.E. & Hegarty, J. (2006). *A community health approach to the assessment of infants and their parents: The CARE programme.* Chichester: Wiley.

Browne, K.D. & Hamilton, C.E. (1998). Physical violence between young adults and their parents: Associations with a history of child maltreatment. *Journal of Family Violence, 13* (1), 59–79.

Browne, K.D., Hamilton-Giachritsis, C.E. & Vettor, S. (2007). *The cycles of violence: The relationship between childhood maltreatment and the risk of later becoming a victim or perpetrator of violence.* World Health Organisation Policy Briefing: Violence and Injury Prevention Programme. Copenhagen: WHO Regional Office for Europe, October, 2007.

Browne, K.D. & Herbert, M. (1997). *Preventing family violence.* Chichester: Wiley.

Burnham, J., Moss, J., deBelle, J. & Jamieson, R. (1999). Working with families of young sexual abusers: Assessment and intervention issues. In M. Erooga & H. Mason (eds), *Children and young people who sexually abuse others: Challenges and responses* (pp. 146–67). London: Routledge.

Butchart, A., Harvey, A.P., Mian, M. & Furniss, T. (2006). *Preventing child maltreatment: A guide to taking action and generating evidence.* World Health Organisation and International Society for Prevention of Child Abuse and Neglect, 2006. Geneva.

Caffaro, J.V. & Conn-Caffaro, A. (2005). Treating sibling abuse families. *Aggression and Violent Behaviour, 19,* 604–23.

Cantwell, H.B. (1988). Child sexual abuse: Very young perpetrators. *Child Abuse and Neglect, 12* (4), 579–82.

Carlson, B.E., Maciol, K. & Schneider, J. (2006). Sibling incest: Reports from forty-one survivors. *Journal of Child Sexual Abuse, 15* (4), 19–34.

Cawson, P., Wattam, C., Brooker, S. & Kelly, G. (2000). *Child maltreatment in the United Kingdom: A study of prevalence of child abuse and neglect.* London: NSPCC.

Craig, L.A. (in press). Controversies in assessing risk and deviancy in sex offenders with intellectual disabilities. *Psychology, Crime & Law.*

Creighton, S.J. (2002). Recognising changes in incidence and prevalence. In K.D. Browne, H. Hanks P. Stratton C.E. Hamilton (eds), *Early prediction and prevention of child abuse: A handbook* (pp. 5–22). Chichester: Wiley.

Crosse, S., Kaye, E. & Ratnofsky, A. (1993). *A report on the maltreatment of children with disabilities.* Washington DC: National Center on Child Abuse and Neglect.

Cyr, M., Wright, J., McDuff, P. & Perron, A. (2002). Intrafamilial sexual abuse: Brother-sister incest does not differ from father–daughter and stepfather–stepdaughter incest. *Child Abuse and Neglect, 26* 957–73.

Davenport, C., Browne, K.D. & Palmer, R. (1994). Opinions on the traumatising effects of child sexual abuse: Evidence for consensus. *Child Abuse and Neglect, 18* (9), 725–38.

Davis, G.E. & Leitenberg, H. (1987). Adolescent sex offenders. *Psychological Bulletin, 101*, 417–27.

Day, K. (1993). Crime and Mental retardation; a review. In K. Howells and C.R. Hollin (eds), *Clinical Approaches to the Mentally Disordered Offender*. Chichester: John Wiley and Sons.

Day, K. (1994). Male mentally handicapped sex offenders. *British Journal of Psychiatry, 165*, 630–9.

Deisher, R., Wenet, G., Paperny, D., Clark, T. & Fehrenbach, P. (1982). Adolescent sexual offense behaviour: The role of the physician. *Journal of Adolescent Health Care, 2*, 279–86.

De Long, A.R. (1989). Sexual interactions among siblings and cousins: Experimentation or exploitation? *Child Abuse and Neglect, 13* (2), 271–9.

Department for Children, Schools Families (2008). *Referrals, assessments and children and young people who are the subject of a child protection plan, England – year ending 31 March 2008*. London: National Statistics, 16 September, 2008 (Ref: SFR 24/2008).

DiGiorgio-Miller, J. (1998). Sibling incest: Treatment of the family and the offender. *Child Welfare, 77* (3), 335–46.

Dolan, M., Holloway, J., Bailey, S. & Kroll, L. (1996). The psychosocial characteristics of juvenile sexually offenders referred to an adolescent forensic service in the UK. *Medicine, Science and the Law, 4*, 343–53.

Elliott, M., Browne, K.D. & Kilcoyne, J. (1995). Child sexual abuse: What offenders tell us. *Child Abuse and Neglect, 19* (5), 579–94.

Epps, K.J. (1991). The residential treatment of adolescent sex offenders. In M. McMurran & C. McDougall (Eds), Proceedings of the DCLP first annual conference. *Issues in Criminological and Legal Psychology, 17 (1)*. Leicester: British Psychological Society.

Erooga, M. & Masson, H. (2006). Children and young people with sexually harmful or abusive behaviours. In M. Erooga & H. Masson (eds), *Children and young people who sexually abuse others (2nd edition): Current developments and practice responses*. London: Routledge.

Finkelhor, D. (1980). Sex among siblings: A survey on prevalence, variety and effects. *Archives of Sexual Behaviour, 9* (3), 171–94.

Finkelhor, D. (1986). *A source book on child sexual abuse*. Beverly Hills: Sage.

Finkelhor, D. (1994). The international epidemiology of child sexual abuse. *Child Abuse and Neglect, 18*, 409–18.

Finkelhor, D. (2008). *Childhood victimization: Violence, crime, and abuse in the lives of young people*. Oxford: OUP.

Finkelhor, D., Hotaling, G., Lewis, I.A. & Smith, C. (1990). Sexual abuse in a national survey of adult men and women: Prevalence, characteristics and risk factors. *Child Abuse and Neglect, 14*, 19–28.

Firth, H., Balogh, R., Berney, T., Bretherton, K., Graham, S. & Whibley, S. (2001). Psychopathology of sexual abuse in young people with intellectual disability. *Journal of Intellectual Disability Research, 45* (3), 244–52.

Flanagan, K. & Hayman-White, K. (1999). *Sexual abuse counselling and prevention program: Five year review of work with victims and adolescent perpetrators of sexual abuse*. Melbourne, Australia: Children's Protection Society.

Furey, E.M. (1994). Sexual abuse of adults with mental retardation: Who and where. *Mental Retardation, 32*, 173–80.

Fyson, R. (2007a). Young people with learning disabilities who sexually harm others: The role of criminal justice within a multi-agency response. *British Journal of Learning Disabilities, 35* (3), 181–7.

Fyson, R (2007b). *Young people with learning disabilities who sexually abuse: Understanding, identifying and responding from within generic education and welfare services. In M.C. Calder (Ed.) Working with children and young people who sexually abuse: Taking the field forward*. Russell House Publishing, Lyme Regis.

Gerhold, C.K., Browne, K.D. & Beckett, R. (2007). Predicting recidivism in adolescent sexual offenders. *Aggression and Violent Behavior, 12*, 427–38.

Gilbert, R., Spatz-Widom, C., Browne, K.D., Fergusson, D., Webb, E. & Janson, S. (2009). Child maltreatment: Burden and consequences in high-income countries. (*The Lancet* Series on Child Maltreatment 1). *The Lancet, 373* (9657), 68–81.

Glasgow, D., Horne, L., Calam, R. & Cox A. (1994). Evidence, incidence, gender and age in sexual abuse of children perpetrated by children: Towards a developmental analysis of child sexual abuse. *Child Abuse Review, 3,* 196–210.

Groth, A.N., Hobson, W. & Garry, T. (1982). The child sexual molester: Clinical observations. In J. Conte and D. Shore (eds) *Social work and child sexual abuse.* New York: Hamworth.

Hamilton, C.E., Falshaw, L. & Browne, K.D. (2002). The link between recurrent maltreatment and offending behaviour. *International Journal of Offender Therapy and Comparative Criminology, 41,* 75–95.

Hayes, S. (1991). Sex offenders. *Australia and New Zealand Journal of Developmental Disabilities, 17,* 220–7.

Hawkes, C., Jenkins, J.A. & Vizard, E. (1997). Roots of sexual violence in children and adolescents. In V. Varma (Ed.), *Violence in children and adolescents* (pp. 84–102). London: Jessica Kingsley.

Hinsberger, D., Griffiths, D. & Quinsey, V. (1991). Detecting counterfeit deviance: Differentiating sexual deviance from sexual inappropriateness. *Rehabilitation Mental Health care Newsletter, 10,* 51–4.

Hoghughi, M.S., Bhate, S.R. & Graham, F. (1997). *Working with sexually abusive adolescents.* London: Sage Publications Limited.

Johnson, T. (1988). Child perpetrators – Children who molest other children: Preliminary findings. *Child Abuse and Neglect, 12* (2), 219–29.

Johnson, T. (1989). Female child perpetrators: Children who molest other children. *Child Abuse and Neglect, 13* (4), 571–85.

Johnson, T. & Friend, C. (1995). Assessing young children's sexual behaviours in the context of sexual abuse evaluations. In T. Ney (Ed.), *True and false allegations of child sexual abuse: Assessment and case management.* NY: Brunner/Mazel.

Kelly, L., Regan, L. & Burton, S. (1991). *An exploratory study of the prevalence of sexual abuse in a sample of 16 to 21 year olds.* London: Child Abuse Studies Unit, Polytechnic of North London.

Kelly, T., Richardson, G., Hunter, R. & Knapp, M. (2002). Attention and executive function deficits in adolescent sex offenders. *Child Neuropsychology, 8* (2), 138–43.

Kendall-Tackett, K., Lyon, T., Taliaferro, G. & Little, L. (2005). Why child maltreatment researchers should include children's disability status in their maltreatment studies: Commentary. *Child Abuse & Neglect, 29,* 147–51.

Langevin, R. & Curnoe, S. (2007). The therapeutic challenge of the learning impaired sex offender. *Sexual Offender Treatment, 2* (1), 1–21.

Langevin, R. & Curnoe, S. (2008). Are the mentally retarded and learning disordered over-represented among sex offenders and paraphilics? *International Journal of Offender Therapy and Comparative Criminology, 52* (4), 401–15.

Lee, J., Jackson, H., Pattison, P. & Ward, T. (2002). Developmental risk factors for sexual offending. *Child Abuse and Neglect, 26* (1), 73–92.

Lindsay, W.R. (2002). Research and literature on sex offenders with intellectual and developmental disabilities. *Journal of Intellectual Disability Research, 46* (1), 74–85.

Lindsay, W.R., Law, J., Quinn, K., Smart, N. & Smith, A.H. (2001). A comparison of physical and sexual abuse: Histories of sexual and non-sexual offenders with intellectual disability. *Child Abuse and Neglect, 25,* 989–95.

Lindsay, W.R., Smith, A.H., Law, J., Quinn, K., Anderson, A., Smith, A., Overend, T. & Allan, R. (2002). A treatment service for sex offender and abusers with intellectual disability: Characteristics of referrals and evaluation. *Journal of Applied Research in Intellectual Disabilities, 15,* 166–74.

McDonald, W.R.,Associates (2005). *Child maltreatment 2003: Reports from the states to the national child abuse and neglect data system*. Washington, DC: US Department of Health and Human Services, Children's Bureau.

McGee, H., Garavan, R., De Barra, M., Byrne, J., & Conroy, R. (2002). The Sexual Abuse and Violence in Ireland (SAVI) Report. Dublin: Dublin Rape Crises Centre and Liffey Press.

Masson, H. & Erooga, M. (1999). Children and young people who sexually abuse others: Incidence, Characteristics and Causation. In M. Erooga and H. Masson (eds), *Children and young people who sexually abuse others (1st Edition): Challenges and responses*. London: Routledge.

Morris, J. (1999). Disabled children, child protection systems and the Children Act, 1989. *Child Abuse Review*, *8*, 91–108.

Morton, N. & Browne, K.D. (1998). Theory and observation of attachment and its relation to child maltreatment: A review. *Child Abuse & Neglect*, *22*, 1093–104.

Mrazek, P., Lynch, M. & Bentovim, A. (1981). Sexual Abuse of Children in the United Kingdom. *Child Abuse & Neglect*, *7*, 147–53.

Murphy, G.H. (2003). Capacity to consent to sexual relationships in adults with learning disabilities. *Journal of Family Planning and Reproductive Health Care*, *29* (3), 148–9.

Murphy, G., Harnett, H. & Holland, A.J. (1995). A survey of intellectual disabilities among men on remand in prison. *Mental Handicap Research*, *8*, 81–98.

Murrey, G.H., Briggs, D. & Davies, C. (1992). Psychopathically disordered, mentally ill and mentally handicapped sex offenders: A comparative study. *Medicine, Science and the Law*, *32*, 331–6.

Nicholas, S., Kershaw, C. & Walker, A. (eds) (2007) Crime in England and Wales 2006/07. London: Home Office.

O'Brian, M.J. (1991). Taking sibling incest seriously. In M. Quinn Patton (Ed.), *Family Sexual Abuse*. California Sage Publications.

O'Callaghan, D. (1998). Practice issues in working with young abusers who ahve learning disabilities. *Child Abuse Review*, *7*, 435–48.

O'Callaghan, D. (1999). Young abusers with Learning Disabilities: Towards better understanding and positive interventions. In M. C. Calder (Ed.), *Working with young people who sexually abuse; new pieces of the jigsaw puzzle*. Dorset: Russell House Publishing.

Pierce, L.H. & Pierce, R.L. (1987). Incestuous victimization by juvenile sex offenders. *Journal of Family Violence*, *2*, 351–64.

Rogers, C.M. & Terry, T. (1984). Clinical intervention with boy victims of sexual abuse. In I.R. Stuart & J.G. Greer (eds), *Victims of sexual aggression: Men, women and children*. New York: Van Nostrand Reinhold.

Rose, J., Jenkins, R., O'Connor, C., Jones, C. & Felce, D. (2002). A group treatment for men with intellectual disabilities who sexually offend or abuse. *Journal of Applied Research in Intellectual Disabilities*, *15*, 138–50.

Rudd, J.M. & Herzberger, S.D. (1999). Brother–sister incest – Father–daughter incest: A comparison of characteristics and consequences. *Child Abuse and Neglect*, *23* (9), 915–28.

Russell, D.E.H. (1983). The incidence and prevalence of intrafamilial and extrafamilial sexual abuse of female children. *Child Abuse and Neglect*, *7*, 133–46.

Russell, D.E.H. (1986). *The secret trauma: Incest in the lives of girls and women*. New York: Basic Books.

Ryan, G. & Lane, S. (1997). *Juvenile sexual offending: Causes, consequences and corrections* San Francisco: Jossey-Bass.

Skuse, D., Bentovim, A., Stevenson, J. *et al*. (1998). Risk factors for the development of sexually abusive behaviour in sexually victimised males. *British Medical Journal*, *317*, 175–9.

Sullivan, P. & Knutson, J. (2000). Maltreatment and disabilities: A population based epidemiological study. *Child abuse & Neglect*, *24*, 1257–74.

Summit, R. (1983). The child sexual accommodation syndrome. *Child abuse and Neglect*, *7*, 177–193.

Swanson, C.K. & Garwick, G.B. (1990). Treatment for low functioning sex offenders: Group therapy and interagency co-ordination. *Mental Retardation, 28,* 155–61.

Thompson, D. & Brown, H. (1997). Men with intellectual disabilities who sexually abuse: A review of the literature. *Journal of Applied Research in Intellectual Disabilities, 10,* 140–58.

Tudiver, J., Broekstra, S., Josselyn, S. & Barbaree, H. (1998). *Addressing the needs of developmentally delayed sex offenders: A guide.* Ottawa: National Clearinghouse on Family Violence (Minister of Public Works and Government Services), Canada.

Veneziano, C. & Veneziano, L. (2002). Adolescent sex offenders: A review of the literature. *Trauma, Violence and Abuse, 3* (4), 247–60.

Vizard, E., Monck, E. & Misch, P. (1995). Child and adolescent sex abuse perpetrators: A review of the research literature. *Journal of child Psychology and Psychiatry, 36* (5), 731–56.

Watkins, B. & Bentovim, A. (1992). The sexual abuse of male children and adolescents: A review of current research. *Journal of Child Psychology and Psychiatry, 33* (1), 197–248.

Wechsler, D. (1984). *Wechsler adult intelligence scale – Revised (WAIS-R).* London: Psychological Corporation.

Wechsler, D. (1999). *Wechsler adult intelligence scale – Third edition (WAIS-III).* London: Psychological Corporation.

Westcott, H. & Jones, D. (1999). The abuse of disabled children. *Journal of Child Psychology and Psychiatry, 40,* 497–506.

Wiehe, V.R. (1997). *Sibling abuse: Hidden physical, emotional, and sexual trauma,* 2nd edn. California: Sage Publications.

Worling, J.R. (1995). Adolescent sibling-incest offenders: Differences in family and individual functioning when compared to adolescent nonsibling sex offenders. *Child Abuse and Neglect, 19* (5), 633–43.

5

Applying the Self-Regulation Model to Sexual Offenders with Intellectual Disabilities

LYNNE ECCLESTON, TONY WARD AND BARRY WATERMAN

INTRODUCTION

The assessment and treatment of sexual offenders has undergone a paradigmatic shift since the beginning of the 1980s moving away from psychoanalytic techniques and behavioural responses such as aversive arousal conditioning and electric shocks. The 1970s witnessed the advent of cognitive behavioural approaches to address the distorted thought processes that sexual offenders used to justify and rationalise their offending and minimise their guilt (Ward, Bickley, Webster, Fisher, Beech & Eldridge, 2006). These treatment strategies have also been modified and applied successfully with intellectually disabled sexual offenders (Lambrick & Glaser, 2004). In general, treatment programmes challenged the cognitive distortions that maintained sexual offenders' pro-offending attitudes and beliefs and focussed on developing victim empathy in an attempt to target victim blaming attitudes and denial of harm to victims (Abel, Blanchard & Becker, 1978). Increasingly, several clinicians and researchers began to argue that the treatment of sexual offenders should be based on understanding the process whereby an individual relapses into another sexual offence (e.g., Pithers, 1990).

By the late 1980s programmes had systematically incorporated relapse prevention (RP), adapted from the addiction research (Marlatt & Gordon, 1985), as the preferred model in the treatment of sexual offenders, including intellectually disabled sexual offenders (Marques, 1982; Pithers, Marques, Gibat & Marlatt, 1983). Within the Risk-Needs framework (see Andrews & Bonta, 1998), the dominant treatment model for sexual offenders culminates in RP. RP strategies focus on teaching sexual offenders to recognise their high-risk situations and other threats to remaining offence-free, and then implementing skills gained from therapy to prevent relapse (Laws, 1999; Pithers, Marques, Gibat & Marlatt, 1983). Lapses can include various offence precursor activities such as deviant fantasising about children, accessing

Assessment and Treatment of Sexual Offenders with Intellectual Disabilities: A Handbook
Edited by Leam A. Craig, William R. Lindsay and Kevin D. Browne
© 2010 John Wiley & Sons, Ltd.

pornographic materials or cruising for potential victims in locations where children congregate (Laws, 2003). Since the 1990s RP has been used as either an all-embracing framework for treatment (e.g., Marques, Nelson, Alarcon & Day, 2000) or as one module, usually in the last phase of treatment, in a multimodal treatment package (Mann, Webster, Schofield & Marshall, 2004; Mann & Thornton, 1998).

In this chapter we provide a brief overview of RP, self-regulation and the Self-Regulation Model (SRM) (Ward & Hudson, 1998) as it applies to the general sexual offender population. We then discuss the application of the SRM to intellectually disabled sexual offenders and present two case studies from a Melbourne study to illustrate the pathways used by this group of offenders. We argue that offenders from this population follow two distinct pathways, and we conclude by briefly discussing implications for treatment.

RELAPSE PREVENTION WITH SEX OFFENDERS

RP was developed in the field of substance abuse research to address the challenging problems that substance abusers faced in their attempts to remain free from addiction in the period after they had received treatment (Ward, Polaschek & Beech, 2006). The theoretical base of RP lies in social learning theory (Bandura, 1986) and focusses on the causal and maintaining factors that prolong an individual's addiction (Keeling & Rose, 2005). The RP model is embedded within a cognitive-behavioural framework and utilises cognitive and behavioural interventions interrelated with lifestyle changes to promote and maintain abstinence from an aberrant behaviour. The success of the RP approach for addictive behaviours instigated the development of relapse models for other challenging behaviours including sexual offending.

Pithers and his colleagues were the first to adapt the RP model for sexual offenders with an emphasis on applying the model to treatment (Marques & Nelson, 1989; Pithers, Marques, Gibat & Marlatt, 1983). Since the 1990s the RP model has dominated treatment approaches for sexual offenders (Marques, Day, Nelson & Miner, 1989; Mann & Thornton, 2000). Although the original RP model was intended to be used as a post-treatment maintenance programme its more common application has been to both treatment and maintenance. The model represented a blueprint of the cognitive, affective and behavioural phenomena related to treatment failure and offered clients a strategic plan to avoid re-offending (Ward, Polaschek & Beech, 2006). The major goal is to help sexual offenders identify the risk factors that precipitate a relapse into offending by teaching them self-management strategies using behavioural, cognitive, educational and social skills. The original model of RP begins with a sexual offender who develops a sense of self-control as he maintains an offence-free lifestyle. His confidence and self-control are stable until he is confronted with a high-risk situation. He then spirals down from abstinence into relapse as he loses self-control. Pithers (Pithers, Marques, Gibat & Marlatt, 1983) noted that sexual offenders can also place themselves in risky situations by using covert planning (apparently irrelevant decisions) that are accompanied by rationalisation and denial (Ward, Polaschek & Beech, 2006).

The next development in Pithers' RP model was to examine the precursors to sexual aggression to identify a common pathway to offending behaviour (Pithers, 1990; Pithers, Cumming, Beal, Young & Turner, 1989). In the revised model relapse was preceded by a negative change in affect followed by difficulties in managing emotions. In the second phase the offender engaged in deviant sexual fantasies, often accompanied by masturbation, which culminated in cognitive distortions, planning and justification for sexually abusive behaviour. The final stage in the pathway is when the offender commits a sexual offence. According to the pathway model lapses can occur during several stages and it is at these critical points that an offender can make an 'adaptive coping response' to avert relapse (Keeling & Rose, 2005; Laws & Ward, 2006).

There is little doubt that the Pithers RP model has had an impact in the treatment and rehabilitation of sexual offenders; however, key researchers in the area have commented that the model has several shortcomings. Laws (1999) points out that although the RP model has been systematically accepted and used since the early 1980s it has not changed demonstrably and has not been well evaluated during that time. Other critics have included Hanson (2000), who challenged the RP model as being too limited in its application to sexual offenders, and Marshall and Anderson (1996), who queried its utility in treatment. These authors later commented that the RP model, albeit comprehensive, contained so many components that sexual offenders may have felt they had unreasonable demands placed on them and that relapse was an almost inevitable occurrence (Laws & Ward, 2006; Marshall & Anderson, 2000). Moreover, Thornton's (1997) main criticism of the RP model was that in line with the dominant risk-needs model of offender rehabilitation (Andrews & Bonta, 1998) there was an over-reliance on identifying risk (Laws & Ward, 2006). Thornton (1997) posited that there were three main difficulties with the RP model. Firstly, he believed the primary focus on deviant behaviour became too compelling and visible to sexual offenders who were tempted to relapse. Secondly, the success of the RP model lay in working with motivated clients, and sexual offenders tend to be unmotivated towards changing their deviant behaviour. Thirdly, he argued that there was too much time invested in identifying risk and discussing coping mechanisms instead of spending more time teaching interventions and coping skills to target the dynamic risk factors that are more relevant to relapse (Laws & Ward, 2006).

Arguably, the major criticism of the Pither's RP model is its adherence to the original Marlatt (1985) 'one size fits all' model of abstinence in that it assumes that all sexual offenders lapse and relapse along a similar pathway (Laws & Ward, 2006). In a single pathway model there is an assumption that all sexual offenders want to remain offence-free and only relapse when they are stressed, unhappy and isolated. Specifically, classic RP models inferred that individuals committed sexual offences because of skills deficits, negative mood states, and/or adverse life events (Ward, Polaschek & Beech, 2006). According to the model, individuals are caught in an 'offence cycle'. Initially, the offender has a negative self-perception, anticipates rejection in relationships, and subjects himself to self-imposed isolation. During this isolated state he engages in sexual fantasies to escape from his negative mood and to create an illusion that he is in control. The fantasies may involve deviant fantasies of having sex with children or forced sex with adults and may be accompanied and reinforced by pornography and masturbation. There may also be evidence of distorted thinking to minimise any guilt the offender experiences associated with engaging in deviant fantasies. The next stage in the cycle is for the offender to plan and then commit the offence. The offence itself serves as a reinforcing event followed by a period of transitory guilt related to the offence. The offender next attempts to restore his self-image and typically engages in additional cognitive distortions to minimise and justify the abuse and to alleviate his guilt and anxiety. At this point the offender is cognisant of his sexual offence, which damages his self-esteem, and the negative feelings he had at the beginning of the cycle re-emerge (ibid.).

Several authors have expressed concern that the single RP model has been widely and uncritically accepted and argued that negative mood states and poor coping strategies alone are inadequate to explain sexual offenders' offence patterns (Hanson, 2000; Laws, 2003; Laws & Ward, 2006; Ward & Hudson, 1998). Ward and Hudson's (1996) major critique of the RP model is that it fails to account for those sexual offenders who make conscious decisions to engage in sexual abuse. Although some offenders' offences are underpinned by 'self-regulatory failure' other offenders demonstrate careful and systematic planning accompanied by positive rather than negative emotional states. Another conceptual weakness that was raised by Ward and Hudson (1996) was the placing of contradictory mechanisms in the RP mode, such as allowing both the abstinence violation effect and immediate gratification to fall between the lapse and relapse (Keeling & Rose, 2005; Ward, Polaschek & Beech, 2006). Ward and his colleagues (Ward, Louden, Hudson & Marshall, 1995) demonstrated that sexual offenders are heterogenous in their offence processes and argued instead for a multiple pathway model. Furthermore, using a grounded theory approach they found that, unexpectedly, child molesters did not co-vary in their use of goals, affect and regulatory style, which prompted the conceptual revision of RP with self-regulation theory (Laws & Ward, 2006).

THE GOOD LIVES MODEL

Ward and Gannon (2006) have recently challenged the efficacy of the RP model (Pithers, Gibat & Marlatt, 1993) and Risk–Need Model of offender rehabilitation (Andrews & Bonta, 1998) in that it is overly focussed on reducing or eliminating an individual's dynamic risk factors without also considering a more holistic approach. This over-reliance on reducing risk has been referred to as a 'pincushion model' (Ward & Gannon, 2006, p. 5) – each risk factor is represented by a pin. The focus in treatment is on removing the pins rather than also concentrating on elevating an individual's adaptive skills and pro-social opportunities and skills inherent in the Good Lives Model (GLM). Ward and his colleagues (Ward & Gannon, 2006; Ward & Brown, 2004; Ward & Marshall, 2004) argue that the GLM has theoretical advantages over the risk–need model of offender rehabilitation. The GLM has the ability to link a set of aetiological assumptions, explicit strategies for motivating offenders, a sound understanding of the internal and external conditions for achieving human goods and well-defined treatment principles and rehabilitation strategies to inform case formulation and treatment planning.

The GLM was first conceptualised by Ward and Stewart (2003) and has continued to be developed into a comprehensive theory of offender rehabilitation (Ward & Marshall, 2004; Ward & Gannon, 2006). The GLM clearly addresses the limitations of the risk–need model for offender rehabilitation (Andrews & Bonta, 1998) and offers an enhancement model that builds on those actions, states of affairs, characteristics, experience and states of mind that are intrinsically beneficial (i.e., primary human goods) to human beings that are therefore sought for their own sake rather than as means to ends (Deci & Ryan, 2000; Emmons, 1996; Emmons, 1999; Schmuck & Sheldon, 2001). The GLM therefore focuses on reducing risk of offending by constructing a balanced, pro-social personal identity and meaningful lifestyle (Lindsay, Ward, Morgan & Wilson, 2007). (For a more thorough exploration of the GLM, see Ward & Stewart, 2003; Ward & Marshall, 2004; Ward & Gannon, 2006;

Ward & Mann, 2004). In essence, if offenders can acquire the internal and external conditions necessary to achieve human needs in adaptive, pro-social ways, they will be less motivated to offend.

The basis of the GLM framework is on enhancing human well-being and quality of life, which is partially determined by an individual's basic needs. Basic needs are innate propensities to engage in certain valued activities that, if not met, result in harm or increased risk of harm in the future. Examples of basic needs include: *relatedness* (an individual's propensity to establish a sense of emotional connectedness to other human beings and seek goals of feeling loved and cared for); *autonomy* (an individual's propensity to self-regulate and organise their experiences, and to function as unified, integrated beings); and *competency* (propensity to establish a sense of mastery over one's environment, to seek challenges and to master them). The fulfilment of these basic needs requires internal and external conditions. Internal conditions refer to psychological characteristics, such as skills, competencies, beliefs, attitudes and values. External conditions refer to social, cultural and interpersonal factors that facilitate the development of the internal psychological characteristics. Examples include education, effective parenting, vocational training, social support and opportunities to pursue important goals. Distortions of these conditions can be viewed as internal and external obstacles that prevent basic needs from being met – Ward and Stewart (2003) have redefined these obstacles as criminogenic needs. Human well-being is therefore derived from the meeting of basic human needs and the existence of the necessary internal and external conditions. The presence of internal and external obstacles results in impaired social and psychological functioning, and hence, a less fulfilling life. Ward and Gannon (2006) have restated the primary goods as: life (healthy living and adaptive functioning); knowledge; excellence in work and play; excellence in agency (self-directedness); inner peace (ability to control stress and emotional turmoil); friendship (intimate and family relationships); community; spirituality (some sense of purpose in life); happiness; and creativity.

According to the GLM a combination of criminogenic needs and dynamic risk factors create a negative life model that leads an individual into sexual offending. Individuals seeking to construct a meaningful life use inappropriate means and maladaptive strategies to achieve their antisocial goals or lack the skills to achieve a GLM (Lindsay, Ward, Morgan & Wilson, 2007). Specifically, sexual offenders need to acquire adaptive and coping skills to replace their maladaptive strategies that lead to offending – focus should be placed on individuals' personal strengths, interests and goals and their living environments (Ward & Gannon, 2006).

Preliminary empirical support for the GLM was reported by Purvis (2005), who found that sexual offenders seek a variety of approach goals (primary goods) when they commit sexual assault. Importantly, she also discovered that offenders engaged in either *direct* or *indirect* routes to their offending behaviour. Offenders who followed a direct pathway tended to seek implicit clusters of goals and strategies that led to the sexual abuse. Sexual goals may become prominent in sexual offenders who are seeking a variety of primary goods. It is feasible that deviant sexual cognitions result from learning and conditioning; however, for some offenders there may be an underlying biological basis. The direct route corresponds to the approach pathways in the SRM (Lindsay, Ward, Morgan & Wilson, 2007; Ward & Gannon, 2006). Conversely, the indirect route to offending occurs when individuals experience some change in their life circumstances, such as a relationship breakdown, and they pursue goods that result in sexual assault. For example, an individual increases his alcohol consumption and seeks a relationship with a child to overcome feelings of loneliness or distress. There is often a chain of events that precedes the sexual offending, and this route relates more to the avoidance pathways in the SRM (Lindsay, Ward, Morgan & Wilson, 2007; Ward & Gannon, 2006).

SELF-REGULATION THEORY

Self-regulation refers to the internal and external processes that allow an individual to participate in goal-directed behaviours across different time periods and in diverse contextual situations (Baumeister & Heatherton, 1996; Ward & Hudson, 2000a).

Goals are key cognitive constructs in self-regulation theory stored as behavioural scripts (Carver & Scheier, 1981). Individuals tap into these behavioural scripts in order to achieve their goals in an optimal manner, including the initial selection of goals, planning, monitoring, evaluation and modification of behaviour. Self-regulation, therefore, is concerned with more than inhibiting or suppressing unwanted behaviour and negative emotions, and can also include the enhancement, maintenance or elicitation of behaviour to promote positive emotional states. In essence, goals originate from basic human needs for autonomy, competence and relatedness (Ryan, 1998) and are desired emotional states or situations that individuals strive to achieve or avoid (Ward & Hudson, 2000b).

Goals can serve completely different functions and Cochran and Tesser (1996) usefully described a distinction between acquisitional (approach) and inhibitory (avoidance) goals. Acquisitional goals involve approach behaviour to increase skills or gain access to a situation, whereas inhibitory goals involve avoidance behaviours to decrease or inhibit a behaviour or situation (Ward & Hudson, 2000a). According to self-regulation theory, inhibitory goals are more difficult to achieve and require considerable cognitive resources to monitor the environment for threats. When an individual is stressed and more vulnerable to intense emotional states self-regulation is likely to be impaired. Emmons (1996) posits that individuals with dominant avoidance goals experience greater levels of psychological distress than individuals who engage in approach goals.

Self-regulation theorists (Baumeister & Heatherton, 1996; Carver & Sheier, 1990) contend that there are three styles of dysfunctional self-regulation within the model that have important implications for the increased likelihood of re-offence for sexual offenders (Keeling & Rose, 2005; Ward & Hudson, 2000a). Firstly, individuals fail to control their cognitions and emotions and exhibit disinhibited behaviour. This type of failed self-regulation is usually accompanied by negative emotional states. Secondly, individuals use ineffective strategies to achieve their goals, which can backfire and can lead to a loss of control or mis-regulation. This style of self-regulation is seen in sexual offenders who use alcohol or deviant fantasies to modulate negative moods or suppress intrusive thoughts. The third style assumes a sexual offender is capable of effective self-regulation but the major problem is goal choice rather than any breakdown in self-regulation processes. To illustrate, a pre-ferential child molester may have very effective goal setting, planning and implementation to achieve his goals but the difficulty in self-regulation lies in his initial goals and distorted values and beliefs. Moreover, he is likely to experience positive rather than negative emotions in achieving his goals and does not view his sexual preferences or lifestyle as problematic (ibid.).

THE SELF-REGULATION MODEL OF RELAPSE PREVENTION

The SRM builds on the earlier descriptive models of Ward and colleagues of the offence process in sexual offenders and theoretical and empirical research on self-regulation (Ward & Hudson, 1998; Ward & Hudson, 2000a; Ward, Louden, Hudson & Marshall, 1995). The SRM constitutes nine phases and four pathways organised around approach and avoidance goals and the strategies sexual offenders use to achieve their goals. Specifically, the four offence pathways are avoidant-passive, avoidant-active, approach-automatic, and approach-explicit. Ward, Yates and Long (2006) contend that the model is fluid in that the relapse process has no timeframe – offenders may move to different phases of the offence chain over time or may remain at a specific phase for a relatively long period before moving to the next phase. As with the classic RP model, offenders can exit the offence process during any phase by implementing appropriate coping strategies (Ward, Polaschek & Beech, 2006). A summary of the phases and pathways and their influence on the offence process of sex offenders follows (see Ward & Hudson, 1998, 2000b for further detail).

Phase 1: Life Event

An individual is attempting to remain abstinent and offence-free when a life event occurs, for example a breakdown in his relationship or stress at work. The individual appraises these life events almost automatically, according to existing beliefs and attitudes, his current needs and goals and the interpersonal context in which they occur. Ward and Hudson (1998, 2000b) suggest that these life events trigger specific patterns of thoughts, emotions and intentions which have been associated with the event or similar events in the past. For example, a breakdown in a relationship can trigger feelings of inadequacy, injured self-esteem and/or a desire to retaliate against what is perceived to be a hostile world.

Phase 2: Desire for Deviant Sex or Activity

The life event and subsequent appraisal of the event results in the desire for deviant sex or maladaptive activities and the presence of emotions related to those desires (Laws & Ward, 2006). Ward and Hudson (1998, 2000b) suggest that the process necessary to reach these goals may be rehearsed covertly, which can lower the offender's inhibitions against indulging in the fantasies. The fantasies may activate memories associated with past offending, which function to prime or increase the accessibility of core dysfunctional beliefs and attitudes. When an offender indulges in sex or sexual fantasies it may also function as a powerful mood regulator and, under stressful circumstances, result in sexual abuse. For example, the affective states that accompany these offence scripts and fantasies may be happiness, sexual arousal, anxiety and anger.

Phase 3: Offence-Related Goals Established

At this stage the offender appraises his maladaptive and deviant desires and makes a decision to establish an offence-related goal. Ward and Hudson (1998, 2000b) contend there are two broad types of relevant goals: avoidance and approach goals. The avoidance goal is associated with a desire to remain offence-free, and the goal is not to achieve a particular state of affairs. The offender is likely to experience negative emotions – for example, fear and anxiety related to the possibility of offending. These types of goals are difficult to implement as there are a number of ways a person can fail to prevent something from happening. Conversely, approach goals reflect an offender's motivation to sexually offend. Offenders may experience positive or negative emotions depending on the underlying aim. For example, if the offender seeks sexual gratification then his affect is likely to be positive, whereas if the aim is to punish or humiliate a victim, then he is likely to experience extremely negative emotions such as anger.

Phase 4: Strategy Selected

During this stage an individual selects a strategy designed to achieve a desired goal. Goals and strategies may not involve an explicit decision but may occur automatically as a result of the activation of offence scripts. Offence scripts are entrenched within an individual's range of behaviours and emerge automatically, often revealing an extensive and prolonged offence history and criminal expertise (Laws & Ward, 2006). The four possible pathways emerge at this stage; avoidant-passive, avoidant-active, approach-automatic and approach-explicit. Consistent with acquisitional and inhibitory goals in self-regulation theory (Cochran & Tesser, 1996), two of the offender pathways are associated with avoidance goals and two are related to approach goals.

Offenders who pursue the *avoidant-passive* pathway display a desire to avoid sexually offending coupled with an inability to prevent this from happening. In self-regulation terms, offenders in this pathway experience under-regulation or disinhibition. When an offender experiences powerful negative emotional states and/or lacks effective coping skills to deal with a stressor in his life he becomes disinhibited or engages in impulsive behaviours that result in loss of control. In essence, offenders in this pathway find it difficult to control their offending because of coping skills deficits, low impulse control and low self-efficacy, and they typically exhibit covert planning (Ward, Polaschek & Beech, 2006).

In the *avoidant-active* or mis-regulation pathway offenders make an active attempt to avoid sexually offending by attempting to control their deviant thoughts, fantasies or negative affective states. Offenders in this pathway are capable of planning, monitoring and evaluating their behaviour but the strategies they employ to exert control are ineffective or counter-productive and they experience a loss of control. The major difference in relapse between the two avoidant pathways is that offenders in this group make an explicit attempt to deal with the threat to restrain from offending. The strategies used are inappropriate and instead of decreasing risk of relapse are more likely to exacerbate the risk factors. For example, an offender may use pornography for masturbatory practices to exhaust offensive sexual desire or to seek relief from anxiety or feelings of rejection. The strategy can backfire and the pornography can increase disinhibition by potentially strengthening the desire for deviant sex and by decreasing regulatory control (Ward, Polaschek & Beech, 2006).

The third pathway *approach-automatic* is also an under-regulation or disinhibition pathway. Offenders follow entrenched behavioural scripts that, combined with impulsivity and rudimentary planning, result in a sexual offence. This pathway is a mirror image of the avoidant-passive relapse pathway in that the offender's goals and strategies are unlikely to be under intentional control and are activated by contextual cues akin to planned impulsiveness (Pithers, 1990; Ward, Polaschek & Beech, 2006). Individuals may experience either a predominant negative or predominant positive affective state. Positive emotions are associated with the anticipated consequences of engaging in deviant sexual or aggressive needs – when offenders attempt to achieve a heightened positive emotional state combined with inappropriate sexual activity they are more likely to relapse.

The final pathway, *approach-explicit*, consists of conscious, explicit planning and elaborate strategies leading to a sexual offending. In this pathway self-regulation is intact and individuals are capable of good self-regulation skills but the goals they are targeting are inappropriate or harmful. For example, they may have inappropriate or maladaptive standards towards sex with children or attitudes towards women (Ward, Polaschek & Beech, 2006). The goals offenders pursue in this pathway intrinsically support and encourage sexual abuse. Early learning experiences may have resulted in offenders perceiving sexual abuse as an acceptable means to a valued goal. Offences can be experienced as positive or negative depending on the valued goal. Moreover, these individuals are not disinhibited, do not lose control, and do not engage in sex to avoid painful negative emotions. If the goal is to maintain or heighten a positive emotional state they may engage in elaborate grooming, for example, to establish an intimate relationship with a child prior to the sexual abuse. Conversely, if the goal is to punish or intimidate someone, for example an adult woman, then the abuse will be accompanied by strong negative emotions such as anger (Laws & Ward, 2006).

In the model, offenders who fit into the two pathways associated with avoidance goals are more likely to experience negative affective states following an offence owing to self-perceived failure. On the other hand, offenders who follow the approach pathways are more likely to assess the offence as successful and experience positive emotions.

Phase 5: High Risk Situation Entered

Contact, or opportunity for contact, occurs in this stage and is influenced by prior explicit or implicit planning or counterproductive strategies (Ward, Polaschek & Beech, 2006). Individuals appraise the situation at this point and determine whether goals will be met. For those offenders who are attempting to control their behaviour (avoidance strategies) a high risk situation represents failure and negative emotions are likely to be dominant. Offenders with approach goals are more likely to experience a high risk situation as successful.

Phase 6: Lapse

The lapse is the stage immediately prior to the sexual offence, such as sharing a sleeping bag with a child on a camping trip. In terms of relapse, the individual has lapsed and intends to engage in sexual activity with a child (Laws & Ward, 2006). Ward, Polaschek and Beech (2006) suggest that it is at this point that individuals who have previously adhered to the avoidant-passive pathway will now exchange their avoidance goals for approach goals. This exchange of goals may be only temporary and indicates an increase in disinhibition combined with lowered self-regulation and control and a preoccupation with sexual gratification. Avoidant-active individuals also fail at attempting to control their deviant sexual cognitions and consequently engage an approach goal. Individuals following the two approach pathways will continue to strive towards goal satisfaction (Ward, Polaschek & Beech, 2006). Individuals with little or no planning who offend by using automatic processes are likely to be impulsive and display aggressive behaviour. Conversely, individuals with explicit approach strategies demonstrate precise planning and management of the situation to achieve their goals. During the lapse stage of the model all offenders are expected to experience positive emotions owing to increased sexual arousal and/or anticipated pleasure and sexual gratification.

Phase 7: Sexual Offence

In this stage of the sexual offence itself an earlier model developed by Ward, Louden, Hudson and Marshall (1995) identified three subcategories underlying the victim–offender relationship during the commission of the offence. These three subcategories are related to different offence styles and impact directly upon the amount of violence used by the offender and the severity of the offence. They are: (i) self-focus in which the offender's needs dominate in response to heightened sexual arousal in a short but highly intrusive offence; (ii) victim-focus in which the offender justifies his behaviour as providing love and care and meeting his victim's needs albeit with undefined duration and level of intensiveness; and (iii) mutual focus, whereby the offender perceives himself in a 'loving reciprocal relationship' with a willing and consensual partner exhibiting an offence style that is of longer duration and typically less intrusive.

In terms of the SRM, Ward, Polaschek and Beech (2006) suggest it is unclear whether such a distinct victim–offender offence pattern emerges. They have inferred, however, that offenders following the avoidant pathways are more likely to fit the self-focused subcategory given that they have become disinhibited and preoccupied with meeting their own needs. These offenders have presumably lost control, and therefore the offence is likely to be violent and intrusive. Conversely, offenders following the approach pathways will use effective strategies in one of two ways, depending on their goals. They will either engage in a mutual relationship and take steps to please the victim (approach-explicit), or humiliate and denigrate the victim (approach-automatic). Ward, Polaschek and Beech (2006) emphasise that chronically accessible goals and interpersonal themes will greatly influence the way the offence is enacted. To illustrate, offenders with entrenched negative attitudes towards women are more likely to use excessive violence or go to great lengths to humiliate and intimidate their victims. Given that all offenders follow the approach pathways, the majority are likely to experience positive affective states, although offenders who expose their victims to intimidation or psychological distress may experience a combination of negative and positive emotions.

Phase 8: Post-Offence Evaluation

The offence itself is followed by an evaluation process. Avoidant pathway offenders are likely to evaluate themselves negatively and experience guilt or shame – a classic abstinence violation effect. Individuals compare their current behaviour with the goal of behavioural inhibition (abstinence), which creates a discrepancy resulting in self-perceived failure. Negative affect is experienced because the offender has not achieved an important goal (Carver & Scheier, 1990; Ward & Hudson, 2000a). If the offender attributes the cause of offending to uncontrollable and stable internal factors, his exposure of the abstinence violation effect is more intrusive and prolonged offending may eventuate. Approach pathway offenders are hypothesised to experience positive affect as a direct result of achieving their goals.

Phase 9: Attitude Toward Future Offending

The final stage in the model relates to the impact of sexual offending on the offender's future intentions and expectations. Offenders with avoidant goals may be determined to remain offence-free and attempt to reassert control or continue mis-regulation. They may, however, continue to offend because they feel incapable of preventing themselves from sexual offending. Other offenders may choose to offend openly if they experience positive affect and then change their goals to follow the approach pathway. Conversely, approach-automatic offenders are likely to have their behavioural offence scripts reinforced and strengthened because of their 'success' (Laws & Ward, 2006). Offenders following the approach-explicit pathway are likely to build on their expertise in sexual offending and continue to refine and develop their abusive strategies accordingly. Offenders with approach goals are less likely to attempt future restraint thanks to the successful achievement of their goals. Ward and Hudson (2000b) contend that whatever offenders learn in a particular offence episode they assimilate into their existing implicit theories, which in turn influences the way future salient life events are interpreted in the future.

SELF-REGULATION AND INTELLECTUALLY DISABLED SEX OFFENDERS

Although RP is a standard part of any treatment approach for intellectually disabled (ID) sexual offenders, the primary focus has been on the method of implementing the concepts underlying RP rather than on the applicability of the RP model itself (Haaven & Coleman, 2000; Keeling & Rose, 2005). Moreover, there has been little prior research on the offence pathways of ID sexual offenders to be able to allocate offenders into different pathways to relapse (Keeling & Rose, 2005). One exception is Courtney, Rose and Mason's (2005) study, which proposed there were eight major categories in the offence process: targeting victim, decision point, offence planning, offence, stopping the offence, reaction to offence and the consequences of being caught. Courtney and associates (ibid.) acknowledge limitations to their study; however, they suggested that the results indicated similarities between the participants of this study and non-disabled sexual offenders, which confers some validity on the use of RP programmes adapted from mainstream sex offender programmes. The next stage in RP for this population for sexual offenders with ID is to investigate whether they can be allocated into the pathways of the SRM – successful allocation would necessarily have important implications for assessment and treatment.

Keeling and Rose (2005) reviewed the growing literature on sexual offenders with ID and hypothesised that these offenders were more likely to offend via one avoidant and one approach pathway: namely avoidant-passive or approach-automatic. They argued that there are shared characteristics between sexual offenders with ID and non-disabled avoidant-passive offenders, including poor self-regulation skills (Nezu, Nezu & Dudek, 1998). Specifically, both groups use ineffective strategies to deal with deviant sexual arousal, lack coping skills, exhibit higher impulsivity (Glaser & Deane, 1999; Lindsay, 2002), low efficacy expectations (Boer, Dorward, Gauthier & Watson, 1995), and engage in apparently irrelevant decisions consistent with lack of insight into their offending. Other shared similarities include low self-esteem, low self-worth and unassertiveness (Keeling & Rose, 2005). Conversely, Keeling and Rose (ibid.) argued that sexual offenders with ID are unlikely to offend via the avoidant-active pathway because this type of offender tends to exhibit some insight into his offending behaviours. The authors posit that offenders with ID rarely display the type of insight that requires recognition of the need to control their deviant thoughts or negative emotions, and they are thus incapable of implementing appropriate coping strategies.

The approach-automatic offender also shares similarities with ID sexual offenders, including impulsivity (Glaser & Deane, 1999) and coping skills deficits (Lane, 1991). Ward and Hudson (2000a) identified the approach-automatic pathway as a mirror image of the avoidant-passive pathway. Both groups of offenders utilise over-learnt behavioural scripts in their offending, use minimal planning and offend over relatively short time periods (Keeling & Rose, 2005). The behavioural scripts develop from prior offence experiences and are likely to be activated without conscious intention by situational or environmental cues (Ward & Hudson, 2000b). It is also feasible that many sexual offences committed by individuals with ID are not reported because of reluctance on the part of family members and residential care workers. Given this potentially high degree of non-reporting, offenders with an ID may have the opportunity to acquire an extensive and coherent repertoire of offence scripts. Keeling and Rose (2005) posited that since offenders' sexual scripts are formed from their life experiences this influences their norms, values, moral and social rules and belief systems. Given that offenders with ID are vulnerable individuals and that many have been victims of sexual abuse it is possible that their sexual scripts have been influenced by this abuse (Lindsay, Law, Quinn, Smart & Smith, 2001). It would therefore be logical to infer that the combination of over-learnt behavioural scripts from previous offending together with sexual abuse experiences suggests that sexual offenders with ID would be more likely to follow the approach-automatic pathway.

Keeling and Rose (2005) hypothesised that sexual offenders with ID would be unlikely to follow the approach-explicit pathway to relapse given that this group of offenders engage in explicit planning and comprehensive offending strategies. They argue that sexual offenders with ID are unlikely to exhibit intact regulation or explicit planning given their high levels of impulsivity, poor control and lack of insight. Notwithstanding, Ward and Hudson (2000b) suggested that early learning experiences – for example, sexual abuse – may form sexual scripts in this group of offenders in that they perceive their sexual behaviour as an acceptable means to an end.

Interestingly, a recent Australian study (Waterman, 2006) investigated the offence process of child sexual offenders with ID residing in the Residential Treatment Program at Disability Forensic Assessment and Treatment Service (formerly known as Statewide Forensic) in Victoria. A grounded theory approach was utilised and analysis reached saturation after 13 interview transcripts were coded. Each offender was allocated to pathways in the SRM. Consistent with Keeling and Rose's (2005) hypothesis six offenders followed the approach-automatic pathway, but contrary to expectations seven offenders followed the approach-explicit pathway. None of the offenders followed the avoidant-passive or avoidant-active pathways. Two case studies are presented below to illustrate the two approach pathways identified in the study.

Case Studies To Illustrate Approach Pathways

Approach-Automatic: John

John is a 50-year-old man who began offending at the age of 20 years. His earlier offences were non-sexual and mainly related to motor vehicle offences and theft. John's first conviction for sexual offences occurred when he was 29 years old and he has subsequently attended court on numerous charges of sexual penetration and indecent assault against minors under the age of 10 years. John's victims have been both intrafamilial and extrafamilial. His gender preference appears to be male children; however, he has offended against female children. All of his victims were sought out in his immediate environment. John has confessed to offences of sexual abuse against other male children for which he has never been apprehended, and he estimates that there have been in excess of 15 victims in his years of offending. He had sexually penetrated and preformed oral sex on the majority of these victims.

John is the third eldest of five siblings but currently has no contact with his family, including his mother who lives interstate. His childhood was characterised by physical and emotional abuse from his father and brothers and he continues to feel a great deal of hostility and anger towards his family. John was made a Ward of the State at 11 years old and spent his late childhood and adolescence in institutional care. John began to receive treatment to address his offending behaviour 14 years ago but he responded poorly to therapy. He was negative and non-compliant and refused to attend sessions, which resulted in re-offending and breaching court orders. Following a two-year prison term he resumed treatment. He continued to demonstrate strong and intense denial of his sexual offending, often blaming others, such as his parents, the police and victims for 'setting him up'. He frequently threatened that he would shoot or run the victims over upon release from custody. His participation in treatment was minimal, he refused to discuss any elements of his offending and maintained the distortion that the seriousness and severity of his behaviour had been exaggerated by police, courts and clinicians working with him. He has little motivation to change and claims this was how he was born, abdicating any personal responsibility for his own situation or behaviours.

John is allocated to the approach-automatic pathway owing to well-entrenched cognitive and sexual scripts that are activated by situational cues to which he responds in an automatic and unregulated manner. For example, John indicated that he

'just went to the park and started talking and I just offended' and

'just went up to one of them, touched them on the breast and that was it'.

When encountering children he responds immediately by touching them, and whenever possible, sexually penetrates them. He targeted vulnerable children in an easily accessible place and received sexual gratification from his offending behaviour. John's behaviour is impulsive and activated by situational cues, typical of this pathway, and he also demonstrates some rudimentary implicit planning. For example, he frequents parks knowing that there would be unsupervised children playing there. He does not take the view that he is being loving and affectionate towards his victims, rather that both parties gain pleasure from the abuse. He externalises his behaviour as purely a reaction to a child's perceived 'provocative' behaviour and minimises the degree of harm that the child experiences from the abuse

Approach-Explicit: Peter

Peter is a 22-year-old man who began offending at the age of 16 years. His history of offending has included convictions for several counts of indecent assault, assault with intent to rape, loitering and attempted rape. Peter's most recent sexual offence occurred in 2001 in a public place. He targeted a young female child (4 years old) unknown to him after he had absconded from residential care. He observed the victim and her mother on previous occasions. He observed the victim's mother liked to use the computer made available to the public. On the occasion of the offence, Peter used the computer to distract the mother so he could gain access to the victim. The duration of the assault was relatively brief. He reportedly also attempted/or achieved actual vaginal and anal penetration. Peter's offences have generally been well planned and on most occasions he has groomed his victims before offending. The majority of offences have been against children or young vulnerable adult women that he has known. Peter's behaviour appears to have escalated in severity over time. He initially sexually assaulted his younger brother in the family home and then offended against young adult females through his day placement.

Peter's mother has a mild level of ID and a history of institutionalisation. She had six children from three separate relationships. Peter's father, her second husband, was an unemployed alcoholic who spent most of his time at home. Peter's father subjected his mother to significant physical and emotional abuse, and she lived in constant fear. She tried to appease Peter's father by complying with his wishes, which included extreme physical and emotional violence towards the children and the sexual molestation of her children, including Peter. There is also a reported episode of the father physically abusing Peter as an infant. Peter was also forced to witness his father rape his sister, made to watch pornography and witness his father's masturbation and self-abuse (i.e. insertion of instruments into his penis and rectum). Peter sexually assaulted his younger brother on several occasions and was removed from the family home when he was 15 years old. He currently has only limited supervised contact with his family because of an intervention order placed by his mother.

Psychometric testing revealed that Peter demonstrated better than average sexual knowledge, although reported marked negative attitudes. His scores also revealed fantasies relating to sadistic sex; problems with aggressive, delinquent behaviours; impulsive hostility; lack of empathy; and indifference to the needs of others. In therapy he minimised the harm he caused to his victims but was clear in regard to the harm inflicted on him and his siblings by his father.

Peter is allocated to the approach-explicit pathway given his approach goals to offending and his explicit and planned behaviour to achieve this goal. He does not desire or attempt to avoid sexual offending and his self-regulation is intact. Contrary to Keeling and Rose's (2005) hypothesis, Peter explicitly plans his offences and there is a pattern of grooming that includes manipulation and coercion of others to gain access to his victims. Peter's history of sexual abuse suggests that he has formed sexual scripts that facilitate his sexual behaviour, which he perceives as acceptable. He specifically targeted a vulnerable 4-year-old child in his most recent offence by luring her away from her mother.

'. . .got to watch the place. And got to know one of the people there who trusted . . . I was there for quite a while.'

'I planned on where I could not being seen. And if there was any sign of anyone just comin' up I could actually get from . . . What I did was shut the door that was three steps down the stairs.'

'And one door was already shut where the Mum could not see, and that was the point where I stand.'

Peter also displayed apparent disregard for the physical and verbal resistance of the victim and the use of verbal aggression to silence the victim. He used cognitive distortions 'she wanted it' and 'she liked it' to justify his actions and does not regard his sexual abuse of others as harmful or abusive.

CONCLUSIONS

Ward, Polaschek and Beech (2006) have clearly demonstrated that 'one size does not fit all' in relation to relapse into offending. There is growing evidence that the SRM of the relapse process can be applied to sexual offenders with ID in addition to non-disabled sexual offenders. Keeling and Rose (2005) postulated, however, that these offenders were more likely to relapse via the avoidant-passive and approach-automatic pathways. Contrary to expectations, Waterman's study (2006) found that this population of sexual offenders could be allocated to both of the approach pathways. A major finding from this study is that sexual offenders with ID are capable of explicit planning in addition to implicit planning and they can be less impulsive and opportunistic than was previously considered. It would appear that for some offenders their goal selection is based on individual preference and motivation consistent with approach-explicit offenders.

Understanding that sexual offenders with ID follow the approach pathways has implications for assessment and treatment. For the approach-automatic offenders, treatment should focus on teaching offenders to identify the specific situations that trigger the desire to offend, such as access to potential victims if they are unable to self-regulate their behaviour. Therapists will need a different therapeutic approach and techniques to treat approach-explicit offenders since they are more likely to be resistant to changing their attitudes, belief systems and behaviours given their reluctance to refrain from sexually offending.

Moreover, as the SRM has been embedded within the GLM, the integration of the two models facilitates effective therapeutic approaches and techniques (Ward, Polaschek & Beech. 2006). It is important to examine the function of the approach goals in sexual offenders with ID – for example, for sexual pleasure and gratification, relatedness and emotional relief. For the approach-automatic offenders, lack of sexual regulation may be the result of a negative mood state or substance abuse. Interventions should therefore focus on elevating mood state and treating substance abuse in addition to addressing cognitive distortions, deviant sexual scripts and high levels of arousal and impulsivity. Conversely, approach-explicit offenders are able to regulate sexual control, but they hold attitudes and beliefs supportive of offending behaviour and actively seek out offending to experience positive emotions. Treatment will be difficult for offenders following this offence pathway as their offending is oriented towards their own self-interest. They will need assistance to work towards non-offending goals within a GLM treatment framework to identify the needs met through offending and assistance in finding alternative ways of acquiring primary goods, such as social and intimate relationships.

The ultimate aim of therapy within this framework is to focus on self-regulation and autonomy concerns and identify offenders ultimate or higher-level goals in life to replace the goals sought in sexual offending. The SRM allows for the provision of responsive treatment by designing treatment programmes around specific offence relapse pathways, which is essential in the treatment of sexual offenders with ID.

REFERENCES

Abel, G.G., Blanchard, G.T., & Becker, J., (1978). An integrated treatment program for rapists. In R. Rada (Ed.), *Clinical aspects of the rapist.* (pp. 161–214). New York, NY: Grune & Stratton.

Andrews, D.A. & Bonta, J. (1998). *The psychology of criminal conduct*, 2nd edn. Cincinnati, OH: Anderson Publishing Co.

Bandura, A. (1986). *Social foundations of thought and action: A social cognitive theory*, Englewood Cliffs, NJ: Prentice Hall.

Baumeister, R.F. & Heatherton, T.F. (1996). Self-regulation failure: An overview. *Psychological Inquiry, 7* (1), 1–15.

Boer, D.P., Dorward, J., Gauthier, C.M., & Watson, D.R. (1995, September). Treating intellectually disabled sex offenders. *Forum on Corrections Research, 7*. Retrieved July 20, 2006, from www.csc-scc.gc.ca/text/pblct/forum/e073/e073j-eng.shtml.

Carver, C.S. & Scheier, M.F. (1981). *Attention and self-regulation: A control-theory approach to human behaviour*. New York: Springer-Verlag.

Carver, C.S. & Scheier, M.F. (1990). Principles of self-regulation: Action and emotion. In E.T. Higgins and R.M. Sorrentino (Eds), *Handbook of motivation and cognition: Foundations of social behaviour* (Vol. 2, pp. 3–52). New York: Guilford Press.

Cochran, W. & Tesser, A. (1996). The 'What the hell' effect: Some effects of goal proximity and goal framing on performance. In L.L. Martin & A. Tesser (Eds), *Striving and feeling: Interactions among goals, affect, and self-regulation* (pp. 99–120). New York, NY: Lawrence Erlbaum.

Courtney, J., Rose, J. & Mason, O. (2005). The offence process of sex offenders with intellectual disabilities: A qualitative study. Birmingham. Unpublished manuscript.

Deci, E.L. & Ryan, R.M. (2000). The 'what' and 'why' of goal pursuits: Human needs and the self-determination of behaviour. *Psychological Inquiry, 11*, 227–68.

Emmons, R.A. (1996). Striving and feeling: Personal goals and subjective well-being. In P.M. Gollwitzer & J.A. Bargh (Eds) *The psychology of action: Linking cognition and motivation to behavior* (pp. 313–37). New York: Guilford.

Emmons, R.A. (1999). *The psychology of ultimate concerns*. New York: Guilford.

Glaser, W. & Deane, K. (1999). Normalization in an abnormal world: A study of prisoners with an intellectual disability. *Journal of Offender Therapy and Comparative Criminology, 43*, 338–50.

Haaven, J.L. & Coleman, E.M. (2000). Treatment of the developmentally disabled sex offender. In D.R. Laws, S.M. Hudson & T. Ward (Eds), *Remaking Relapse Prevention with Sex Offenders: A Sourcebook* (pp. 369–88). Sage: Thousand Oaks, CA.

Hanson, R.K., (2000). What is so special about relapse prevention? In D.R. Laws, S.M. Hudson & T. Ward (Eds), *Remaking relapse prevention: A sourcebook* (pp. 27–38). Thousand Oaks, CA: Sage Publications.

Keeling, J.A. & Rose, J.L. (2005). Relapse prevention with intellectually disabled sexual offenders. *Sexual Abuse: A Journal of Research and Treatment, 17*, 407–23.

Lambrick, F. & Glaser, W. (2004). Sex offenders with an intellectual disability. *Sexual abuse: A journal of research and treatment, 16*, 381–92.

Lane, S.L. (1991). Special offender populations. In G.D. Ryan & S.L. Lane (Eds), *Juvenile sexual offending: Causes and consequences* (pp. 229–32). Lexington: Lexington Press.

Laws, D.R. (1999). Relapse Prevention: The state of the art. *Journal of Interpersonal Violence, 14*, 285–302.

Laws, D.R. (2003). The rise and fall of relapse prevention. *Australian Psychologist, 38*, 22–30.

Laws, D.R. & Ward, T. (2006). When one size doesn't fit all: The reformulation of relapse prevention. In W.L. Marshall, Y.M. Fernandez, L.E. Marshall & G.A. Serran (Eds), *Sexual offender treatment: Controversial issues*. John Wiley & Sons, Chichester, England.

Lindsay, W.R. (2002). Research and literature on sex offenders with intellectual and developmental disabilities. *Journal of Intellectual Disability Research, 46*, 74–85.

Lindsay, W.R. Law, J., Quinn, K., Smart, N. & Smith, A. H. W. (2001). A comparison of physical and sexual abuse histories: Sexual and non-sexual offenders with intellectual disability. *Child Abuse and Neglect, 25* (7), 989–95.

Lindsay, W.R., Ward, T., Morgan, T. & Wilson, I., (2007). Self-regulation of sex offending, future paths and the good lives model: Applications and problems. *Journal of Sexual Aggression, 13,* 37–50.

Mann, R.E. & Thornton, D. (1998). The evolution of a multi-site treatment program for sexual offenders. In W.L. Marshall, Y.M. Fernandez, S.M. Hudson & T. Ward (Eds), *Sourcebook of treatment programs for sexual offenders.* New York: Plenum.

Mann, R.E. & Thornton, D. (2000). An evidence-based relapse prevention program. In D.R. Laws, S.M. Hudson, & T. Ward (Eds), *Remaking relapse prevention with sex offenders* (pp. 341–52). California: Sage.

Mann, R.E., Webster, S.D., Schofield, C. & Marshall, W.L. (2004). Approach versus avoidance goals in relapse prevention with sexual offenders. *Sexual Abuse: A Journal of Research and Treatment, 16,* 65–75.

Marlatt, G.A. (1985). Relapse prevention: Theoretical rationale and overview of the model. In G.A. Marlatt, & J.R. Gordon (Eds) *Relapse prevention: Maintenance strategies in the treatment of addictive behaviors* (pp. 3–70). New York: Guilford Press.

Marlatt, G.A. & Gordon, J.R. (1985). *Relapse prevention: Maintenance strategies in the treatment of addictive behaviors.* New York, NY: Guilford.

Marques, J.K. (1982, March). *Relapse prevention: A self-control model for the treatment of sex offenders.* Paper presented at the 7th Annual Forensic Mental Health Conference, Asilomar, CA.

Marques, J.K., Day, D.M., Nelson, C. & Miner, M.H. (1989). The sex offender treatment and evaluation project: California's relapse prevention program. In D.R. Laws (Ed.), *Relapse prevention with sex offenders* (pp. 247–67). New York: Guilford.

Marques, J.K. & Nelson, C. (1989). Understanding and preventing relapse in sex offenders. In M. Gossop (Ed.), *Relapse and addictive behaviour.* New York, NY: Tavistock/Routledge.

Marques, M. J. K., Nelson, C., Alarcon, J.M. & Day, D.M. (2000). Preventing relapse in sex offenders: What we learned from SOTEP's experimental program. In D.R. Laws, S.M. Hudson, & T. Ward (Eds), *Remaking relapse prevention with sex offenders* (pp. 321–340). Thousand Oaks, CA: Sage.

Marshall, W.L. & Anderson, D. (1996). An evaluation of the benefits of relapse prevention programs with sexual offenders. *Sexual Abuse: A Journal of Research and Treatment, 8,* 209–21.

Marshall, W.L. & Anderson, D. (2000). Do relapse prevention components enhance treatment effectiveness? In D.R. Laws, S.M. Hudson, & T. Ward (Eds), *Remaking relapse prevention with sex offenders* (pp. 341–52). California: Sage,

Nezu, C.M., Nezu, A.M. & Dudek, J.A. (1998). A cognitive behavioral model of assessment and treatment for intellectually disabled sexual offenders. *Cognitive and Behavioral Practice, 5,* 25–64.

Pithers, W.D. (1990). Relapse prevention with sexual aggressors: A method for maintaining therapeutic gain and enhancing external supervision. In W.L. Marshall, D.R. Laws, & H.E. Barbaree (Eds), *Handbook of sexual assault: Issues, theories and treatment of the offender* (pp. 343–61). New York, NY: Plenum.

Pithers, W.D., Cumming, G.F., Beal, L.S., Young, W. & Turner, R. (1989). Relapse prevention: A method for enhancing behavioral self-management and external supervision of the sexual aggressor. In B. Schwartz (Ed.), *Sex offenders, Issues in treatment* (pp. 292–310), Washington DC: National Institute of Corrections.

Pithers, W.D., Marques, J.K., Gibat, C.C. & Marlatt, G.W. (1983). Relapse prevention: A self-control model of treatment and maintenance of change for sexual aggressives. In J. Greer & I.R. Stuart (Eds), *The sexual aggressor: Current perspectives on treatment* (pp. 214–34). New York: Van Nostrand Reinhold.

Purvis, M. (2005). Seeking a good life: Human goods and sexual offending. Unpublished manuscript. The University of Melbourne.

Ryan, R.M. (1998). Commentary: Human psychological needs and issues of volition, control and outcome focus. In J. Heckhausen & C.S. Dweck (Eds), *Motivation and self-regulation across the lifespan* (pp. 114–33). New York: Cambridge University Press.

Schmuck, P. & Sheldon, K.M. (Eds) (2001) *Life goals and well-being*. Toronto, Ontario: Hogrefe & Huber Publishers.

Thornton, D. (1997). Is relapse prevention really necessary? Paper presented at the Sixteenth Annual Research and Treatment Conference of the Association for the Treatment of Sexual Abusers, Arlington, VA.

Ward, T. & Gannon, T.A. (2006). Rehabilitation, etiology, and self-regulation: The comprehensive good lives model of treatment for sexual offenders. *Aggression and Violent Behavior, 11*, 77–94.

Ward, T. & Brown, M. (2004). The good lives model and conceptual issues in offender rehabilitation. *Psychology, Crime & Law, 10*, 243–57.

Ward, T. Hudson, S.M. (1996). Relapse prevention: A critical analysis. *Sexual Abuse: A Journal of Research and Treatment, 8*, 177–200.

Ward, T. & Hudson, S.M. (1998). A model of the relapse process in sexual offenders. *Journal of Interpersonal Violence, 13*, 700–25.

Ward, T. & Hudson, S.M. (2000a). A self-regulation model of relapse prevention. In D.R. Laws, S.M. Hudson & T. Ward (Eds), *Remaking relapse prevention with sex offenders: A sourcebook*, pp. 79–101. London: Sage Publications.

Ward, T. & Hudson, S.M. (2000b). Sexual offenders' implicit planning: A conceptual model. *Sexual Abuse: A Journal of Research and Treatment, 12* (3), 189–202.

Ward, T., Louden, K., Hudson, S.M. & Marshall, W.L. (1995). A descriptive model of the offence chain for child molesters. *Journal of Interpersonal Violence, 10*, 452–72.

Ward, T. & Mann, R. (2004). Good lives and the rehabilitation of offenders: A positive approach to treatment. In A. Linley & S. Josephs (Eds), *Positive psychology in practice* (pp 598–616). John Wiley & Sons.

Ward, T. & Marshall, W.L. (2004). Good lives, etiology and the rehabilitation of sex offenders: A bridging theory. *Journal of Sexual Aggression, 10*, 153–69.

Ward, T., Polaschek, D. L. L., & Beech, A.R., (2006). *Theories of Sexual Offending*. Chichester, England: John Wiley & Sons.

Ward, T. & Stewart, C. (2003). Criminogenic needs and human needs: A theoretical model. *Psychology, Crime & Law, 9*, 125–43.

Ward, T., Yates, P.M. & Long, C.A. (2006). *The self-regulation model of the offence and relapse process: Volume 2: Treatment*. Victoria, BC, Canada: Pacific Psychological Associate Corporation.

Waterman, B. (2006). Child sex offenders with an intellectual disability: A descriptive model of the offence process. The University of Melbourne. Unpublished manuscript.

PART TWO

Diagnostic Assessment and Comorbidity

6

Psychiatric Illness, Pervasive Developmental Disorders and Risk

FABIAN HAUT AND ELEANOR BREWSTER

INTRODUCTION

Medical interest in intellectual disabilities (ID) first developed in France with the work of the physician Itard (1774–1838) and his pupil Seguin (1812–80). They introduced teaching for people with ID, where previously it had been the mainstream opinion that it was hopeless to attempt to treat 'idiots' (Porter, 1997). With the Enlightenment these pessimistic views were set aside and a spirit of optimism prevailed. This was pioneered by Seguin, who believed that training and colony living would enable people with ID to develop to a point where they could return to mainstream society.

In 1886, as a result of this developing interest in the care of people with ID, the Idiots Act was passed in the UK (Anon., 1887). This led, over subsequent decades, to the building of special asylums with same conditions for admission for the intellectually disabled as for people with mental illness. Initially these institutions focused on education, training and rehabilitation. Later, concerns developed about public safety and the risks caused by contact with people with ID. Eugenics gained in popularity, and, with it, fears that the 'feeble minded' would damage society by spreading undesirable genetic characteristics. Intellectually disabled people were seen as lacking in moral sense, 'Every feeble-minded person, especially the high-grade imbecile, is a potential criminal, needing only the proper environment and opportunity for the development and expression of his criminal tendencies' (Fernald, 1912). In response to societal concerns about safety, in 1913 the Mental Deficiency Act was passed. This allowed for statutory institutional or community care under guardianship or license. It addressed contemporary social concerns about people with ID by allowing the 'feeble minded' to be detained in hospital.

From 1931 to 1938 Professor Lionel Penrose undertook the 'Colchester Survey', a piece of research based on the residents of a Colchester asylum. This work, examining the biological

Assessment and Treatment of Sexual Offenders with Intellectual Disabilities: A Handbook
Edited by Leam A. Craig, William R. Lindsay and Kevin D. Browne
© 2010 John Wiley & Sons, Ltd.

causes of ID laid the foundations for medical interest in this area (Penrose [1949] 1963). At first it was suggested that people with a learning disability would be less likely to develop mental illness as it was held that deficits in intelligence would help prevent the person experiencing the normal stressors of life (Schneider, 1959). Later work has shown that people with ID are susceptible to mental illness, in some cases at a higher rate than the general population (Borthwick-Duffy & Eyman, 1990).

This chapter describes the prevalence of mental illness in people with ID in general terms and also with reference to offending behaviour (sexual and otherwise). The diagnosis and treatment of the most common mental illness is detailed and developmental disorders, for example autism and attention deficit hyperactivity disorder (ADHD), discussed. Finally, we discuss the impact on risk of offending and recidivism through the treatment of mental illness.

PREVALENCE OF MENTAL ILLNESS

Determining the prevalence of mental illness in people with ID is fraught with difficulty. The prevalence found varies depending on the method of study used. The geographical and cultural characteristics of the population studied and the diagnostic criteria employed will also be relevant. Many early studies used patients from asylums, giving a skewed idea of prevalence compared to population-based sampling. Some of the most important work in this area is described and the results illustrated in Table 6.1.

Cooper, Smiley, Morrison, Williamson and Allan (2007) investigated people with ID living in Glasgow. This involved identifying all people thought by relevant agencies to have ID and then excluding those with an IQ over 70, leaving 1,023 participants (a rate of 3.33 per 1,000 general adult population). After screening assessments, all people thought to be possibly, probably or definitely mentally ill were seen by a Learning Disability psychiatrist. Case notes were reviewed and a corroborative history taken. If appropriate, a diagnosis of psychiatric illness was made on the basis of clinical interview and various assessment tools. Diagnoses were made with reference to the three main classificatory systems the *Diagnostic criteria for psychiatric disorders for use with adults with learning disabilities/mental retardation* (DC-LD) (Royal College of Psychiatrists, 2001), *International classification of diseases* (ICD)-10 (WHO, 1992) and *Diagnostic and statistical manual, fourth edition, text revision* (DSM-IV-TR) (APA, 2000).

Deb, Thomas and Bright (2001a) studied a population-based group of 101 adults in south Wales, using the Mini Psychiatric Assessment Schedule for Adults with a Developmental Disability (PAS-ADD) (Prosser, Moss, Costello, Simpson, Patel & Rowe, 1998) as a screening tool and then the full PAS-ADD interview for those identified by the Mini PAS-ADD as being cases. The figures for psychiatric illness included only participants with enough verbal communication to complete the Mini PAS-ADD. This study excluded autism and ADHD as diagnosis because of the difficulties of obtaining a reliable developmental history. Behaviour disorders were estimated in a separate, subsequent publication (Deb, Thomas & Bright 2001b).

Taylor, Hatton, Dixon and Douglas (2004) completed a study in the north of England with 1,155 participants who were either hospital residents or known to care management. The purpose of this work was to provide normative data for the PAS-ADD. The PAS-ADD is a screening tool rather than a diagnostic instrument and so is designed to be over-inclusive. Therefore, this study cannot be directly compared to studies which reach diagnosis by way of a clinical interview.

Table 6.1 Studies on the prevalence of psychiatric disorders in people with ID

	Corbett (1979)	Lund (1985)	Cooper and Bailey, 2001	Deb (2001a, b)	Taylor (2004)	Cooper (2007)	Regier (1988)	Smiley (2007)	Regier (1988)
Size of Group (n =)	402	302	207	101	1,155	1,023	18,571	651	18,571
Type of Study	Point Prevalence	Point Prevalence	Point Prevalence	Point Prevalence	Point Prevalence	Point Prevalence	Point Prevalence	2-year Incidence	Lifetime Prevalence
Patient Group/Diagnosis	ID	ID	ID	ID	ID	ID	General Adult	ID	General Adult
Diagnosis									
Psychotic Disorder	6.2	1.3	2.7	7.8	2.7	4.4	0.7	1.4	1.5
Affective Disorder	4.0	1.7	6.0	5.5	14*	6.6	5.1	8.3	8.3
Personality Disorder	}25.4	10.9	–	1.1	–	1.0	0.5**	–	2.5[b]
Problem Behaviour		–	15.1	60.4	–	22.5	–	4.6	–
Anxiety Disorder		2.0***	7.2	7.8	–	3.8	7.3***	1.7	14.6
Obsessive Compulsive Disorder	–	–	2.5	–	–	0.7	–	0	0
Organic Disorder	–	3.6	3.9	–	–	2.2	–	1.5	–
Alcohol/Substance Use	–	0	1.3	–	–	1.0	3.8	0.3	16.4
Pica	–	–	–	–	–	2.0	–	0.2	–
Sleep Disorder	–	–	–	–	–	0.6	–	0	–
ADHD	–	–	–	–	–	1.5	–	–	–
Autistic Spectrum Disorder	8.2	3.6	6.8	–	–	7.5	–	–	–
Other Mental Ill-Health	1.3	–	–	–	–	1.4	–	0.2	–
Mental Ill-Health	46.3	28.1	37.0	14.4	20.1	40.9	15.4	16.3	32.2

*Includes all affective and neurotic disorders
**Includes only antisocial personality disorder
***Includes obsessive compulsive disorder

Cooper and Bailey (2001) conducted a population-based study of 207 adults with ID in Leicestershire; participants were drawn from a learning disabilities register. Patients were assessed by means of the Present Psychiatric State-Learning Disabilities (PPS-LD) (Fitzgerald, 1998) and the Disability Assessment Schedule. Developmental level was assessed with the Vineland Social Maturity Scale (Sparrow, Balla & Cichetti, 1984); psychiatric diagnoses in the participants were classified using the ICD-10 derived Diagnostic Criteria for Research (DCR) (WHO, 1993), with some modifications. Corbett (1979) completed a population-based study with 402 adult participants. These were people in contact with Learning Disability services in Camberwell. This study used ICD-8, a non-operationalised diagnostic criteria, and the exact method of diagnosis is unclear. Participants were found by initially screening case files for disturbed behaviour or a recorded psychiatric diagnosis. Some participants in the study had an IQ over 70.

Lund (1985) examined a group of 302 adults drawn from a register of the Danish National Service for the Mentally Retarded. Lund made his diagnosis using the Medical Research Council Handicap, Behaviour and Skills Schedule (MRC-HBS). The HBS schedule was derived from observation of symptoms displayed by a group of 38 patients, and so may not have been completely comprehensive. Modified DSM-III criteria were used, though the exact nature of the modification is not discussed. The author carried out all patient interviews, though the method of assessing patients is less comprehensive than more recent work. This study used a maximum IQ of 85 as criterion for inclusion.

The Smiley et al. (2007) study was a follow up of Cooper, Smiley, Morrison, Williamson and Allan (2007) and 651 of the original group of 1,023 were reassessed. The PAS-ADD was used with a modified (lowered) threshold and was followed by an interview with a psychiatrist for cases. This study also used details of demographics and personal history in an attempt to establish predictive factors for mental illness.

Regier et al. (1988) examined the one-month prevalence of mental illness, interviewing 18,571 people. This was done by sampling in 5 'catchment areas' in the USA and then used probability sampling to select adults within these areas. The study was designed to over-sample elderly and ethnic minority groups. The DSM-III derived National Institute of Mental Health (NIMH) Diagnostic Interview Schedule (DIS) was used as the case identification instrument.

From these studies and the results in Table 6.1 it is clear there are significant issues with mental illness for people with ID. The prevalence of schizophrenia and other non-affective psychosis is considerably higher in people with ID than in the general adult population.

Levels of affective disorder (e.g., depression, bipolar affective disorder) appear similar to that found in the general population. However, this may be an underestimate since, despite the fact that these studies were based upon diagnoses by experienced clinicians, there are high levels of 'problem behaviour' in people with ID, a category with no readily comparable general adult counterpart which encompasses various types of disordered behaviour. This leads to the question of whether those who fit within diagnostic criteria for depression are, by virtue of the definition, the only people who could be said to be depressed, or whether depression is currently incompletely defined, leaving present diagnostic criteria concomitantly, deficient. The diagnosis of depression is challenging, especially in people with limited verbal ability.

The level of substance abuse, of both alcohol and illicit drugs, is much lower in the ID population than the general population. This probably reflects a generally lower level of access to these substances. The increased prevalence of illness appears to be the result of both increased incidence rates (the occurrence of new episodes of psychiatric ill-health) and also a longer duration of episodes of ill health (Smiley *et al.*, 2007).

There are a number of possible explanations for the increased susceptibility of individuals with ID to psychiatric illness. The ID and the mental illness may have a shared causation, or the factors leading to the ID may predispose to mental illness; for example, perinatal brain damage may leave the brain susceptible to mental illness. Psychological factors such as an altered and possibly dysfunctional parent–child relationship may lead to difficulties with the child's self-esteem. Neglect and physical or sexual abuse may be important risk factors for the development of psychiatric disorder in persons with ID. Social factors such as lack of a consistent family home or difficulties with social relationships and finding appropriate employment may also be of importance.

OFFENDING IN PEOPLE WITH INTELLECTUAL DISABILITIES

Determining the prevalence of ID in offenders is difficult as many studies have relied on offenders' own reports of ID by inquiring after a history of special schooling or reading difficulties. Additionally, there are difficulties in the way alleged offences perpetrated by people with ID progress through the criminal justice system. This may impact on the prevalence of convicted offenders who have an ID.

Hodgins (1992) used data from a Swedish cohort of all 15,117 people up until the age of 30 who had been born in Stockholm in 1953 and were still residing there 10 years later. This study compared data for convictions, and supplies information in the form of odds ratios rather than absolute numbers (Table 6.2). People with ID were at increased risk of having a criminal record, with a three-fold increase in risk for men and a nearly four-fold increase in risk for women. There are difficulties in generalising the results of this study because of the overly inclusive definition of ID, the exclusion of people to whom more than one category would have applied (which thereby excluded everyone with a significant comorbidity) and also the very high percentage of people said to have a conviction (30 per cent of the general population).

When attempts are made to develop a more formal view of a person's level of intelligence, this apparent excess of ID reduces. Murphy, Harnett and Holland (1995) surveyed a sample of 157 men remanded to prison. Although 33 of those interviewed stated they had had reading problems, ID or had been to a special school, on formal testing, none of these men had an IQ below 70. Winter, Holland and Collins (1997) surveyed people arrested who self-reported having difficulty reading or special educational provision. Of 212 offenders screened,

Table 6.2 Cohort study – mental disorder, intellectual disability and substance abuse in convicted participants (Hodgins, 1992)

Category	Men (odds ratio)	Women (odds ratio)
Major Mental Disorder	2.56 (95% CI 1.66–3.97)	5.02 (95% CI 2.78–9.06)
Other Mental Disorder	1.15 (95% CI 0.69–1.93)	1.67 (95% CI 0.91–3.05)
Intellectual Deficiency	3.12 (95% CI 2.17–4.49)	3.73 (95% CI 2.00–6.94)
Substance Abuse	20.37 (95% CI 12.12–34.26)	32.34 (95% CI 21.11–49.53)

47 admitted to difficulty reading or special schooling. Of the 21 people who then agreed to be included in the study only two had an IQ below 70. Bluglass (1966) in his MD thesis studied a group of 300 post-conviction prisoners. He carried out assessments of psychiatric status and intelligence (using Ravens Progressive Matrices and the Mill Hill vocabulary scale) finding that 2.6 per cent were 'mentally retarded'.

It can be seen that when objective measurements of intelligence are used the proportion of offenders with ID is roughly similar to levels of ID in the general population. However, this broad figure may conceal more subtle differences in offending by individuals with and without ID. When people with an ID commit a crime they may be less able to conceal the crime or their involvement in it. There are also obstacles in the passage of cases through the criminal justice system, when the alleged offender has learning disabilities. It is not unusual to find that although people with ID have been assessed as posing a high risk and have been involved in a number of alleged offences either they have not been reported to the police, they have not been charged or the prosecution has been abandoned for a variety of reasons.

There may also be a bias in the type of research carried out. Research in the field of ID tends to be carried out by people from a healthcare as opposed to a criminal justice background. This may therefore inadvertently emphasise differences between offenders with ID and the general population (Simpson & Hogg, 2001).

MENTAL ILLNESS OF OFFENDERS WITH INTELLECTUAL DISABILITIES

Overall it is thought that approximately one-third of offenders with ID also suffer from psychiatric illness. Day (1994) completed a retrospective survey of the psychiatric case notes of 47 male ID patients referred for antisocial sexual behaviour. Of the sample, 32 per cent of the men had a psychiatric diagnosis. Lindsay *et al.* (2004a) evaluated a community ID offender service over the period 1990–2001. Thirty-two per cent of the patients who had committed sexual offences had a diagnosis of major mental illness, while in a cohort of non-sexual offenders with an ID 33 per cent had attracted a diagnosis of major mental illness.

Lund (1990) used the Danish Central Criminal register to extract data on the number of mentally retarded offenders serving statutory care orders on two census days, in 1973 and 1984. Of the registered offences 20.9 per cent were sexual, and in 12.9 per cent a sexual offence was the sole offence with which the person had been charged. The psychiatric diagnoses of the offenders are reported in Table 6.3.

Table 6.3 Psychiatric diagnoses of sample in the study by Lund, 1990

Diagnosis	Offenders (%)	Controls (%)
Schizophrenia	1.4	1.3
Affective Disorders	2.8	1.7
Dementia	–	3.6
Autism	–	7.6
Other Psychosis	–	1.0
Neurosis	–	2.0
Behaviour Disorder	87.5	10.9

Over the time period of this study (1973–84) there was a reduction in the number and type of care orders made. This reflects a trend towards deinstitutionalisation and normalisation. There was a reduction in the proportion of people with a borderline IQ who became more likely to be subject to standard penal disposal.

Brewster, Willox and Haut (2008) examined 137 pre-trial court reports performed by ID services with regards to the alleged offenders' fitness to plead. Information about psychiatric diagnosis was collected. Overall 21 per cent of people with ID also carried an ICD-10 diagnosis of mental disorder.

SEXUAL OFFENDERS WITH INTELLECTUAL DISABILITIES

There is said to be little specific link between sexual offending and psychiatric illness (Chiswick, 1983). Mental illness has a similar prevalence in sexual offenders as it has in non-offenders with ID. Studies have given rates of approximately one-third of sexual offenders having a psychiatric diagnosis (Day, 1994; Lindsay *et al.*, 2004a). People with ID were not over-represented in a group of sexual offenders or in a group of general offenders (Langevin & Curnoe, 2008). Langevin and Curnoe (ibid.) investigated 2,286 male sex offenders and paraphilics and 241 non-sex offenders, assessing cognitive functioning through formal assessments. The absolute level of sexual offending in people with ID is not known. Deb *et al.* (2001b), in the study of 101 people with ID in south Wales detailed earlier in this chapter, examined behavioural disorders; 'sexual delinquency' was described in 3.9 per cent of cases. The definition of sexual delinquency was not further clarified.

There are differences in the way that offenders with ID and non-ID offenders are treated. A sample from a secure hospital (Baker & White, 2002) examined characteristics of 53 sex offenders detained in maximum security institutions. The offenders were categorized by diagnosis. The four main groups were: mental handicap, mental illness, mental illness with comorbid personality disorder and personality disorder. Compared to the other groups the sex offenders with ID typically had more previous uncharged sex offences, more previous uncharged violent offences and a higher number of victims. None of this group of offenders with ID had a comorbid psychiatric illness.

PEOPLE WITH INTELLECTUAL DISABILITY AS VICTIMS OF SEXUAL OFFENDING

It is likely that sexual offending is in some cases a learnt behaviour, a consequence of previous abuse. A person with an ID is more likely to be a victim than a perpetrator of abuse. Prevalence rates for sexual abuse in people with ID are likely to be subject to under-reporting, but published prevalence rates vary from 8–83 per cent (Peckham, 2007). This is higher than comparative measures for the general population. Sexual offenders with ID have more frequently previously been a victim of sexual abuse than have people with ID convicted for non-sexual offences (Lindsay, Law, Quinn, Smart & Smith, 2001; Thompson & Brown, 1997).

ASSESSMENT AND DIAGNOSIS OF PSYCHIATRIC ILLNESS

The psychiatric assessment of a person with ID involves a modified version of a standard psychiatric assessment. This includes eliciting, if possible, a full psychiatric history, including a more comprehensive developmental history than is usually found in general adult psychiatric assessments. A collateral, corroborative history from a family member or other carer is essential. A mental state examination seeking evidence for the presence or absence of psychiatric symptomatology is performed followed by a full physical examination and evaluation. Depending on the information gained in the history and examination there may be a need for further investigations – for example, laboratory-based investigation of blood or urine samples, X-ray or CT or MRI scanning. If there is a question of organic brain changes, for example, suspicion of epileptic activity, then an EEG may be obtained.

Difficulties in the Psychiatric Assessment of a Person with Intellectual Disabilities

Some of the assessment factors for a person with ID are similar to those of a non-ID person. However, the processes for gathering information are often very different, and when interviewing a person with an ID there are aspects over which additional care must be taken. When someone is known to have an ID there is a risk that psychiatric or emotional symptoms may be seen as being a representation of the intellectual impairment rather the result of mental illness; this is called diagnostic overshadowing (Reiss, Reiss, Levitan & Szyszko, 1982). Questions must be asked in a way which reflects the person's level of understanding. It is important to check the consistency of the information given by asking the same question in different ways to confirm the internal validity of the account obtained. A person with an ID may be suggestible, and so care should be taken to ask open questions where possible and be mindful of the patient's wish to please by providing the answer they think is desired. The level of a person's ID can have a pathoplastic effect on the way the mental illness presents itself.

The level of detail obtained may be reduced as the person may lack the verbal skills needed to express what are often complicated ideas. In this situation, observation of the person's behaviour assumes greater significance. The evaluation of possible psychotic symptoms requires caution. In a person of average intelligence delusions are described as having an 'unshakable' quality, whereby reasoned persuasion will not alter the belief. A person with an ID may be more easily dissuaded from the belief but will repeatedly return to it. Psychotic symptoms may reflect the developmental level of the person and so may be relatively unsophisticated and lacking detail (Sovner, 1986). Ideas which appear to show evidence of paranoia may be based in reality, reflecting the fact that people with ID are often exploited or abused. They might also result from misinterpretation of a situation by the intellectually disabled person.

Developmentally appropriate behaviour may also lead to a suspicion of mental illness; for example, soliloquy when a person reprises or rehearses important events. This is a common behaviour even in people of non-impaired intelligence but if done in public it can give the impression that the person is responding to hallucinations. Obtaining a corroborative history may be more difficult when the person is cared for by paid carers. Problems with high staff turnover may mean that the account given lacks a long-term perspective. If a number of carers are involved in providing care then individual carers may have observed different behaviours.

Carers are not always educated in the symptoms and signs of mental illness and so may not be aware of what would be considered relevant information. They may report symptoms that are obvious – for example, aggression, self-injurious behaviour – but not realise the significance of more subtle changes, such as social withdrawal.

While many people with a mild ID will be able to give enough of an account of their illness for standard diagnostic criteria to apply, more severely affected people may require a modification of the usual approach, with less reliance on verbal communication. In view of this, a separate diagnostic criteria for people with ID was developed by the Royal College of Psychiatrists. The DC-LD (Diagnostic Criteria-Learning Disabilities) was developed (Royal College of Psychiatrists, 2001). More recently the DSM-IV criteria were similarly adapted for use in people with ID (Fletcher, Loschen, Stavrakaki, & First, 2007).

TREATMENT ISSUES

Treatment of specific psychiatric disorders will be detailed below. In general terms, treatment of psychiatric disorder in people with an ID follows the same principles as treatment within the general population. People with ID are said to be more susceptible to side effects of psychotropic medication than are the general population, and as a consequence treatment should be introduced at a low dose and increased slowly. There should be regular monitoring for side effects and the lowest effective dose should be used for the shortest possible time. Treatment with psychotropic medication should usually be given for a specific diagnosis rather than as a behavioural control.

Schizophrenia

There is evidence that schizophrenia is significantly more prevalent in people with ID than in people of average IQ. It has a prevalence rate of 4.4/10,000 (Cooper, Smiley, Morrison, Williamson & Allan, 2007). The symptoms of schizophrenia are traditionally divided into 'positive' and 'negative' symptoms. Positive symptoms include hallucinations, delusions, abnormal thought processes and a feeling of loss of control over body, thoughts or emotions. Negative symptoms include a loss of interest and motivation, also poverty of thought and speech content. While positive symptoms are usually the more superficially striking feature, in the long term it is often the negative symptoms which will be more disabling. Positive symptoms, especially command hallucinations, are concerning to psychiatrists working with people who suffer from a psychotic illness and have committed a sexual offence. However the relationship of these symptoms and sexual offending is complex. Smith and Taylor (1999) examined 84 restricted hospital order in-patients in England and Wales who had committed an index contact sex offence against a woman. They found that at the time of the index offence 80 men were acutely psychotic and half of them had positive symptoms relating to their offence. Factors such as the individual's resistance to comply with command hallucinations and situational variables were thought to determine whether an assault actually occurred. Bjorkly (2002a) reviewed the literature with regards to psychotic symptoms and violence directed towards others. His review showed that 'distress factors' such as low self-esteem, high levels of anxiety and anger have an aggravating effect on persecutory delusions and appear to enhance the risk of persecutory delusions being acted upon. Persecutory delusions per se were found to be associated with an increased risk of violence in some patients. There was also some evidence to suggest that perceived emotional threat and intent control override (TCO) is a risk factor for violence. TCO, a term coined by Link and Stueve (1994), describes a perceived threat of harm from others, that one's thoughts are not one's own and that they were put into one's head and are controlled by others. Bjorkly (2002b) suggested that while command hallucinations were not of themselves dangerous, there was increased tendency to comply with voices ordering acts of violence towards others. They could therefore be conducive to violent behaviour. Evidence, however, was felt to be inadequate overall and further studies to investigate the link of psychotic symptomatology and violent offending behaviour are needed.

Smith, Quinn and Lindsay (2000) found that sexual offences committed by people with ID and psychotic illness tended to occur in the early part of the illness, when more positive, florid symptoms were not evident or the emerging psychotic illness had not been recognised. This has also been shown to be the case with mainstream sex offenders with schizophrenia (Craissati & Hodes, 1992). It is clear that adequate, early treatment in the emergence of a psychotic illness is of great importance; however, besides optimising pharmacological treatment there is also the need for specific psychological interventions aimed at sexually offending behaviour to optimise treatment outcomes and risk management.

Pharmacological treatment of schizophrenia primarily involves the use of antipsychotic medication. This may be either a 'typical' antipsychotic (e.g., Haloperidol, Chlorpromazine, or an 'atypical' antipsychotic (e.g., Olanzapine, Risperidone, Clozapine). The difference between typical and atypical antipsychotics is defined by the greater ability of typical antipsychotics to induce catalepsy in rats. Though typical and atypical antipsychotics are usually presented as separate categories of drugs in reality they range along a spectrum on which Clozapine is the most 'atypical'. There is no clear difference in the effectiveness of typical and atypical medication, with the exception of Clozapine, which is the most effective antipsychotic. Despite its effectiveness, Clozapine is reserved for cases when treatment with two other antipsychotics (at least one of which is an atypical) has failed. Clozapine increases the risk of patients developing a potentially fatal white blood count abnormality (agranulocytosis) and so it requires regular monitoring. When atypical antipsychotics were introduced they quickly became the first-line drug for the treatment of psychosis as they do not predispose to the development of extra-pyramidal side effects and dystonias. However, in recent years it has been shown that this is balanced by the tendency of atypical antipsychotics to lead to difficulties with weight gain and glucose and lipid elevations, the 'metabolic syndrome'. People with an ID may find it especially difficult to moderate this by restricting their dietary intake, though physical activity and dietary modification have been shown to be effective in this group (Drahelm, Williams & McCubbin, 2002; McKee, Bodfish, Mahorney, Heeth & Ball, 2005).

Depression

Around 1 in 20 ID people will meet diagnostic criteria for depression at any one time (Cooper, Smiley, Morrison, Williamson & Allan 2007). Depression is a mental illness characterised by a lowered mood, reduced enjoyment of life and fatigue. Changes may occur in the way the person's body functions, with insomnia or unsatisfying sleep, loss of appetite and reduced libido, and thoughts of suicide may also arise. Making a diagnosis of depression in people with an ID can be difficult. People with an ID may have limited verbal skills and so the emphasis will then lie on detecting behavioural changes, which may be subtle. They may include lowered or irritable mood, tearfulness, lack of interest in activities that are usually enjoyed, social withdrawal, increased aggression and tantrums, reduced concentration and indecisiveness, a loss of energy, disrupted sleep or appetite or weight change, reduced self-care, reduced speech, agitated or slowed down body movements (Cooper & Collacot, 1996).

Treatment of depression in a person with an ID proceeds along similar lines to that of a person of average IQ. An antidepressant would be a typical first line therapy. This would usually be with a drug from the selective serotonin reuptake inhibitors (SSRI) group of antidepressants. If initial antidepressant therapy is ineffective, subsequent treatment either involves substituting the antidepressant initially with a second SSRI and then with an antidepressant with an alternative mechanism of action or augmenting the antidepressant with a mood stabiliser, another antidepressant or an antipsychotic.

Psychological therapies have a more limited role in ID than in General Adult Psychiatry. The evidence base supporting psychotherapeutic approaches to emotional problems in people with ID remains limited (Wilner, 2005)

Electroconvulsive therapy (ECT) is an option for treatment resistance or when a rapid response is needed. ECT appears to be as effective and safe for people with a ID as it is for the general population (Cutajar & Wilson, 1999; Reinblatt, Rifkin & Freeman, 2004). Although depressive disorders can manifest themselves as aggression or violence in people with an ID, which can lead to involvement with police and criminal justice services, there is no evidence that depression plays a major part in the aetiology of sexual offending behaviour in people with ID.

Bipolar Affective Disorder

Bipolar affective disorder is a condition which causes prolonged episodes of abnormal mood, either depression or hypomania and mania. Mania refers to symptoms that impact on social functioning, where as hypomania is a less severe form of abnormally elevated mood. During episodes of lowered mood the presentation will be that of depression. When the mood is abnormally elevated, this could present as either euphoria or as irritation. There may be physical overactivity and a reduced need for sleep. The person may feel their thoughts are moving especially fast. They may have many ideas, which typically involve a self-aggrandising theme.

Bipolar disorder can be subdivided into four categories; Bipolar 1; Bipolar 2; Bipolar Affective Disorder, Not Otherwise Specified; and Cyclothymic Disorder. In Bipolar 1 the person experiences mania while in Bipolar 2 the person affected has not had a manic episode but instead experiences hypomania. Bipolar Affective Disorder, Not Otherwise Specified relates to the presence of major depressions and episodes that almost but do not quite reach the criteria for hypomania. Cyclothymic Disorder is characterised by hypomania and mild depression alternating together, though with changes occurring over the course of a few days mood states are less prolonged than in classical bipolar disorder.

Rapid Cycling Bipolar Affective Disorder

This is a sub-classification that can apply either to Bipolar 1 or 2. If the patient has at least four major depressive, manic, hypomanic or mixed episodes over a 12-month period they are described as having rapid cycling bipolar affective disorder (Dunner & Fieve, 1974). Estimates of the proportion of people with rapid cycling bipolar affective disorder vary depending on the setting. Dunner and Fieve (ibid.) found that 13 per cent of attendees at a lithium clinic were rapid cycling. In a sample that included both inpatients and outpatients with bipolar affective disorder 20 per cent were rapid cycling (Kukopulos, Reginaldi, Laddomada, Floris, Serra & Tondo, 1980). Of a group of people with bipolar affective disorder and treatment resistance 37 per cent were rapid cyclers (Cole, Scott, Ferrier & Eccleston, 1993). In people with an ID, men are likely to have an earlier onset of affective illness than women and are more likely to be rapid cycling. (Vanstraelen & Tyrer, 1999). In people with an ID rapid cycling bipolar affective disorder is associated with an earlier age of onset than either people with rapid cycling disorder without ID or people with non-rapid cycling bipolar affective disorder and a learning disability. Shorter and more frequent episodes occurred in those suffering from more severe forms of ID.

There is little evidence linking bipolar affective disorder to serious sexual offending behaviour in people with ID. Loss of inhibition because of manic or hypomanic mood states might lead to public order offences, theft and assault. Smith, Quinn and Lindsay (2000) compared 19 offenders with an ID, 16 offenders with ID and diagnosed with schizophrenia and 115 people with ID without any diagnosis of major mental disorder. People with a diagnosis of hypomania were less likely to re-offend than people without psychiatric disorder, suggesting that treatment of the mood disorder had an effect on re-offending. Although individuals with mood disorder were less likely to commit a sexual offence and had a reduced risk of re-offending this was not the case with regards to offences against children, where the re-offending rate was similar to individuals with ID alone.

Raymond, Coleman, Ohlerking, Christenson and Miner (1999) assessed 45 males with paedophilia who were participating in residential or outpatient treatment programmes. The individuals were assessed for presence of psychiatric disorder and 31 per cent were felt to fulfil diagnostic criteria for DSM-IV mood disorders with 4 per cent fulfilling diagnostic criteria specific to bipolar disorder. Although numbers were small there seems to be no direct link between bipolar affective disorder and paedophilia.

Treatment of bipolar affective disorder involves using mood stabilising medication. This would be either a traditional mood stabiliser (e.g., lithium) or an anticonvulsant licensed for this purpose. Since 2008 certain antipsychotics e.g., Quetiapine have been licensed in the UK for use in bipolar affective disorder. If a person with bipolar affective disorder becomes depressed then the mood stabiliser can be augmented with an antidepressant. In this case tricyclic antidepressants should be avoided because of the risk of promoting a switch into mania or the onset or maintenance of rapid cycling. Treatment of rapid cycling bipolar illness follows the same principles as treatment of mainstream patients. Rates of response to treatment are similar in people with an ID to those in the general adult population. People with rapid cycling bipolar affective disorders tend to have a poorer response to lithium, and this may be especially true in ID (Vanstraelen & Tyrer, 1999).

Personality Disorder

Personality disorders are severe disturbances in the personality and behavioural tendencies of the individual which are not the direct result of disease, damage or other insult to the brain or of another psychiatric disorder. They usually involve several areas of the personality and are nearly always associated with considerable personal distress and social disruption.

They usually manifest in childhood or adolescence and continue throughout adulthood. As the DC-LD points out diagnosis is made on the basis of the severity/intensity of the traits rather than on psychopathological abnormalities of form, so in some ways the dividing line between normal personality and personality disorder could be considered arbitrary (Royal College of Psychiatrists, 2001). Various studies have looked at the prevalence of personality disorder in people with an ID. Estimates range considerably, from 1 per cent (Cooper, Smiley, Morrison, Williamson & Allan, 2007) to 28 per cent (Lidher, Martin, Jayaprakash & Roy, 2005) or 31 per cent (Khan, Cowan & Roy 1997) in community samples. Ballinger and Reid (1987) did not make a formal personality disorder diagnoses but found that in a group of ID hospital inpatients 22 per cent had a marked personality abnormality and 56 per cent had features of abnormal personality. In an inpatient sample with mild to moderate ID and severe challenging behaviour 92 per cent of patients with whom interviews were carried out met the criteria for personality disorder (Flynn, Matthews & Hollins, 2002).

Studies involving the general adult population (based on a sample of primary care patients with chronic psychiatric needs) have estimated personality disorder as being present in 3–8 per cent (Cooper, 1965) and in 33.9 per cent of people with conspicuous psychiatric morbidity (Casey, Dillon & Tyrer, 1984). In a person with an ID the presence of a personality disorder could have a decisive bearing on whether that person is able to live independently in the community. Despite this, and also the high prevalence of ID found in research studies, there appears to be a reluctance to allocate a personality disorder diagnosis to a person with ID in the course of normal clinical practice. This may be the result of a perception that a diagnosis of personality disorder would be additionally stigmatising to a person in an already disadvantaged situation. However, a diagnosis is often needed before services and benefits can be accessed, and so there may be a detriment to patients in allowing concerns about stigma to inhibit the clinician from making a diagnosis that may otherwise be beneficial to the patient (Zigler & Burack, 1989)

Personality disorder, especially antisocial personality disorder and psychopathy within general forensic patients, has attracted a lot of attention and appears, especially in relation to rape, to be a risk factor. Additionally, antisocial traits together with deviant sexual interest appear to be associated with sexual recidivism (Hanson & Morton-Bourgon, 2005). Antisocial traits have also been identified as risk factors for recidivism in people with ID who had sexually offended. Lindsay, Elliot and Astall (2004) completed a retrospective study on 52 male sex offenders, of whom 18 had re-offended or were strongly suspected of having re-offended. Antisocial attitude emerged as a significant predictor for recidivism. Antisocial personality disorder was found in 22 per cent of 164 individuals with ID and forensic needs (Lindsay *et al.*, 2007).

There is no specific pharmacological treatment for people who have personality disorder. There is a body of evidence to suggest that mood stabilising medication and low dose antipsychotic medication have a beneficial impact on impulse control and in reducing inappropriate behaviour.

Substance Use

Alcohol use or consumption are, in general terms, at a similar or reduced level in people with an ID compared with their use in the general population (Krischef & Di Nitto, 1981). Huang (1981) assessed and compared the use of alcohol by adolescents with an ID (n = 190) to its use by a group of adolescents without ID (n = 187). Information was collected through a verbally administered questionnaire and alcohol users were defined as having consumed alcohol at least twice in the preceding year. Of the sample, 32 per cent of students with ID were found to be 'users' compared to 59 per cent of individuals in the control group. There was evidence to suggest that the individuals with ID were more susceptible to social influences.

Krischef (1986) surveyed 214 adults with predominantly mild ID living in the community and found that about half of the participants had used alcohol in their lifetime and about 10 per cent reported daily alcohol use. With regards to substance abuse problems within people with ID, prevalence rates vary according to diagnostic criteria used and population studied. Sturmey, Reyer, Lee and Robek (2003) estimated that from 0.5 per cent to 2 per cent of people with ID in the UK and the US may have a substance misuse disorder, with alcohol being the main substance of abuse. Taggart, McLaughlin, Quinn and Milligan (2006) examined substance misuse in people with ID in Northern Ireland. Individuals were identified through community teams working with people with ID. Sixty-seven adults with ID were identified as misusing substances resulting in substantial problems. Taking the limitations of the study into account this gives a prevalence rate of 0.8 per cent. Alcohol was reported to be misused by all of the users with about 20 per cent also misusing illicit drugs and prescribed medication. More than a third of people identified were reported to have come to the attention of criminal justice services with male users (56.7 per cent) more likely to engage in offending behaviour than female users (30 per cent).

Studies assessing the prevalence of alcohol and substance misuse in offender populations and offenders with psychiatric disorders tend to identify an increased prevalence of alcohol problems and drug use (Coid, Hickey, Kathan, Zhang & Yang, 2007; Davidson, Humphreys, Johnstone & Owens, 1995). In people with ID who offended, 65 per cent have been reported by family members of having alcohol and/or drug problems (Cockram, Jackson & Underwood, 1998). McGillivray and Moore (2001) assessed 30 participants with ID in the Statewide Forensic Program in Australia by questionnaire measuring knowledge of alcohol and illicit drugs and pattern of use. Sixty per cent reported that they had been under the influence of alcohol, illicit drugs (6.6 per cent) or both (20 per cent) just prior to committing the offence suggesting some relationship between substance misuse and involvement by individuals with ID in the criminal justice system. Alcohol and substance misuse in people with ID may be an emerging factor contributing to the aetiology of offending behaviour in people with ID although Lindsay, Steele, Smith, Quinn, and Allan (2006) found that male sexual offenders had lower rates of alcohol and substance abuse than other male and female offenders.

PERVASIVE DEVELOPMENTAL DISORDERS

Pervasive developmental disorder (PDD) is a term referring to the group of heterogeneous conditions that comprise the spectrum of autistic disorders. They are characterised by a core triad of impairments:

1. qualitative impairments in reciprocal social interactions;
2. qualitative impairments in communication (verbal and non-verbal);
3. restricted, repetitive and stereotyped patterns of interest and behaviour.

It is useful clinically to regard these disorders as lying on a spectrum. However, there may, within this spectrum, be differences in terms of aetiology, clinical presentation and prognosis. There are classifications within the autistic spectrum – for example, classical autism (Kanner, 1943) which has the symptoms described above with onset before the age of 3, and Asperger's Syndrome, which is distinguished from classical autism by not having any clinically significant delay to language. High functioning autism is the term often applied when the IQ is over 70.

The prevalence of autism is uncertain. It was initially believed that the prevalence of autism was 2–5/10,000 children, though more recent studies have suggested higher rates (Gillberg & Wing, 1999). The rate of autism is currently believed to be around 10 per 10,000, and the prevalence of pervasive developmental disorders 27.5 per 10,000 (Williams, Higgins & Brayne, 2006). Studies have variously suggested that the prevalence of autism is between 0.7 and 72.6 per 10,000 (Fombonne, 2003). The prevalence figures seem to increase over time. The reasons for this increase are not clear. They may reflect a genuine rise in the prevalence of autism, but they may also be the result of improved awareness and diagnostic services, changes in study design and acceptance that autism can be comorbid with other conditions, or indeed that autistic spectrum disorders (ASD) may occur without a deficit in IQ. The rate of autism found in prevalence studies varies according to the diagnostic criteria used (ICD-10 or DSM-IV), the age of children tested, and the location of the study (Williams, Higgins & Brayne, 2006).

Autism and Mental Illness

The relationship between autism and schizophrenia is controversial. There are studies that have reported a link between schizophrenia and autism, particularly in people with a pre-pubertal onset of psychotic symptoms (Sverd, 2003). In a study of 85 adults with Asperger's syndrome, Tantam (1991) reported that 30 patients (35 per cent) met criteria for a psychiatric disorder other than a developmental disorder. Of these patients, 18 (21 per cent of the total study population) showed psychosis: 4 had mania, 4 had mania alternating with depression, 4 experienced hallucinations, 1 had epileptic psychosis, 2 had depressive psychosis, and 3 were diagnosed as having schizophrenia. Of the remaining 12 patients, 2 showed OCD (one of these patients experienced hallucinations) and 11 showed depression and anxiety, alone or together. Some of the cases of depression were severe and associated with delusions and suicidal thinking. One patient showed catatonic stupor.

Offending and Sexual Offending in Autistic Spectrum Disorders

Tantam (1988) studied 60 individuals, with a mean age of 24 years (range 16–65 years), with lifelong eccentricity and social isolation, 46 of whom he diagnosed as having ASD. Nearly half of the subjects had been involved in antisocial behaviour and nearly a quarter had committed a criminal offence. Six patients showed morbid fascination with violence or socially proscribed behaviour. One subject had sadistic fantasies about women and another subject attacked a woman after writing increasingly aggressive accounts of his sexual feelings. Three subjects engaged in indecent exposure and one attempted rape. Other subjects perpetrated serious assaults on younger children. Aggressive assaults were often unexplainable in terms of an individuals' motivation. The most common type of assault was on a member of the family, usually the mother, and often the cause was trivial.

Scragg and Shah (1994) found an increased prevalence (1.5 per cent) of Asperger's syndrome among the male inpatient population at Broadmoor special hospital over the population prevalence, suggesting a possible association between Asperger's syndrome and violence. Siponmaa, Kristiansson, Jonson, Nyden and Gillberg (2001), in re-examining case records of 126 young offenders assessed by a forensic psychiatry department in Stockholm, identified 30 per cent of the individuals with a possible diagnosis of PDD, including 4 per cent with a definite diagnosis of Asperger's syndrome and concluded that Asperger's syndrome was ove-represented in forensic psychiatry. An association between PDD and arson was found, which was the only significant relationship between type of offence committed and diagnosis.

There is limited research looking at people with ASDs who sexually offend (Kohn, Fahum, Ratzoni & Apter, 1998). Sexual offending in this group may be related to difficulty in understanding 'theory of mind': the independent thought and behaviour of other people.

Barry-Walsh and Mullen (2004) detailed five case histories of offenders with Asperger's syndrome. They state that each of the offences is understandable in terms of the patient's diagnosis. One of the cases involved sexual offending, which was felt to result from the interplay between the patients Asperger's syndrome and his developing libido. They high-lighted the lack of appreciation a person with Asperger's syndrome may have for the consequences of his or her actions.

Proctor and Beail (2007) compared 25 male offenders with ID to 25 male non-offenders, also with ID, and measured their performance on two empathy and three theories of mind tasks. Offenders performed better than non-offenders on a second order theory of mind task and on emotion recognition, suggesting than offenders with ID have better theory of mind and empathy ability than non-offenders with ID.

Woodbury-Smith, Clare, Holland, Kearns, Staufenberg, and Watson (2005) produced a case control study designed to indicate if the cognitive impairments of people with ASD are associated with their vulnerability to offending. It was found that, compared with non-offenders with ASD, offenders showed a significantly greater impairment in recognition of emotional expressions of fear, but no difference in theory of mind, executive function and recognition of facial expressions of sadness. It was suggested that this might reflect a real difference in neuropsychological phenotypic expression, in that some people with ASD may also be comorbid for developmental disorders of antisocial behaviour, and that this might be related to their greater propensity to offend.

Attention Deficit Hyperactivity Disorder

The prevalence of ADHD is higher in people with ID than in the general population (Epstein, Cullinan & Gadow, 1986; Fox & Wade, 1998; Rutter, Graham & Yule, 1970). The prevalence of symptoms increases with the severity of the ID (O'Brien, 2000). A study of children (Epstein, Cullinan & Gadow, 1986), some with an ID and some with average IQ, found that levels of hyperactivity were 17.8 per cent for girls and 21.4 per cent for boys with an ID in comparison with 3.5 per cent and 4.4 per cent respectively for girls and boys in the average IQ group. In a study of adults with ID, ranging from severe to profound (Fox & Wade, 1998), 55 per cent were found to have inattentive type ADHD and 15 per cent had hyperactive/impulsive type ADHD. The prevalence of ADHD was higher in males, and in those with lower IQ or poorer adaptive function. In people with an ID the presence of ADHD may be missed. ADHD is diagnosed on the basis of severity of behaviour rather than on the presence or absence of unique symptoms. Inattention and difficulty sustaining meaningful behaviour are common in people with ID. The diagnosis of ADHD should only be applied if the symptoms are of a degree that would be unusual once the level of ID has been taken into account.

ADHD has known association with offending behaviour. Moffit and Silva (1988) reported that close to 60 per cent of individuals who had a diagnosis of ADD had become delinquent by the age of 13. Satterfield and Schell (1997) followed up young adult males who had been diagnosed as hyperactive between the ages of 6 and 12. Eighty-nine participants were matched on age, IQ and social class to a non-hyperactive control group. Young men who had been diagnosed as hyperactive were at an increased risk for juvenile and adult criminality. The risk of becoming an adult offender was found to be associated with conduct problems in childhood and serious antisocial behaviour in adolescence. Rabiner, Coie, Miller-Johnson, Boykin, and Lochman (2005) followed up an initial sample of 622 African-American males and interviewed the participants on a two-yearly basis between the ages of 12 and 22. Individuals were categorised into three groups: persistent aggressive offenders, adolescent-only aggressive offenders and never aggressive, depending on whether they self-reported a felony assault in adolescence and/or adulthood. An association was found between ADHD and aggressive offences in adolescents as well as adults. There is little evidence specifically with regards to ADHD and sexual offending in people with ID. It is noteworthy that although one of the diagnostic criteria of ADHD relates to impulsiveness, impulsiveness alone does not appear to be a major factor in the aetiology of people with ID who sexually offend (Parry & Lindsay, 2003).

MANAGEMENT

It is important that sexual offences thought to involve perpetrators with ID are dealt with through normal criminal justice means. This means that a person should be convicted only if the evidence meets the legal threshold of 'beyond reasonable doubt'. More informal approaches may lead to someone's liberty being restricted because of suspicions that may have developed about their behaviour but for which there is sufficient proof to secure a conviction. One study looked at attitudes of staff and police to offending behaviour in people with ID and found a high tolerance for offending behaviour. Seventeen of 20 group establishments would not always report a rape or sexual assault to the police (Lyall, Holland & Collins 1995). Formal approaches, for example, convictions for previous incidents, makes it easier for the various agencies involved in a person's care to understand the potential seriousness of the person's behaviour. Finally, convictions for sexual offences, and subsequent sentencing, may place a compulsion on the perpetrator to comply with treatment.

As already discussed, there is little to link specific psychiatric diagnoses with sexual offences, and they do not appear to be any more prevalent in people convicted of sexual offences than in those convicted of mainstream offences. Effective treatment of a comorbid psychiatric condition may help to reduce a person's offending behaviour, particularly if it is driven by mental illness. It is important, though, to be alert to the possibility that treatment may worsen offending behaviour by enabling the person to conceal their thoughts and to plan offences.

CONCLUSIONS

People with ID are, for a number of reasons, at elevated risk of experiencing psychiatric illness and other problem behaviours. The pattern of incidence and prevalence of different disorders varies but shows a clearly increased risk of psychotic illness. The comparative figures for affective disorder are less clear, and it seems likely that this is, at least in part, because of the difficulty of assigning a psychiatric diagnosis in a person with an ID and the possibility that disordered behaviour is simply accepted, rather than being viewed as a possible presentation of mental illness. If the behaviour of someone with an ID suddenly worsens or changes then psychiatric illness should be suspected as a possible reason. There should be a careful evaluation of the person's mental and physical state, their environment and level of support. The psychiatric assessment of a person with ID must be careful and thorough.

Any mental illness should, of course, be treated. This would usually follow similar principles to the treatment of mental illness in the general population, but with consideration given to a higher vulnerability to side effects compounded by the difficulty in determining if side effects are present. Psychological treatment of mental illness also requires modification of the approach taken in the general adult population, with emphasis given to behavioural methods rather than a strictly cognitive approach.

People with ID and mental illness are not over-represented in the offending population; however, mental illness and ID can have an influence on the likelihood of a person offending. People with ID are an important group who require a specialised approach, which acknowledges their communication needs, the pertinent risk factors and the potential for ongoing emotional and social development. Sexual offending does not generally appear to be related to mental illness, either in the general population or in those with ID. In individual cases, however, the presence or absence of mental illness may be an important modifier of risk.

REFERENCES

American Psychiatric Association. (2000). *DSM-IV-TR: Diagnostic and Statistical Manual of Mental Disorders*. American Psychiatric Association.

Anon. (1887). Idiots Act, 1886. *Journal of Mental Science, 33*, 103–8.

Baker, M. & White, T. (2002). Sex offenders in high-security care in Scotland. *Journal of Forensic Psychiatry, 13* (2), 285–97.

Ballinger, B., & Reid, A. (1987). Personality Disorder in mental handicap. *Psychological Medicine, 17* (4), 983–7.

Barry-Walsh J. B., & Mullen, P. E. (2004). Forensic Aspects of Asperger's Syndrome. *Journal of Forensic Psychiatry & Psychology, 15* (1), 96–107.

Bjorkly, S. (2002a). Psychotic symptoms and violence towards others - a literature review of some preliminary findings Part 1. Delusions. *Aggression and Violent Behaviour, 7*, 617–31.

Bjorkly, S. (2002b). Psychotic symptoms and violence towards others - a literature review of some preliminary findings. Part 2: Hallucinations. *Aggression and Violent Behaviour, 7*, 605–15.

Bluglass, R. (1966). A psychiatric study of Scottish convicted prisoners. MD Thesis. University of St Andrews, Scotland.

Borthwick-Duffy, S. A. & Eyman, R. K. (1990). Who are the dually diagnosed? *American Journal on Mental Retardation, 94*, 586–95.

Brewster, E., Willox, E. G. & Haut F. (2008). Assessing fitness to plead in Scotland's learning disabled. *The Journal of Forensic Psychiatry and Psychology, 19* (4), 597–602.

Casey, P. R., Dillon, S. & Tyrer, P. J. (1984). The diagnostic status of patients with conspicuous psychiatric morbidity in primary care. *Psychological Medicine, 14* (3), 673–81.

Chiswick, D. (1983). Sex crimes. *The British Journal of Psychiatry, 143*, 236–42.

Cockram, J., Jackson, R. & Underwood, R. (1998). People with an ID and the criminal justice system: The family perspective. *Journal of Intellectual and Developmental Disability, 23* (1), 41–56.

Coid, J., Hickey, N., Kathan, N., Zhang, T. & Yang, M. (2007). Patients discharged from medium secure forensic psychiatry services: Reconvictions and risk factors. *The British Journal of Psychiatry, 190*, 223–9.

Cole, A. J., Scott, J., Ferrier, I. N. & Eccleston, D. (1993). Patterns of treatment resistance in bipolar affective disorder. *Acta Psychiatrica Scandinavica, 88*, 121–3.

Cooper, B. (1965). A Study of One Hundred Chronic Psychiatric Patients Identified in General Practice, *The British Journal of Psychiatry, 11*, 595–605.

Cooper, S. A. & Bailey, N. M. (2001). Psychiatric disorders amongst adults with learning disabilities: Prevalence and relationship to ability level. *Irish Journal of Psychological Medicine, 18*, 45–53.

Cooper, S. A. & Collacott, R. A. (1996). Depressive episodes in adults with learning disabilities. *Irish Journal of Psychological Medicine, 13*, 105–13.

Cooper, S. A., Smiley, E., Morrison, J., Williamson, A. & Allan, L. (2007). Mental ill-health in adults with ID: Prevalence and associated factors. *The British Journal of Psychiatry, 190*, 27–35.

Corbett J. (1979). Psychiatric morbidity and mental retardation. In F. E. James and R. P. Snaith (Eds), *Psychiatric Illness and Mental Handicap* (pp. 11–25). London. Gaskell Press.

Craissati, J. & Hodes, P. (1992). Mentally ill sex offenders: The experience of a regional secure unit. *The British Journal of Psychiatry, 161*, 846–9.

Cutajar, P. & Wilson, D. (1999). The use of ECT in ID. *Journal of ID Research, 43*, 421–7.

Davidson, M., Humphreys, M. S., Johnstone, E. C. & Owens, D. G. C. (1995). Prevalence of psychiatric morbidity among remand prisoners in Scotland. *The British Journal of Psychiatry, 167* (4), 545–8.

Day, K. (1994). Male mentally handicapped sex offenders, *The British Journal of Psychiatry, 165*, 630–9.

Deb, S., Thomas, M. & Bright, C. (2001a). Mental disorder in adults with ID: I. Prevalence of functional psychiatric disorder among a community-based population aged between 16 and 64 years. *Journal of ID Research, 45*, 495–505.

Deb, S. Thomas, M. & Bright, C. (2001b). Mental disorder in adults with ID. 2: The rate of behaviour disorders among a community–based population aged between 16 and 64 years. *Journal of ID Research, 45*, 506–14.

Drahelm, C. C., Williams, D. P. & McCubbin, J. A. (2002). Physical activity, dietary intake, and the insulin resistance syndrome in nondiabetic adults with mental retardation. *American Journal on Mental Retardation, 107* (5), 361–75.

Dunner, D. L. & Fieve, R. R. (1974). Clinical factors in lithium carbonate prophylaxis failure. *Archives of General Psychiatry, 30* (2), 229–33.

Epstein, M. H., Cullinan, D. & Gadow, K. D. (1986). Teacher ratings of hyperactivity in learning disabled, emotionally disturbed and mentally retarded children. *Journal of Special Education, 20*, 219–29.

Fernald, W. E. (1912). The burden of feeble-mindedness. *Journal of Psycho-Asthenic, 17*. Available at www.disabilitymuseum.org/lib/docs/1208.htm.

Fitzgerald, B. (1998). *Reliability and validity of the present psychiatric state-learning disabilities (PPS-LD).* Abstracts of the Penrose Society Spring Meeting, 7.

Fletcher, R., Loschen, E., Stavrakaki, C. & First, M. (2007). *Diagnostic manual - ID: A textbook of diagnosis of mental disorders in persons with ID.* Kingston, New York: NADD Press.

Flynn, A., Matthews, H. & Hollins, S. (2002). Validity of the diagnosis of personality disorder in adults with learning disability and severe behavioural problems: Preliminary study. *The British Journal of Psychiatry, 180*, 543–6.

Fombonne, E. (2003). Epidemiological surveys of autism and other pervasive developmental disorders: an update. *Journal of Autism and Developmental Disorders, 33,* 365–82.

Fox, R. A. & Wade, E. J. (1998). Attention deficit hyperactivity disorder among adults with severe and profound mental retardation. *Research in Developmental Disabilities, 19,* 275–80.

Gillberg, C. & Wing, L. (1999). Autism: Not an extremely rare disorder. *Acta Psychiatrica Scandinavica, 99,* 399–406.

Hanson, R. K. & Morton-Bourgon, K. E. (2005). The characteristics of persistent sexual offenders: A meta-analysis of recidivism studies. *Journal of Consulting and Clinical Psychology, 73* (6), 1154–63.

Hodgins, S. (1992). Mental disorder, intellectual deficiency and crime. Evidence from a birth cohort. *Archives of General Psychiatry, 49* (6), 476–83.

Huang, A. M. (1981). The drinking behaviour of the educable mentally retarded and the non retarded students. *Journal of Alcohol and Drug Abuse, 26,* 41–9.

Kanner, L. (1943). Autistic disturbances of affective contact. *Nervous Child, 2,* 217–50.

Kendall, K. A. (2004). *Female offenders and developmental disabilities: A critical review.* In W. R. Lindsay J. L. Taylor & P. Sturmey (Eds), *Offenders with Developmental Disabilities* (pp. 265–88). Chichester: John Wiley & Sons.

Khan, A., Cowan, C. & Roy, A. (1997). Personality disorders in people with learning disabilities: A community survey. *Journal of ID Research, 41* (4), 324–30.

Kohn, Y., Fahum, T., Ratzoni, G. & Apter, A. (1998). Aggression and sexual offense in Asperger's syndrome. *Israel Journal of Psychiatry and Related Sciences, 35* (4), 293–9.

Krischef, C. H. (1986). Do the mentally retarded drink? A study of their alcohol usage. *Journal of Alcohol and Drug Education. 31,* 64–70.

Krischef, C. H. & Di Nitto, D. M. (1981). Alcohol use among mentally retarded individuals. *Mental Retardation, 19,* 151–5.

Kukopulos, A., Reginaldi, D., Laddomada, P., Floris, G., Serra, G. & Tondo, L. (1980). Course of the manic depressive cycle and changes caused by treatments. *Pharmakopsychiatry, 13,* 156–67.

Langevin, R. & Curnoe, S. (2008). Are the mentally retarded and learning disordered overrepresented among sex offenders and paraphilics? *International Journal of Offender Therapy and Comparative Criminology, 52* (4), 401–15.

Lidher, J., Martin, D. M., Jayaprakash, M. S. & Roy, A. (2005). Personality disorders in people with learning disabilities: Follow-up of a community survey. *Journal of ID Research, 49,* 845–51.

Lindsay, W. R., Elliot, S. & Astell, A. (2004). Predictors of Sexual Offence Recidivism in Offenders with ID. *Journal of Applied Research in ID, 17* (4), 299–305.

Lindsay, W. R., Law, J., Quinn, K., Smart, N. & Smith A. H. (2001). A comparison of physical and sexual abuse: Histories of sexual and non-sexual offenders with ID. *Child abuse & neglect, 25* (7), 989–95.

Lindsay, W. R., Smith, A. H., Law, J., Quinn, K., Anderson, A., Smith, A. & Allan, R. (2004a). Sexual and nonsexual offenders with intellectual and learning disabilities: A comparison of characteristics, referral patterns, and outcome. *Journal of Interpersonal Violence, 19* (8), 875–90.

Lindsay, W. R., Smith, A. H. W., Quinn, K., Anderson, A., Smith, A., Allan, R. & Law, J. (2004). Women with ID who have offended: Characteristics and outcome. *Journal of ID Research, 48* (6), 580–90.

Lindsay, W. R., Steele, L., Smith, A. H. W., Quinn, K., & Allan, R. (2006). A community forensic ID service: Twelve year follow up of referrals; analysis of referral patterns and assessment of harm reduction. *Legal and Criminological Psychology, 1* (1), 113–30.

Lindsay, W. R., Steptoe, L., Hogue, T. E., Taylor, J. L., Mooney, P., Haut, F., Johnston, S. & O'Brien, G. (2007). Internal consistency and factor structure of personality disorders in a forensic ID sample. *Journal of Intellectual and Developmental Disability, 32* (2), 134–42.

Link, B. & Stueve, A. (1994). Psychotic symptoms and the violent/illegal behaviour of mental patients compared to community controls. In J. Monahan, & H. Steadman (Eds), *Violence and Mental Disorder* (pp. 137–59). Chicago: University of Chicago Press.

Lund, J. (1985). The prevalence of psychiatric disorder in mentally retarded adults. *Acta Psychiatrica Scandinavica*, *72*, 563–70.

Lund, J. (1990). Mentally retarded criminal offenders in Denmark. *The British Journal of Psychiatry*, *156*, 726–31.

Lyall, I., Holland, A. J. & Collins, S. (1995). Offending by adults with learning disabilities and the attitudes of staff to offending behaviour: Implications for service development. *Journal of ID Research*, *39*, 501–8.

McGillivray, J. A. & Moore, M. R. (2001). Substance use by offenders with mild ID. *Journal of Intellectual and Developmental Disability*, *26* (4), 297–310.

McKee, J. R., Bodfish, J. W., Mahorney, S. L., Heeth, W. L. & Ball, M. P. (2005). Metabolic effects associated with atypical antipsychotic use in the developmentally disabled. *Journal of Clinical Psychiatry*, *66* (9), 1161–8.

Moffit, T. E. & Silva, P. A. (1988). Self-reported delinquency, neuropsychological deficit, and history of attention deficit disorder. *Journal of Abnormal Child Psychology*, *16*, 553–69.

Murphy, G. H., Harnett, H. & Holland, A. J. (1995). A survey of ID amongst men on remand in prison. *Mental Handicap Research*, *8*, 81–98.

O'Brien, G. (2000). Learning disability. In C. Gillberg & G. O'Brien (Eds), '*Developmental Disability and Behaviour*' Clinics in Developmental Medicine (No. 149, pp. 12–26). London: MacKeith Press.

Parry, C. J. & Lindsay, W. R. (2003). Impulsiveness as a factor in sexual offending by people with mild ID. *Journal of ID Research*, *47* (6), 483–7.

Peckham, N. G. (2007). The Vulnerability and sexual abuse of people with learning disabilities. *British Journal of Learning Disabilities*, *35* (2), 131–7.

Penrose, L. S.[1949] (1963). *The Biology of Mental Defect*. 2nd edn. New York, NY: Grune and Stratton, Inc.

Porter, R. (1997). *The Greatest Benefit to Mankind*. 2nd edn. London: Harper Collins.

Proctor, T. & Beail, N. (2007). Empathy and theory of mind in offenders with ID. *Journal of Intellectual & Developmental Disability*, *32* (2), 82–93.

Prosser, H., Moss, S., Costello, H., Simpson, N., Patel, P. & Rowe, S. (1998). Reliability and validity of the Mini PAS-ADD for assessing psychiatric disorders in adults with intellectual disability. *Journal of Intellectual Disability Research*, *42*, 264–72.

Rabiner, D. L., Coie, J. D., Miller-Johnson, S., Boykin, A. S. M. & Lochman, J. E. (2005). Predicting the persistence of aggressive offending of African American males from adolescence into young adulthood. *Journal of Emotional and Behavioural Disorders*, *13* (3), 131–40.

Raymond, N. C., Coleman, E., Ohlerking, F., Christenson, G. A. & Miner, M. (1999). Psychiatric comorbidity in pedophilic sex offenders. *The American Journal of Psychiatry*, *156* (5), 768–88.

Regier, D. A., Boyd, J. H., Burke, J. D., Rae, D. S., Myers, J. K., Kramer, M., Robins, L. N., George, L. K., Karno, M. & Locke, B. Z. (1988). One-month prevalence of mental disorders in the United States. *Archives of General Psychiatry*, *45*, 977–86.

Reinblatt, S. P., Rifkin, A. & Freeman, J. (2004). The efficacy of ECT in adults with mental retardation experiencing psychiatric disorders. *The Journal of ECT*, *20* (4), 208–12.

Reiss, S., Levitan, G. W. & Szyszko J. (1982). Emotional disturbance and mental retardation: Diagnostic overshadowing. *American Journal of Mental Deficiency*, *86* (6), 567–74.

Royal College of Psychiatrists (2001). *DC-LD: Diagnostic criteria for psychiatric disorders for use with adults with learning disabilities/mental retardation*. London: Gaskell Press.

Rutter, M., Graham, P. & Yule, W. (1970). *A neuropsychiatric study in childhood: Clinics in developmental medicine, nos 35/36*. London: William Heinemann Medical Books Ltd.

Satterfield, J. H. & Schell, A. (1997). A prospective study of hyperactive boys with conduct problems and normal boys: Adolescent and adult criminality. *Journal of the American Academy of Child and Adolescent Psychiatry*, *36* (12), 1726–35.

Schneider, K. (1959). *Clinical Psychopathology*. New York, NY: Grune and Stratton, Inc.

Scragg, P. & Shah A. (1994). Prevalence of Asperger's syndrome in a secure hospital. *The British Journal of Psychiatry, 165* (5), 679–82.

Simpson, M. K. & Hogg, J. (2001). Patterns of offending among people with ID: A systematic review. Part I: Methodology and prevalence data. *Journal of ID Research, 45,* 384–96.

Siponmaa, L., Kristiansson, M., Jonson, C., Nyden, A. & Gillberg, C. (2001). Juvenile and young adult mentally disordered offenders: The role of child neuropsychiatric disorders. *Journal of the American Academy of Psychiatry and the Law, 29,* 420–6.

Smiley, E., Cooper, S. A., Finlayson, J., Jackson, A., Allan, L., Mantry, D., McGrother, C., McConnachie, A. & Morrison, J. (2007). Incidence and predictors of mental ill-health in adults with ID: Prospective study. *The British Journal of Psychiatry, 191,* 313–19.

Smith, A. H. W., Quinn, K. & Lindsay, W. R. (2000). Influence of mental illness on the presentation and management of offenders with learning disabilities. *Journal of ID Research, 44,* 360–1.

Smith, A. D. & Taylor, P. J. (1999). Serious sex offending against women by men with schizophrenia: Relationship of illness and psychotic symptoms to offending. *The British Journal of Psychiatry, 174* (3), 233–7.

Sovner, R. (1986). Limiting factors in the use of DSM-III criteria with mentally ill/mentally retarded persons. *Psychopharmacology Bulletin, 22* (4), 1055–9.

Sparrow, S. S., Balla, D. A. & Cichetti, D. V. (1984). A revision of the Vineland Social Maturity Scale by E. A. Doll. American Guidance Service, Inc., MN.

Sturmey, P., Reyer, H., Lee, R. & Robek, A. (2003). *Substance related disorders in persons with mental retardation.* Kingston, NY: NADD.

Sverd, J. (2003). Psychiatric disorders in individuals with pervasive developmental disorder. *Journal of Psychiatric Practice, 9,* 111–27.

Taggart, L., McLaughlin, D., Quinn, B. & Milligan, V. (2006). An exploration of substance misuse in people with ID. *Journal of ID Research, 50* (8), 588–97.

Tantam, D. (1988). Lifelong eccentricity and social isolation. II: Asperger's syndrome or schizoid personality disorder? *The British Journal of Psychiatry, 153,* 783–91.

Tantam, D. (1991). Asperger's syndrome in adulthood. In U. Frith (Ed.), *Autism and Asperger's syndrome* (pp. 147–83). Cambridge: Cambridge University Press.

Taylor, J. L., Hatton, C., Dixon, L. & Douglas, C. (2004). Screening for psychiatric symptoms: PAS-ADD Checklist norms for adults with ID. *Journal of ID Research, 48,* 37–41.

Thompson, D. & Brown, H. (1997). Men with ID who sexually offend: A review of the literature. *Journal of Applied Research in ID, 10,* 140–58.

Vanstraelen, M. & Tyrer, S. P. (1999). Rapid cycling bipolar affective disorder in people with ID: A systematic review. *Journal of ID Research, 43,* 349–59.

Williams, J. G., Higgins, J. P. & Brayne, C. E. (2006). Systematic review of prevalence studies of autism spectrum disorders. *Archives of Disease in Childhood, 91* (1), 8–15.

Wilner, P. (2005) Psychotherapeutic interventions in learning disability. *Journal of Intellectual Disability Research, 49* (1), 73–85.

Winter, N., Holland, A. J. & Collins, S. (1997). Factors predisposing to suspected offending by adults with self reported learning disabilities. *Psychological Medicine, 27* (3), 595–607.

Woodbury-Smith, M. R., Clare, I. C. H., Holland, A. J., Kearns, A., Staufenberg, E. & Watson, P. (2005). A case-control study of offenders with high functioning autistic spectrum disorders. *Journal of Forensic Psychiatry & Psychology, 16* (4), 747–63.

World Health Organization. (1992). *ICD-10: The ICD-10 Classification of Mental and Behavioural Disorders: Clinical Descriptions and Diagnostic Guidelines.* Geneva World Health Organization.

World Health Organization (1993). *The ICD-10 classification of mental and behavioural disorders: Diagnostic criteria for research.* Geneva: World Health Organization.

Zigler, E. & Burack, J. A. (1989). Personality development and the dually diagnosed person. *Research in Developmental Disabilities, 10* (3), 225–40.

7

Sexual and Gender Identity Disorders in People with Intellectual Disabilities

DOROTHY M. GRIFFITHS, PAUL FEDOROFF AND DEBORAH RICHARDS

INTRODUCTION

The *Diagnostic and statistic manual, fourth edition, text revision* (DSM-IV-TR) is the standard for psychiatric diagnostic criteria in North America. Individuals who present with sexual and gender identity disorders (GID) are identified according to these criteria. However, concerns have been raised since the 1990s that these criteria may be routinely misapplied when diagnosing persons with ID. In response to the concern about the misapplication of the DSM-IV-TR criteria to persons with ID, the National Association for the Dually Diagnosed (NADD) and the American Psychiatric Association joined forces to adapt the criteria and publish guidelines for clinicians regarding their application to this population (Fletcher, Loschen, Stavrakaki & First, 2007a, 2007b).

This chapter discusses sexual and GIDs identified within the DSM-IV-TR under three distinct sections: sexual dysfunctions, GIDs and paraphilias. It reviews how these criteria are applied to persons with ID.

SEXUAL DYSFUNCTIONS

Psychosexual disorders were first listed in 1980 in the *Diagnostic and statistical manual, third edition* (DSM-III), the manual widely used by most health care professionals in North America. Since that first initial listing an individual that is consistent with the diagnostic criteria for sexual dysfunction can now identify the problem as a medical issue similar to that of other mental disorders outlined in this manual.

Assessment and Treatment of Sexual Offenders with Intellectual Disabilities: A Handbook
Edited by Leam A. Craig, William R. Lindsay and Kevin D. Browne
© 2010 John Wiley & Sons, Ltd.

According to the *Diagnostic and statistical manual*, fourth edition, revised (*DSM-IV-TR*) the definition of sexual dysfunction includes the following principles:

- whenever more than one sexual dysfunction is present, all are recorded;
- no attempt is made to specify a minimum frequency or range of settings, activities or type of sexual encounter in which the dysfunction occur;
- the clinician takes into account such factors as age and experience of the individual, frequency and chronicity of the symptom, subjective distress and effect on other areas of functioning;
- words such as 'recurrent or persistent' in the diagnostic criteria indicate need of clinical judgement;
- if sexual stimulation is inadequate in focus, intensity or duration the diagnosis of sexual dysfunction involving excitement or orgasm is not made.

While recognising those principles, the DSM-IV-TR, defines each sexual dysfunction under *Sexual Desire Disorders* (hypoactive sexual desire disorder and sexual aversion disorder); *Sexual Arousal Disorders* (female sexual arousal disorder and male erectile disorder); *Orgasmic Disorders* (female orgasmic disorder [formerly inhibited female orgasm], male orgasmic disorder [formerly inhibited male orgasm], and premature ejaculation); *Sexual Pain Disorders* (dyspareunia and vaginismus); and *Other Sexual Dysfunctions* (sexual dysfunction as a result of a general medical condition, substance misuse or not otherwise specified).

The Diagnostic manual-intellectual disability (DM-ID) explains that, historically, the identification criterion for the DSM-IV-TR did not consider sexual dysfunctions as a topic of concerns for individuals with ID in comparison to the non-ID population (Fletcher, Loschen, Stavrakaki & First, 2007b). This lack of diagnosis could be attributed to marginalisation and sexual oppression along with the limited sexual rights people with disabilities have experienced (Richards *et al.*, 2008). However, when health care professionals are determining a diagnosis that may in fact be a sexual dysfunction, individuals with ID can and should be clinically diagnosed regardless of Axis II evidence of mental retardation. The authors (Fletcher, Loschen, Stavrakaki & First 2007b) from the DM-ID stated there is limited literature when sexual dysfunction is accompanied with ID. A clinician typically relies on several variables in the non-ID population; however, this may not be available or easily sought when examining an individual with ID. The DM-ID lists seven factors which may conceal the identification of a diagnosis: lack of communication skills and sexual language; limited sexual knowledge; limited sexual experiences; that sexuality is often ignored in persons with ID; people with ID are seen as asexual; erotophobia; and the sexual response cycle.

Lack of Communication Skills and Sexual Language

The DM-ID explains that people with ID who have limited verbal skills can have difficulty in expressing their sexuality because of communication differences. Since general language skills are often delayed it can be safely assumed that the ability to discuss sexual concerns will also be impaired. People with ID are frequently misunderstood or simply may not have the language skills to communicate their needs, feelings, opinions and desires (Ruiter, 2000). The following

Case 1 example will demonstrate how a sexual dysfunction disorder can go undetected when a person has limited verbal communication.

Case 1

A 38-year-old woman with cerebral palsy and an ID has been married to her long-time partner for one year. She has no verbal skills and therefore uses facilitated communication methods. Speaking with her counsellor it was discovered that the couple has not been sleeping together. The counsellor came to learn that they had not had sexual intercourse either. She then referred this couple to the sex educator/counsellor who discovered that each time they attempt to become intimate, the woman experiences extreme pain and stops all physical contact with her husband.

During a visit to her gynaecologist it was discovered she had never had a pelvic exam because of her level of anxiety at the onset of the examination. The doctor did not want to upset her as she was non-verbal and he had no way of communicating the steps of the procedure with her. After a thorough examination by the gynaecologist and a referral to a psychiatrist and information gathering from the woman by using her communication board, she was diagnosed with dyspareunia.

The DSM-IV-TR defines dyspareunia as a sexual pain disorder, a subcategory of sexual dysfunction. The pain must be persistent or recurrent and cause marked distress or interpersonal difficulty. The woman in the case example fits the DSM-IV-TR criteria. This diagnosis may well have gone undetected without persistent and ongoing communication among several parties and, most importantly, providing the woman herself the opportunity to explain through her communication tool.

Limited Sexual Knowledge

According to McCabe and Cummins (1996), people with ID showed lower levels of knowledge in most areas of sexuality with the exception of menstruation and body parts. Additionally, Konstantareas and Lunsky (1997) found that people with ID showed less ability to define a sexual activity regardless of the level of functioning, group or gender, thereby demonstrating a need for sexuality knowledge. Koller (2000) states that there are several barriers that limit people's ability to understand their sexuality that include social myths, insufficient knowledge and training opportunities, personal discomfort and limited access to available and appropriate educational resources. Watson, Griffiths, Richards and Dykstra (2002) state that sexuality training for people with ID has been neglected and that few people with ID are given learning opportunities. McCabe (1994) states that people with ID have rarely been provided comprehensive sex education, and that, therefore, when the information is provided it is typically meant to address problems rather than to build healthy sexuality. Griffiths *et al.* (1996) determined that the retention of sexual information can become problematic for individuals with ID if it is not repetitive in nature. It can therefore be concluded that it is necessary to present recurring information on an ongoing basis in order for the retention of sexual information to become imbedded in the daily awareness of the individual. The following Case 2 example will demonstrate a successful diagnosis along with a positive treatment plan to support the multiple needs that enable a woman with an ID with hopes to be sexual and free of the distress.

Case 2

A 28-year-old woman with an ID recently became involved in a relationship with a man of a similar age. Everything seemed to be moving along in terms of their relationship when one day the woman seemed to be upset with him and appeared withdrawn. She confided in one of the staff that her boyfriend kept touching her and she did not like it. Her staff asked her if she would like to talk to a counsellor about this and she agreed.

After several visits to the therapist it was discovered she had limited information about sexuality and could benefit from sex education classes. As well, she disclosed having been sexually abused as a child. The therapist recommended that she seek medical attention. Firstly, a gynaecological examination was conducted to rule out a vaginal infection, and, secondly, a psychiatric assessment was made as it was possible that she was experiencing a condition called vaginismus. Therapy was continued as well as sex education classes, which included sexual abuse prevention to decrease the likelihood of further abuse of this woman.

Sobsey and Mansell's (1994) extensive research verified increased incidence of sexual abuse among people with ID. Therefore, conditions such as vaginismus should be a considered factor when there is discomfort and anxiety expressed in the progression of sexual relationships for this population. According to the DSM-IV-TR, the first criterion for the diagnosis of vaginismus is the spasm of the muscles in the outer third of the vagina that are involuntary and recurring or persistent. The symptoms must cause physical or emotional distress, or, in particular, problems with relationships. A traumatic childhood experience, such as sexual molestation, is thought to be a possible cause of vaginismus.

Limited Sexual Experiences

There is limited research in recognition of the sexual experiences of people who have ID, although there have been a number of studies which have investigated the level of abuse experienced by people with disabilities (McCabe & Schreck, 1992). It has been found that people with ID need to acquire the knowledge and experience of a comprehensive range of positive sexual activities, the context in which these occur and the factors that are involved in the decision to participate in consensual sexual contact. The Case 3 example presents the outcome of someone with an ID who has been limited in their sexual experiences.

Case 3

A couple who have ID married after dating for approximately 8 years. They seemed to be a happy couple. One day the female came to her support worker to discuss her relationship with her husband. The woman had limited language skills and a lack of sexual knowledge but made all efforts to relay her story. The question she posed to the support worker was whether or not it was time for her and her husband to begin having sexual intercourse given that they were now married.

The support worker was taken aback as she had assumed they had been having a sexually intimate relationship for years, although had never had any discussion to verify this. The couple became involved with a sex educator/counsellor. This gave them the opportunity to learn and acquire the sexual knowledge to enhance their sexual relationship. Through this they were able to begin to explore their sexuality with one another. It was eventually

> discovered that the husband had erectile dysfunction with an associated feature of decreased subjective sense of sexual excitement and pleasure.

Phillips (2000) states that sexuality is complex from a medical perspective as it entails neurologic, vascular and endocrine systems. However, according to the Sex Information and Education Council of the United States (SIECUS) sexuality includes sexual knowledge, beliefs, attitudes, values and behaviours of individuals. Individually, sexuality integrates family, societal and spiritual beliefs as well as being influenced by age, health, personal circumstances and historical factors such as past sexual experiences and abuse. Furthermore, sexual activity involves current interpersonal relationships. These sexuality complexities linked to ID in a person increases the chances of a diagnosis of sexual dysfunction.

Sexuality is Often Ignored in Persons with Intellectual Disabilities

The research from Held (1993) and McCabe and Schreck (1992) indicates a clear need for people with ID to have their sexual needs listened to as well as their emotional and physical experiences. According to Corbett, Shurberg, Klien and Bregante (1989) women with ID possess the sexual desires and actions of women in general. Therefore, these women require information about their sexuality. When a person is not listened to, there is potential risk of a sexual dysfunction going undetected, as is shown by the following, Case 4, example.

Case 4
A 45-year-old man with an ID of mild cognition has been apparently sexually active for many years. Staff have reported that he presents as being frustrated and angry. In particular, reports have indicated these moods are possibly related to his relationship with his girlfriend as he appears exceptionally moody after spending time with her.   According to reports and files there is no indication this man has had any type of sociosexual education or relationship counselling. The question of whether he has good knowledge of sexuality has been raised. Is there a possibility that his frustration could be because of a male erectile disorder or premature ejaculation leaving him frustrated and angry after making attempts to be intimate with his girlfriend? If he has not had any formal sex education and lacks the understanding of the sexual response cycle and his sexual functioning he is at risk of not receiving adequate treatment.

The Valencia Declaration of Sexual Rights (1999) includes the right to sexual health and the right to wide, objective and factual information and education on human sexuality. It is essential that people with ID be given adequate and accurate sexual information to enable them to have healthy sexual lives filled with positive experiences of their choice (Richards, Miodrag & Watson, 2006). The right to sex education would give an individual the understanding of his own sexual health.

People with Intellectual Disabilities are Seen as Asexual

People with ID have not been identified in the same way as others sexually. Because of this societal attitude, sexual needs have been ignored, often because of the perception that people with ID were asexual (Di Giulio, 2003; Karellou, 2003; King & Richards, 2002,

Richards, Miodrag & Watson, 2006). According to Neiderbuhl and Morris (1993), health care professionals stereotype people with ID as being asexual, as well as lacking the same relationship and sexual wants and desires as people without disabilities. Griffiths (1999) discusses the sexual 'mythconceptions' of people with ID and concludes that people with ID are often perceived as eternal children and therefore asexual even though these individuals develop their secondary sexual characteristics at about the same rate as non-disabled people (with the exception of individuals who may have genetic or endocrine disorders that effect sexuality). The Case 5 example demonstrates the concerns that may erupt through seeing individuals as childlike throughout their adult life.

Case 5

A petite 40-year-old woman is regarded as a child most of the time by the majority of people, primarily because of her size, limited verbal skills and ID. Although she is able to muddle through the childlike treatment from others it has also created another problem for her. Because she is seen as a child she is not seen as a sexual being, and therefore her support network has not made efforts to provide her with sex education, relationship enhancement or sexual abuse prevention.

The lack of training made her vulnerable to sexual abuse, which occurred between the ages of 20 and 30 years. Since she had no encouragement to seek out intimate relationships, she has been missing out on this very important aspect of her life. Her support staff members describe her as having low self-worth. She has been diagnosed with depression and is being treated pharmacologically. It is not known if this woman has a sexual dysfunction, however it could be assumed that she is at an increased risk.

Griffiths, Richards, Fedoroff and Watson (2002) state that people with ID are at an increased risk of sexual abuse often leading to a mental health diagnosis. This abuse is often ignored or ineffectively assessed and treated causing a potential aftermath which can lead to severe mental health risks.

Erotophobia

It has been suggested that the sexual experiences of individuals with ID may have been so suppressed, controlled or punished that individuals may be conditioned to respond with a negative reaction to anything sexual (Hingsburger, 1992). Hingsburger continues by stating that this erotophobic behaviour includes fear of one's own genitals, a negative reaction to any discussion, pictures or act involving sexual things, denial and anger over their own developing sexuality, self-punishment following sexual behaviour and a conspiracy of denial. Thus, individuals with ID may experience a differential conditioning to their sexuality as a result of punishment and fearful experiences. This may alter their response to normal sexual experiences and may lead to sexual repression (see Case 6).

Case 6

Ron a 26-year-old man moved into a group home operated under a local agency. Until then he had lived at home with his family, who describe themselves as strong, moral Christian people, which included holding very firm opinions around issues of sexuality. The group home was offering sexuality training and staff thought this may be an opportunity for the man to gain some understanding of his own sexuality as he has shown an interest in one of the ladies at the home. It was their understanding that he had very limited knowledge. After each class staff began to notice that Ron was aggressive and appeared very angry, behaviours which were not common for him. As the classes progressed, the behaviours became more intense. A psychologist began working with Ron. It was revealed that Ron's father had used forms of corporal punishment when found Ron masturbating. This mostly took place during his adolescent years. As a result of the control and punishment from masturbating, Ron experienced emotionally negative reactions to the sexuality classes he was attending.

According to Griffiths, Richards, Fedoroff and Watson (2002), agencies that support individuals with ID often do not teach or permit sexual activity because of a lack of policies recognising the importance of providing people with the education, knowledge and opportunity to have healthy sexual lives free of punishment and oppression.

The Sexual Response Cycle

People who have ID require some knowledge of the sexual response cycle in order for the clinician to rely on personal accounts. This can also aid in determining a difficulty or interruption in the sexual response cycle. Further investigation may be necessary in order to make a clinical diagnosis if the person is not aware of the sexual response cycle. Relying solely on the individual may result in a misdiagnosis or no diagnosis. The DM-ID (Fletcher, Loschen, Stavrakaki, & First, 2007b) identified particular problems that people with ID may experience while considering the sexual response phases:

- *Desire*: Clinicians need to be sensitive to concerns about sexual desire. Sexual desire problems often come to the clinician's attention because of concerns of the sexual partner. In the case of individuals with ID, complications are often raised by support workers, though inhibited sexual desire is rarely seen as a problem. This may lead to a failure of adequate attention to the problem(s).
- *Excitement*: The clinician needs to use language with which the patient is familiar; therefore, it would be useful to have the support person involved in the interview to assist in interpreting the level of understanding the person with an ID has, what terms they are acquainted with, interpretation of language, etc. The clinician may want to use educational DVDs, graphics and pictures as visual cues.
- *Orgasm*: Again, the use of educational DVDs, graphics and pictures as a way to describe what is occurring during the orgasm phase may be extremely helpful. The use of vernacular terms for orgasm ('coming', etc.) may benefit the individual to respond more accurately to the clinicians interview.
- *Resolution*: Since fatigue, tiredness and relaxation, are common reactions during this phase, the person with an ID may be more likely to respond to everyday language as opposed to making a statement about the effects of the resolution state of a sexual response phase.

Unless discussion of sexual health for people with ID has meaning, the actual sexual activity behaviours of this group will not be understood (Servais, 2006). There seems to be a lack of information through research and other data sources, which creates difficulty in understanding the sexual activity and sexual experiences of this population (ibid.). This may imply a lack of importance placed on a medical diagnosis of sexual dysfunction.

Fletcher, Loschen, Stavrakaki and First (2007b) noted that clinicians investigating the possibility of sexual dysfunction in people who have an ID need to use atypical approaches to gain a greater understanding of the problem. They go on to say that the importance of building a rapport with the individual, using language with which the person is most accustomed and familiar, understanding their sexual knowledge and communicating with the people supporting the individual with a disability can allow for an accurate assessment and successful outcomes. Although there are several factors to be considered in the determination of a diagnosis of sexual dysfunction for individuals with ID the DM-ID concurs with the DSM-IV-TR criterion and no adaptations were needed.

GENDER IDENTITY DISORDERS

DSM-IV-TR and ICD-10 criteria for these disorders are very similar. Diagnostic criteria for 'Gender identity in children' (DSM: 302.6) are equivalent to those for 'Gender identity disorder of childhood' (ICD: F64.2). Criteria for 'Gender identity disorder in adolescents or adults' (DSM: 302.85) are also equivalent to those for 'Transsexualism' (ICD: F64.0) but the DSM also subdivides 302.85 by the designation of 'sexual attraction to males', 'to females', 'to both sexes', or to 'neither sex'. The sub-designations do not have separate diagnostic codes. Both classifications also include a designation for patients who do not meet full criteria for the other diagnoses: 'Gender identity disorder not otherwise specified' (DSM: 302.6) or 'Gender identity disorder unspecified' (ICD: F64.9). The ICD criteria also include a 'research category': 'Dual-role transvestism' (F64.1), characterised by cross-dressing in order to experience 'temporary membership in the opposite sex' in the absence of any sexual motivation for the cross-dressing or desire for 'permanent change to the opposite sex' (World Health Organization, 1993).

In both classification systems the cardinal features are persistent cross-gender identification combined with persistent discomfort with assigned gender role. Therefore, in order to meet criteria for a GID the person must be capable of the following: (i) formation of a persistent gender identity, (ii) ability to recognise alternative gender identities, (iii) ability to reject the current gender identity in favour of an alternative one, (iv) ability to recognise and reject gender roles.

Gender identity has been defined as 'the sameness, unity, and persistence of one's individuality as male, female, or ambivalent, in greater or lesser degree, especially as it is experienced in self-awareness and behaviour'; *gender role* has been defined as 'everything that a person says and does to indicate to others and to the self the degree that one is either male or female, or androgynous; it includes but is not restricted to sexual arousal and response' (Money, 1973, 1994; Torgrimson & Minson 2005; Money & Ehrhardt, 1972). The two concepts have also frequently been combined in the term 'gender-identity/role (G-I/R): 'gender identity is the private experience of gender role, and gender role is public manifestation of gender identity' (Money, 1985b). The aetiology of problems with G-I/R are unknown (Fedoroff & Blanchard, 2000) so diagnosis is based on observed patterns of behaviour and the elicitation of symptoms via interview of the patient and, with permission, those who know the patient well. For a diagnosis of GID, the following DSM criteria A and B are required (American Psychiatric Association, 2000).

Criteria A: Strong and persistent cross-gender identification (not merely a desire for any perceived cultural advantages of being the other sex). In children, this must be manifested by four or more of the following criteria:

1. repeated stated desire to be, or insistence that he or she is, the other sex;
2. in boys, preference for cross-dressing or simulating female attire; in girls, insistence on wearing only stereotypical masculine clothing;
3. strong and persistent preferences for cross-sex roles in make-believe play or persistent fantasies of being the other sex;
4. intense desire to participate in the stereotypical games and pastimes of the other sex;
5. strong preference for playmates of the other sex.

In the DSM, adolescents with GID have the following symptoms:

1. stated desire to be the other sex
2. frequent passing as the other sex
3. desire to live or be treated as the other sex, or
4. the conviction that he or she has the typical feelings and reactions of the other sex

Criteria B: 'A persistent discomfort with his or her sex or sense of inappropriateness in the gender role of that sex' (p. 581). Again, additional specific criteria are applied to children concerning any of the following:

In boys

1. assertion that the penis or testes are disgusting or will disappear
2. assertion it would be better not to have a penis
3. aversion to rough and tumble play
4. rejection of male stereotypical toys, games and activities

In girls

1. rejection of urinating in a sitting position
2. assertion that she will grow a penis
3. assertion that she does not want to grow breasts or menstruate
4. marked aversion toward 'normative' feminine clothing

In adolescents and adults

1. preoccupation with 'getting rid of' primary and secondary sex characteristics
2. preoccupation with other procedures to physically alter sexual characteristics to simulate the other sex
3. belief that he or she was born the wrong sex

Both the ICD and DSM exclude diagnosis of GID in the case of an individual with a physical intersex condition. The DSM requires that the condition cause significant distress while the

ICD requires that the condition be accompanied by a wish to 'make one's body as congruent as possible with one's preferred sex through surgery and hormonal treatment'.

Issues arising from application of the diagnostic criteria listed above to individuals with ID are reviewed in Table 7.1.

The composite case of Ms A, while technically meeting ICD and DSM criteria for GID or transsexualism, would clearly be misdiagnosed if either were assigned. While the DSM explicitly excludes diagnosis of GID in cases in which the person wishes for a sex change on the basis of perceived social advantage these diagnostic decisions are often blurred in patients with ID. Similar diagnostic difficulties can arise, for example, in men with ID who may have been raised in all-male institutions presided over by women or who have been subjected to sexual abuse or punishment that involved 'humiliation' by being cross-dressed or assigned female roles.

The fact is that the ability to accurately differentiate between assigned and possible sex roles and not only to reject them but to seek psychiatric or surgical reparation is difficult for many with ID. This task is made more difficult because of the higher incidence of intersex syndromes in people with ID. Given the issues reviewed above, the following recommendations are made:

1. Clinicians should be aware of both over-diagnosis and under-diagnosis of GID.
2. In situations in which the question is raised, clinicians should investigate both the patient's wishes and the wishes of care providers.
3. Proceed with caution. GID is a lifelong condition that is not life-threatening. Most recommendations include at least a two-year 'real-life' test in which the patient fully assumes the G-I/R of the opposite sex before irreversible recommendations are made (e.g., 'sex reassignment' surgery).
4. Investigate and exclude other explanations: over-valued ideas, mood disorders, delusional disorders, intersex conditions.
5. Recognise and respect the courage of any individual who presents with problems concerning such a fundamental issue as sexual and gender identity.

PARAPHILIAS

The word 'paraphilia' is derived from the Latin word meaning 'love of the unusual' (Money, 1985a). However, the diagnostic criterion for paraphilia according to the DSM-IV-TR involves for a period of at least six months (American Psychiatric Association, 2000) the following: "recurrent, intense sexually arousing fantasies, sexual urges, or behaviours generally involving

1. non-human objects
2. the suffering or humiliation of oneself or one's partner, or
3. the suffering or humiliation of children or other non-consenting persons" (p. 522).

Paraphilia can involve but is not limited to exhibitionism, fetishism, frotteurism, paedophilia, sexual masochism, sexual sadism, transvestic fetishism, voyeurism and paraphilia not otherwise specified (APA, 2000).

Table 7.1 Illustrative hypothetical case of GID

Criteria	Case	Comment
A strong and persistent cross-gender identification (not merely a desire for any perceived cultural advantages of being the other sex).	Ms A is referred because she insists in being called 'Mr' or 'Dr'	People with ID are more likely to confuse labels or presumed social advantage; also more likely to generalize
Repeated stated desire to be or insistence that one is of the other sex.	She says she is a man	Investigation is warranted into what being a man means. Ms A says it means being a doctor
Insistence on wearing only stereotypical masculine clothing	Wants to wear pants and a holster; wants her head shaved; would also like a stethoscope	Says Dr X is bald too and he likes guns and to play golf
Persistent fantasies of being the other sex	Day dreams of being a doctor 'just like Dr X'	Ms A becomes angry when told that women can be doctors 'Dr X is not gay'
Stereotypical games and pastimes of the other sex	Wants to 'play doctor' in a non-sexual sense	Again, insists that being female and a doctor are not consistent
Strong preference for playmates of the other sex	Raised in a foster home with 6 boys	Prefers the company of males, 'especially ones like Dr X'
Rejection of urinating in a sitting position	Wishes to use the men's restroom	'Dr X never uses the women's room'
Assertion that she will grow a penis	Thinks any woman could be a doctor if they had one	'Dr X has one, I will too'
Assertion that she does not want to grow breasts or menstruate	Although adult, has never menstruated	Has Turner's syndrome and fetal alcohol syndrome
Marked aversion toward normative feminine clothing	Refuses to wear skirts or a bra	Asks repeatedly for a white lab coat

- *Exhibitionism* (exposure of the genitals) and *Frotteurism* (touching and rubbing against a non-consenting person) are often considered less serious offences than *sexual assault* or *paedophilia*, but can have a devastating emotional impact on the victim.
- *Sexual masochism* involves sexual arousal in response to images of being humiliated, beaten or bound by others. In most cases, masochistic acts involve enticing a partner to use humiliating or harmful methods as part of the sexual act. However, one of the most dangerous forms of masochism, which has been noted in persons with ID, is *hypoxyphilia* (or *autoerotic asphyxia*) (S. Hucker, personal communication) This paraphilia involves the use of objects, which may include a noose or a plastic bag, to temporarily decrease the oxygen to the brain. This behaviour can occur with a partner or alone.
- *Sexual sadism* involves sexual arousal to images where the victim is psychologically or physically made to suffer. Sexual sadism presents on a continuum of dangerousness from bondage to infliction of harm or death. This behaviour varies in how it develops; however, it generally is accepted that it first manifests itself in early adulthood.
- *Paedophilia* involves sexual activity with a child younger than 13 years of age by a perpetrator who is older than 16 years of age, and in which the victim is at least 5 years younger chronologically than the perpetrator. Paedophilia can be demonstrated in a number of ways, including exposure, touching, fondling, masturbating, performance of fellatio or cunnilingus on the child or penetration with finger, objects or penis. Some paedophiles are sex-specific and age-specific in their attraction whereas others are not. Other individuals engage in this behaviour only within their own family (*incest*).

In the population at large, sexual victimisation of children (under 18 years) involving exhibitionism, paedophilia, or *voyeurism* is among the most frequently reported of sexual crimes.

Incidence of Paraphilias in People with Intellectual Disabilities

A full range of deviant sexual arousal patterns and cognitive distortions, from fetishism to paedophilia, have been reported among persons with ID (Murphy, Coleman & Abel, 1983a; Day, 1997). The incidence of sexual offences committed by persons with ID varies greatly depending on the study. There is research that suggests that persons with ID are disproportionately represented among the population of sexual offenders (Shapiro, 1986; Steiner, 1984; Langevin, 1992). However, Griffiths, Watson, Lewis and Stoner (2004) caution that much of the incidence research is based on prison populations, which may be more reflective of the increased arrest and conviction rates of this population rather than the actual incidence.

As Case 7 illustrates, there is increased likelihood of apprehension, confession, self-incrimination, respond to leading questions in people with ID and less likelihood that they will understand the legal process, have appropriate legal defence, plea-bargain or understand the implications of their statements (Abel & Rouleau, 1990; Brown & Courtless, 1971; McGee & Menolascino, 1992; Murphy, Coleman & Haynes, 1983b; Santamour & West, 1978).

Case 7

In a well-publicized case in Montreal, a man confessed to the sexual assault of a woman and was sentenced to jail. After several years he was released, and he then confessed to another rape. This time DNA evidence showed that he had not committed the second assault. Upon investigation of the DNA evidence that was available in the first case but never examined it was uncovered that he had not committed the first crime either. Although the man had a dual diagnosis of ID and a mental health problem, his confession was never questioned.

Analysis and review of the literature on men with ID is complicated by variable definitions of what is meant by the term 'intellectual disability' (Griffiths & Fedoroff, 2008). This distinction is not merely semantics: failure to use standardised criteria has resulted in conclusions that may not be warranted and which makes comparisons between studies problematic. For example, in a large meta-analytic review of studies reporting IQ scores in sex offenders (Cantor, Blanchard, Robichaud & Christensen, 2005) involving 236 samples consisting of a total of 25,146 sex offenders and controls, the authors concluded that 'IQ relates primarily to the presence of paedophilia among sexual offenders and that differences in samples' scores reflect differing proportions of genuinely paedophilic offenders occurring within those samples' (p. 564). However, analysis of the reported data indicates that the weighted mean average IQ of all adult offenders was above 90 (i.e., within one standard deviation of the population average of 100 on the WAIS). The difference between adult sexual offenders and non-sexual offenders was only about 5 IQ points. Therefore, even this large review of studies on sex offenders and intelligence cannot be viewed as a study of offenders with ID.

A second common problem in the literature is the use of non-standardised definitions of ID. For example, one widely cited study investigating the relationship between paedophilia and 'mental retardation' in fact used a combination of offenders who had ID and those who were borderline. Moreover, the classification was based on the interviewer's 'global estimate' of intelligence on a 6-point scale: 1 = retarded, 2 = borderline, 3 = dull normal, 4 = average, 5 = bright normal, 6 = superior intelligence (Blanchard et al., 1999). Similarly, in the standardisation sample used to construct the Violence Risk Appraisal Guide 'offenders with intellectual disabilities' was defined as men with an IQ under 85 (Quinsey, Book & Skilling, 2004).

Lindsay (2002), in a review of the research and literature on sex offenders with ID, concluded that there is no clear evidence that there is either an over- or an under-representation of people with ID who sexually offend. This latter position appears to represent the current state of research evidence on incidence.

Diagnosis of Paraphilia in Persons with Intellectual Disabilities

Few modifications to the criteria of paraphilia are necessary for the ID population. However, caution should be used when applying the criteria to individuals who have more significant ID. Some individuals who are or have experienced atypical living experiences, such as institutionalisation, might engage in behaviour that may on the surface look like paraphilia but may have an aetiology that is not driven by the recurrent and intense sexual urges and fantasies required in the diagnostic criteria. The diagnostic criteria provide an accurate description of the sexual offences of some individuals with ID but may be inaccurate for others. Some authors have claimed that there may be two categories of offenders with ID: Type I represents offenders who are similar to the non-disabled offenders and appear to fit the label of paraphilia; Type II Offenders, although sexually inappropriate in their behaviour, are not deviant per se but, rather, commit more 'minor or nuisance offences' (Day, 1997, p. 279). It has been hypothesised that Type II Offenders may commit a sexual offence for reasons other than the ongoing urges or fantasies that typify paraphilia. Sexual behaviours that appear to be paraphilia but that after clinical evaluation can be better explained by a rival hypothesis are often referred to as 'counterfeit deviance' (Hingsburger, Griffiths & Quinsey, 1991) (see Chapter 2). The DSM-IV-TR diagnostic guidelines caution that for people with ID, where there might be a 'decrease in judgment, social skills, or impulse control that, in rare instances, leads to unusual sexual behaviour' that is distinguishable from a paraphilia (American Psychiatric Association, 2000, p. 568).

Typically, diagnoses are founded on the typography of an offence and do take into account other factors that might relate to the experiences of people with ID, experiences that could contribute to the commission of an offence that might be not related to the presence of a paraphilia. Among this population, there is a higher experience of abuse (Gilby, Wolf & Goldberg, 1989; Griffiths, Quinsey & Hingsburger, 1989), poor self-esteem (Lackey & Knopp, 1989), lack of sociosexual knowledge and experience (Hingsburger, 1987) and poor social problem-solving skills (ibid.), all of which can contribute to a false diagnosis of a paraphilia.

Inappropriate or age-inappropriate behaviour learned through abuse might appear natural to the individual with ID who has been afforded no appropriate sexual education, personal experience or social opportunity to learn otherwise. Learned institutional sexual behaviour, though appearing inappropriate within the context of the community, might have functionality within the culture of the institution. Additionally, there might be genetic influences that could instigate behaviours symptomatic of a paraphilia which might have medical or biomedical factors that cause or contribute to the presentation of symptoms that could be mislabelled as a paraphilia.

Hingsburger, Griffiths and Quinsey (1991) provided case examples of sexual misbehaviour of people with ID that were often the product of experiential, environmental or medical factors rather than of a paraphilia. A careful differential diagnosis, based on an evaluation of the individual's environment, sociosexual knowledge and attitudes, learning experiences, partner selection, courtship skills and biomedical influences is required to differentiate a paraphilia from counterfeit deviance. Such misbehaviour can result from a lack of privacy (structural), modelling, inappropriate partner selection or courtship, lack of sexual knowledge or moral training or a maladaptive learning history or medical or medication effects. The sexual development of persons with ID is often shaped by a lack of normative learning experiences, segregation, imposed restrictions, lack of privacy, abuse, medication that can affect sexual drive, a lack of sex education and social attitudes that either infantilise or demonise their sexuality (Griffiths, Quinsey & Hingsburger, 1989). These factors may leave the individual vulnerable to engage in an inappropriate sexual behaviour.

A behaviour such as public exposure could certainly be explained as *exhibitionism* if the person is motivated by the desire to expose himself or herself in public. However, other hypotheses have been generated for this behaviour within ID clients. For example;

- Mary pulled up her skirt while on the bus and began to grab at her crotch in what was described as an angry masturbation. Upon investigation, Mary described having 'horrible itch'. She had a vaginitus. Mary had no intense sexual desire or fantasy related to her exposure. Her behaviour was functional and occurred because of a lack of impulse control and training regarding private and public.

- John had lived his entire life in an institutional setting; within months of moving to the community he pulled out his penis in a public washroom and began to show it to the men who came in to use the facilities. John was not seeking to shock the individuals but performing a ritual of courting that he had learned in the facility.
- Alex has Tourette's Disorder. One of his complex motor tics involving grabbing at his genitalia.
- Peter lived in an institutional environment where privacy was not respected nor taught. He is now living in the community. He drops his pants when he needs to go to the bathroom to signal his discomfort; however, he does so whether in private or public. This behaviour could be misinterpreted as a paraphilia rather than simply a lack of pro-social learning.

Examples such as these demonstrate how diagnostic criteria such as exhibitionism should be distinguished from exposure behaviour arising from a lack of sociosexual knowledge regarding public and private, institutionally learned behaviour; abuse learned behaviour; or a response to a medical discomfort.

Research in the general population has identified risk factors and influences that appear to be associated with paraphilic behaviours. Vulnerability influences can be psychological (deficit anger control skills, deficit social skills or a lack of empathy skills), biomedical (mental illness, neurological disorders, physical problems or a behavioural phenotype) or socio-environmental (restricted opportunity for sexual expression). Many of the vulnerabilities associated with paraphilia are also associated with ID. As a result it may appear that they may have increased risk of demonstrating a paraphilia; however, it has been questioned whether the presentation of a seemingly paraphilic behaviour in persons with ID is always mitigated by the fantasies and urges associated with the paraphiliac behaviour or other variables. For example,

- Could the paedophiliac behaviour be explained as a result of a history of punishment and restriction to age-appropriate interactions rather than to sexual preference or because the individual is unable to discriminate self, a child and an appropriate sexual partner? An assessment of the individual's ability to identify self, a child and an appropriate sexual partner is important to determine if the behaviour is complicated by challenges in age discrimination.
- Could the sexual masochism and sadism be related to abusive learning experiences and not be associated with fantasies, sexual urges or behaviours?
- Could apparent voyeurism be a lack of knowledge regarding private, public or social norms? The behaviour might represent a learned institutional behaviour or curiosity.

The DSM-IV-TR manual suggests that a differential diagnosis should include exploration of the following areas: Does the behaviour of the offender represent a sexual pattern that is not preferred? Are the sexual behaviours present only when there is an active mental disorder? Are the behaviours isolated and not part of a recurrent pattern? Was the age of onset later in life? They suggest that an affirmative answer on these issues can be indicative of sexual behaviours that might be motivated by factors other than a paraphilia.

Biomedical Influences

Because persons with ID may not be able to explain or convey their medical or mental health needs in the same way as non-disabled persons their behaviour often gives clues to a discomfort. However, when the behaviours are sexual they are often misunderstood (see Case 8).

Case 8
Alice was found inserting a florescent light into her vagina. The staff immediately jumped to the conclusion that she was masturbating and she was told that this was 'dirty and not right'. She was made to wash her hands repeatedly. Several days later a consultant came to the home for another reason and was told the story. The consultant asked if Alice had ever had problems with vaginal or yeast infections. The consultant examined the medications that Alice had been on recently and realised that one of the side effects of the medication was yeast infection. A visit to the doctor yielded appropriate medication for the yeast infection.

Similarly, mental health challenges may be misinterpreted as sexual problems. Langevin (1992) noted that one in ten sex offenders have a coexisting mental health problem, yet persons with ID are even more likely than the general population to experience a coexisting mental health problem (Nezu, Nezu & Dudeck, 1998), see Case 9.

Case 9
Jason has begun to touch individuals in a sexual manner at his school. He grabs at the private parts of young girls and the teacher. His behaviour was considered 'purposefully sexual' until the psychologist noted that along with this new behaviour, Jason was constantly moving, displaying very pressured speech patterns and had rapid flights of ideas. She investigated with his mother about his sleep patterns and found that he had not been sleeping. A referral to a psychiatrist resulted in a diagnosis of mania, which when treated resulted in the elimination of all symptoms including sexual touching (Griffiths & Fedoroff, 2008).

Another possible biomedical influence on certain sexualised behaviours may relate to genetic syndromes. Some syndromes that either cause or are associated with ID may present with behavioural phenotypes that topographically appear as paraphilia. The expression of the inappropriate sexual behaviour might not be directly related to the disability but to an aspect of the behavioural pheonotype. In the example in Case 10, below, Peter has Smith-Magenis syndrome.

Case 10
Peter is referred for sexual stimulation with objects and frotteurism. He inserts various objects into his rectum and rubs his hands and feet up against others. His care providers have begun to dress him in overalls and have secured the zipper so he cannot get at himself. Peter has caused life threatening injury to himself. He also engages in what his staff called 'aggressive hugging'. He also has been known to strip his clothes off at will. A programme of intrusive behavioural procedures was being considered before the staff decided to refer him to a clinician with expertise in sexual paraphilia and ID.

At first glance, it may appear that Peter has a paraphilia. A clinician, who had expertise in ID immediately noted his distinctive physical features. He had a flat head and mid face, broad nasal bridge, a distinctive upper lip shaped like a 'cupid's bow', fair hair and complexion, large teeth and short small hands. When he talked his voice was deep and hoarse and when he walked he had a 'stork-like' appearance. The clinician asked about his vision (nearsighted), other forms of self-injury (picking at/pulling at fingernails and toenails, hand biting or head banging), other examples of polyembolokoilamania (orifice stuffing) and sleep disturbances (frequent awakenings at night and early wake-up with narcolepsy-like episodes during day). She asked if he was attention-seeking and craved one-to-one interactions, often competing with others for attention, many times by repeating the same questions over and over. She noted that in the consultation he was engaging, endearing, full of personality and had a good sense of humour. Her initial hypothesis that he has Smith-Magenis Syndrome was confirmed when his staff answered her question about whether he self-hugs when excited affirmatively (a 'spasmodic upper body squeezing tic thing, with facial grimacing'). Although Smith-Magenis Syndrome is rare (1 in 25,000 to 1 in 50,000 live births), a clinician who works with persons with ID who engage in sexual problems will be very likely to see several individuals with this syndrome because the symptoms are so often mistaken for sexual paraphilia. Persons with Smith-Magenis often engage in polyembolokoilamania (the inserting of objects into orifices, such as ears or mouth as well as anus or vagina). These latter expressions of orifice stuffing are typically interpreted to be a sexual act rather than as behaviour associated with the syndrome. Although the function of this behaviour is unknown there is no evidence to date to indicate that this behaviour is sexual (Griffiths, Richards, Fedoroff & Watson, 2002). The rubbing and orifice stuffing are likely the result of peripheral neuropathy. The disrobing is the result of extreme tactile sensitivity. And the hugging is an involuntary reaction when excited.

There are a number of challenging behaviours that might be considered paraphilic but may be the result of behavioural phenotypes and genetic disorders; these behaviours might be a feature of that disorder, or they might be a self-stimulatory challenging behaviour. Behaviours such as anal gouging and vaginal or penile stimulation fall into these categories. It can be difficult to judge in any single case whether these behaviours are sexual. In addition, the sexual gratification might be a secondary aspect of the challenging behaviour. Alternatively, the sexual gratification might have arisen serendipitously from the self-stimulatory or challenging behaviour, and, as a result of intrinsic reinforcement with pleasant feelings, it might have become a primary motivation.

Genetic syndromes may also have a significant influence on how the person processes information, adapts to situations and is able to inhibit impulses, in other words their psychological responses to events.

Psychological Influences

Lack of adequate understanding of acceptable social and sexual interactions can cause individuals to behave inappropriately. Limited social contact with the opposite gender because of same-sex residences might lead heterosexual individuals to express themselves sexually with individuals of the same sex. Lack of privacy in residences increases the risk that the individual will express his or her sexuality publicly. Individuals with ID are more vulnerable than are non-disabled people to such psychological factors, which might be associated with counterfeit deviance.

The psychological factors that can contribute to counterfeit deviance include, but are not limited to, a lack of social skills or sociosexual knowledge, institutionally learned sexualised behaviour and communication problems. Moreover, the lack of typical sexual learning and the nature of sexual and relationship experiences generally afforded by society to individuals with ID has also been found to correlate to expressions of sexuality that were inappropriate and sometimes labelled deviant. Individuals with ID are more likely to experience repressive, abusive and culturally distorted sexual learning, which can contribute to inappropriate expressions of their sexuality. Some of the common psychological influences have to do with cognitive challenges, histories of abuse and a lack of sociosexual knowledge.

Cognitive Challenges

The cognitive challenges of the person with ID can also play a role in the presentation of a behaviour that might appear as a paraphilia. Often individuals who present with challenging sexual behaviours are given a test of intelligence. Although this measure can provide information regarding the individual's general cognitive functioning and particular strengths and weaknesses in learning such a test is often misapplied to predict the person's overall functioning and sexual development. A test of intelligence does not provide information regarding adaptive functioning or what adaptations need to be made to support the person's functioning. Moreover, the mental age, as identified in a test of intelligence, does not predict overall functioning or sexual interest or knowledge. Mental age is indicative of the age equivalence of others who answered a comparable number of questions on the test. It is predictive of academic achievement, and in some global way it might describe the typical outcomes for individuals so labelled, but in no way accounts for life experience or learning. A 40-year-old man with a mental age of 5 has 40 years of life experience and learning and the physical and sexual development of a 40-year-old man, and he is in no way comparable to a 5-year-old child in any real-life dimensions.

However, the cognitive abilities of the individual may play a mitigating role in the exhibition of a particular sexual behaviour. For example, Griffiths and Fedoroff (2008) described a young man who repeatedly masturbated in the living room. He was redirected to his bedroom and instructed that the bedroom was the appropriate location for such behaviour; he immediately returned to the living room and began to engage in the behaviour again. One conclusion would be that he was sexually aroused from the reaction he received from the female staff and residents. On the other hand, an alternate hypothesis was tested to see if he needed the presence of some visual aid (for example, the presence of the women) to gain arousal. Clinicians tested the rival hypothesis by providing him access in his bedroom to posters of women in bathing suits from the swimsuit edition of *Sports Illustrated*. From that time on he remained in his room to masturbate. Instruction was also provided so that he understood why his previous behaviour was considered inappropriate and offensive to the women. A simple testing of an alternative hypothesis quickly allowed the determination of a paraphilia to be put aside.

Sexual Abuse

Sexual abuse has been estimated to be one-and-half times more likely for persons with ID than other members of society (Doucette, 1986), and the experience of sexual trauma has been linked to an increased incidence of sexual abuse in later life. Most individuals who have experienced childhood sexual abuse do not develop paedophilia; conversely, most individuals who sexually offend against female children were not themselves sexually abused. Nonetheless, for some offenders there is a correlation between the age of onset of fantasy-driven sexual aggression and the age of their own abuse, the duration of their abuse and the level of invasiveness of the abuse (Pithers, 1993). Hingsburger (1987) reported on a group of individuals with ID who had been institutionalised and who had experienced childhood molestation or coercive sexual activity who later committed similar acts against individuals who were younger and more vulnerable.

Lindsay, Law, Quinn, Smart and Smith (2001) reviewed the patterns of physical and sexual abuse in offenders with ID comparing those who offended sexually (n = 46) with those who offended non-sexually (n = 48). After conducting comprehensive assessments of the experiences of childhood sexual and physical abuse they found that 37 per cent of the sexual offenders and 12.7 per cent of the nonsexual offenders had been sexually abused, whereas 13 per cent of the sexual offenders and 33 per cent of the non-sexual offenders had experienced non-sexual physical abuse. They concluded that sexual abuse in childhood was a significant variable in the history of sexual offenders, whereas physical abuse was more prevalent in the history of non-sexual offenders; nonetheless, they concluded that a history of abuse does not invariably lead to offending behaviour, nor is it sufficient as an explanation of the abuse–offence cycle.

It has been suggested that there are several possible reasons why people with ID might be more likely to be vulnerable to the traumagenic effects of abuse. Firstly, their abuse is often repeated. Secondly, their abuse remains largely unidentified, sometimes disbelieved, rarely reported or processed through the legal system and typically untreated. Thirdly, the individual is generally unable to escape the conditions or environment or victimiser associated with the event. Fourthly, the person is less likely to experience positive sexual experiences to compare to the abusive event or events.

Sexual Knowledge

Recent research has shown that, on average, adults with ID know less about sexuality and sexual abuse than do teenagers and young adults without disabilities (Murphy, 2003; Griffiths & Lunsky, 2003). However, sex education was able to make a significant difference. Recent clinical examples demonstrate that a lack of education regarding sexually appropriate and responsible behaviour represents a critical vulnerability for the development of sexually inappropriate behaviour (see Griffiths, 2002). However, it would be erroneous to assume that all persons with ID who demonstrate sexually inappropriate behaviour do so because of a lack of sexual knowledge.

Hingsburger, Griffiths and Quinsey (1991) presented case examples of people with ID for whom the treatment for certain inappropriate sexual behaviours was sex education alone. Other cases, however, represent more clinically complex interventions in which sex education is often a critical vulnerability for the development of the inappropriate sexual expression and is one of the main components of effective intervention (Griffiths, Quinsey & Hingsburger, 1989; Griffiths, 2002). The evaluation of the sociosexual knowledge and attitudes of sexual offenders with ID is critical in making a differential diagnosis of a paraphilia.

Lunsky, Frijters, Griffiths, Watson and Williston (2007) noted that clinical experience would suggest that paraphilics with ID do not engage in sexual offending behaviour because of a lack of knowledge or experience, but for the same reasons that paraphiliacs without disabilities engage in sexually offending behaviours. Individuals with ID who appropriately fit the category of paraphilia often have more advanced sexual knowledge than other persons with ID and are fully cognisant of the social norms and sanctions of the behaviour for which they have been charged. However, a study by Lunsky and colleagues (ibid.) indicates that a lack of sexual knowledge can play a role in some offences and that only a careful differential diagnosis will reveal if the offence is motivated by the sexual urges and fantasies consistent with paraphilia or some other mitigating factors. The theory posed by Day (1994) and Hingsburger, Griffiths and Quinsey (1991) states that there are two distinct groups of individuals with ID who offend sexually. The first group commits sexual crimes similar to those of the non-disabled paraphiliac sexual offenders. This group may have greater knowledge than another individual with ID. The second subgroup of individuals with ID who commit a sexual offence may be more appropriately classified as counterfeit deviant due to having great gaps in their socio-sexual knowledge and little knowledge of appropriate norms, boundaries or the law.

Social Influences

In the environments where traditionally people with ID have been supported sexual activity is generally severely restricted or punished. Day (1997) has suggested that the high rates of sexual offence behaviour committed by people with ID may be reflective of the generally repressive and restrictive attitudes toward the sexuality of people with disabilities. Many agencies still hold written or unwritten policies that fail to recognise the sexuality of the people they serve or that prohibit and even punish sexual expression, appropriate or inappropriate, consenting or not. Consequently, there is no differential response for individuals who engage in consenting appropriate sexual expression from those who engage in coercive non-consensual expression. The only difference pragmatically is that inappropriate or non-consenting sexual behaviour might have less of a probability of being detected by staff (see Case 11).

Case 11

Jason was referred for being a sexual predator. He had sexual relations with a woman at the workshop. The woman was not capable of giving informed consent for sexual intercourse. The incident was opportunistic because he did not know the woman and enticed her into the washroom where he had sexual intercourse with her. The staff from the group home where he lived suggested that he had a pattern of sexual predatory behaviour.

A comprehensive history of Jason revealed a very different story. Jason was placed in a group home by his parents because he had developed a crush on a girl at his school. There had been no problem but the parents were concerned about Jason's burgeoning sexuality and so placed him in a setting with a strict policy against any sexual contact.

Jason lived at the group home for several years during which he became very attached to another resident. They were inseparable and at some point their friendship became sexual. The woman was immediately moved and Jason was sent for sex education. He then became known as a person to watch and he was placed on constant staff-watch in his residence.

Several years later he met a woman at his workplace and again developed a strong attachment. The relationship was mutual and it became sexualised. She was removed, as was his other friend, and he was sent to social skills training (because he had had sex at work). He was now on full watch at his workplace.

A third similar event occurred at a recreation programme many years later that resulted in him being on 24-hour watch and he was referred for therapy.

Several months after this incident, while at the workshop, he wandered off from his one-to-one staff and it was during this time that he enticed the young woman into the washroom. She had not resisted and appeared to be agreeable to the encounter, but she was not able to give legal consent.

Is this a pattern of a sexual predator? No, it is the behaviour of a young man who wanted to be intimate with a woman. The first three relationships were mutual and consensual but were considered inappropriate by the agency. His relationship was ended and he was punished by sanctioning and therapeutic intervention. The final incident was indeed inappropriate because her consent ability was questionable; however, the agency had created a scenario where his only option for sexual contact would be to take advantage of a moment when he could be free of his individual surveillance. The agency had created a sexual opportunist. He wanted a relationship but the agency would not allow it. Although he had mistakenly chosen an individual who could not give legal consent, she had agreed that it was fine. He was not a predator but a very frustrated young man who needed an environment that respected his sexuality.

Edgerton (1973) suggested that people with ID demonstrate no more sexually inappropriate behaviour than non-disabled people if they are provided a normative learning experience. Hingsburger (1992) suggested that the sexual experiences of persons with ID have been so suppressed, controlled or punished that the individuals could be conditioned to a negative reaction tendency to anything sexual. This conditioning can alter their response to the instigating factors for normal sexual experiences. In some cases, the person might shift to response patterns that appear abnormal. In addition, the erotophobia might alter an individual's response to interviewing and phallometric testing, which could account for the differential patterns of some people with ID that were observed by Murphy *et al.* (1983a).

CONCLUSIONS

In this chapter, the authors have attempted to demonstrate how additional cautions should be applied when utilising the DSM-IV-TR criteria with persons with ID. Application to this population requires knowledge of the nature of the disabling condition the person experiences and the impact of their life experiences on the commission of the offence. The reader is referred to Griffiths (2002) for additional reading on this topic.

REFERENCES

Abel, G.G. & Rouleau, J. (1990). The nature and extent of sexual assault. In W. Marshall, D.R. Laws & H. E. Barbaree (Eds), *Handbook of sexual assault.* (pp. 9–21). New York: Plenum Press.

American Psychiatric Association (2000). *Diagnostic and statistical manual of mental disorders, fourth edition, text revision.* Washingon: APA.

Blanchard, R., Watson, M.S., Choy, A., Dickey, R., Klassen, P., Kuban, M. et al. (1999). Pedophiles: Mental retardation, maternal age, and sexual orientation. *Archives of Sexual Behaviour, 28,* 111–27.

Brown, B.S. & Courtless, R.F. (1971). *Mentally retarded offender*. Washington, DC: National Institute of Mental Health, Center for Studies of Crime and Delinquency.

Cantor, J.M., Blanchard, R., Robichaud, L.K. & Christensen, B.K. (2005). Quantitative reanalysis of aggregate data on IQ in sexual offenders. *Psychological Bulletin, 131*, 555–68.

Corbett, K. (1987). The role of sexuality and sex equity in the education of disabled women. *Peabody Journal of Education, 64* (4), 198–212.

Corbett, K., Shurberg, S., Klein, J. & Bregante, L. (1987). The role of sexuality and sex equity in the education of disabled women. *Peabody Journal of Education; Sex Equity and Sexuality in Education, 64* (4).

Day, K. (1994). Male mentally handicapped sex offenders. *British Journal of Psychiatry, 165*, 630–9.

Day, K. (1997). Clinical features and offence behaviour of mentally retarded sex offenders: A review of research. In R.J. Fletcher & D. Griffiths (Eds), *Congress proceedings – International Congress II on the dually diagnosed.* (pp. 95–9). Kingston: NADD Press.

Di Giulio, G. (2003). Sexuality and people living with physical or developmental disabilities: A review of key issues. *The Canadian Journal of Human Sexuality, 12*, 53–68.

Doucette, J. (1986). *Violent acts against disabled women*. Toronto: DAWN Canada.

Edgerton, R. (1973). Socio-cultural research considerations. In F.F. de la Cruz & G.G. La Veck (Eds), *Human sexuality and the mentally retarded.* (pp. 240–49). New York: Brunner/Maze.

Fedoroff, J.P. & Blanchard, R. (2000). Is sex re-assignment surgery ethical? In D. Goldbloom (Ed.), *Psychiatry rounds 4.* (pp. 1–8). Toronto: Snell Medical Communication Inc.

Fletcher, R., Loschen, E., Stavrakaki, C. & First, M. (2007a). *Diagnostic manual – intellectual disability (DM-ID): A textbook of diagnosis of mental disorders in persons with intellectual disability.* Kingston, NY: NADD Press.

Fletcher, R., Loschen, E., Stavrakaki, C. & First, M. (2007b). *Diagnostic manual – intellectual disability: A clinical guide for diagnosis of mental disorders in persons with intellectual disability*. Kingston, NY: NADD Press.

Gilby, R., Wolf, L. & Goldberg, B. (1989). Mentally retarded adolescent sex offenders: A survey and pilot study. *Canadian Journal of Psychiatry, 34*, 542–8.

Griffiths, D. (1999). Sexuality and people with developmental disabilities: Myth, conceptions and facts. In I. Brown & M. Percy (Eds), *Developmental disabilities in Ontario.* (pp. 443–51). Toronto: Front Porch Publishing.

Griffiths, D. (2002). Sexual aggression. In W.I. Gardner (Ed.), *Aggression and other disruptive behavioural challenges: Biomedical and psychosocial assessment and treatment.* (pp. 525–398). Kingston, New York: NADD Press.

Griffiths, D., Baxter, J., Haslam, T., Richards, D., Stranges, S. & Vyrostko, B. (1996). Building healthy boundaries: Considerations for reducing sexual abuse. (pp. 143–48). *National Association for Dual Diagnosis Annual Conference Proceedings.* New York: National Association for the Dually Diagnosed.

Griffiths, D. & Fedoroff, P. (2008). Persons with intellectual disabilities who sexually offend. In F.M. Saleh, A.J. Grudzinksas & J.M. Bradford (Eds), *Sex offenders: Identification, risk assessment, treatment and legal issues.* New York: Oxford University Press.

Griffiths, D. & Lunsky, Y. (2003). *Socio-Sexual Knowledge and Attitude Assessment Tool (SSKAAT-R).* Wood Dale, IL: Stoelting Company.

Griffiths, D., Quinsey, V.L. & Hingsburger, D. (1989). *Changing inappropriate sexual behaviour: A community based approach for persons with intellectual disabilities.* Baltimore: Paul H. Brookes Publishing.

Griffiths, D., Richards, D., Fedoroff, P. & Watson, S. (2002). Sexuality and mental health issues. In D. Griffiths, C. Stavrakaki & J. Summers (Eds), *Dual diagnosis: An introduction to the mental health needs of persons with developmental disabilities.* Sudbury, ON, Canada: Habilitative Mental Health Resource Network.

Griffiths, D., Richards, D., Fedoroff, P. & Watson, S. (2003). Sexuality and mental health in persons with developmental disabilities. In D. Griffiths, C. Stavrakaki & J. Summers (Eds), *An introduction to the mental health needs of persons with developmental disabilities*. Mental Health Resource Network, Ontario. Canada.

Griffitths, D.M., Ware, J., Haslam, T., Richards, D., Vyrostko, B. & Stranges, S.(n.d.). Healthy boundaries: Sexual abuse prevention. Welland and District Association for Community Living unpublished research document.

Griffiths, D., Watson, S., Lewis, R. & Stoner, K. (2004). Research in sexuality and intellectual disability. In E. Emerson, C. Hatton, T. Parmenter & T. Thompson (Eds), *Handbook of methods of research and evaluation in intellectual disabilities*. London: Wiley.

Held, K.R. (1993). Ethical aspects of sexuality of persons with mental retardation. In M. Nagler (Ed.), *perspectives on disability: text and readings on disability*. 2nd edn. Palo Alto, CA: Health Markets Research.

Hingsburger, D. (1987). Sex counselling with the developmentally handicapped: The assessment and management of seven critical problems. *Psychiatric Aspects of Mental Retardation Reviews*, *6*, 41–6.

Hingsburger, D. (1992). Erotophobic behaviour in people with intellectual disabilities. *The Habilitative Mental Healthcare Newsletter*, *11*, 31–4.

Hingsburger, D., Griffiths, D. & Quinsey, V. (1991). Detecting counterfeit deviance: Differentiating sexual deviance from sexual inappropriateness. *The Habilitative Mental Healthcare Newsletter*, *10*, 51–4.

Karellou, J. (2003). Laypeople's attitudes towards the sexuality of people with learning disabilities in Greece. *Sexuality and Disability*, *21*, 65–84.

King, R. & Richards, D. (2002). Sterilization and birth control. In D. Griffiths, D. Richards, P. Fedoroff & S.L. Watson (Eds), *Ethical dilemmas: Sexuality and developmental disability*. Kingston, NY: NADD Press.

Koller, R. (2000). Sexuality and adolescents with autism. *Sexuality and Disability*, *18* (2), 125–35.

Konstantareas, M.M. & Lunsky, Y. (1997). Sociosexual knowledge, experience, attitudes and interests in individuals with autistic disorder and intellectual delay. *Journal of Autism and Intellectual Disorders*, *27*, 397–413.

Lackey, L.B. & Knopp, F.H. (1989). *A summary of selected notes from the working sessions of the First National Training Conference on the Assessment and Treatment of Intellectual Disabled Juvenile and Adult Sexual Offenders*. Orwell, VT: Safer Society Press.

Langevin, R. (1992). A comparison of neuroendocrine abnormalities and genetic factors in homosexuality and in pedophilia. *Annals of Sex Research*, *6*, 67–76.

Lindsay, W.R. (2002). Research and literature on sex offenders with intellectual and developmental disabilities. *Journal of Intellectual Disabilities Research*, *46*, (Suppl 1), 74–85.

Lindsay, W.R., Law, J., Quinn, K., Smart, N. & Smith, A.H. (2001). A comparison of physical and sexual abuse: Histories of sexual and non-sexual offenders with intellectual disability. *Child Abuse and Neglect*, *25*, 989–95.

Lunsky, Y., Frijters, J., Griffiths, D., Watson, S.L. & Williston, S. (2007). Sexual knowledge and attitudes of men with intellectual disabilities who sexually offend. *Journal of Intellectual and Developmental Disability*, *32* (2), 74–81.

McCabe, M.P. (1994). *Sexual knowledge, experience, feelings and needs scale for people with intellectual disability (Sex Ken-ID)*. 4th edn. Burwood, Australia: Deakin University.

McCabe, M. & Cummins, R. (1996). The sexual knowledge, experience, feelings, and needs of people with mild intellectual disability. *Education and Training in Mental Retardation and Developmental Disabilities*, *31* (1), 13–21.

McCabe, M. & Schreck, A. (1992). Before sex education: An evaluation of the sexual knowledge, experience, feelings and needs of people with mild intellectual disabilities. *Australia and New Zealand Journal of Developmental Disabilities*, *18* (2), 75–82.

McGee, J. & Menolascino, F.J. (1992). The evaluation of defendants with mental retardation in the criminal justice system. In R.W. Conley, R. Luckasson & G.N. Bouthilet (Eds), *The criminal justice system and mental retardation: Defendants and victims*. Baltimore: Paul.H. Brookes.

Money, J. (1973). Gender role, gender identity, core gender identity: Usage and definition of terms. *Journal of American Academy of Psychoanalysis*, 397–402.

Money, J. (1985a). *The destroying angel*. Buffalo, NY: Prometheus press.

Money, J. (1985b). Gender: History, theory and usage of the term in sexology and its relationship to nature/nurture. *Journal of Sex and Marital Therapy*, *11*, 71–9.

Money, J. (1994). The concept of gender identity disorder in childhood and adolescence after 39 years. *Journal of Sex and Marital Therapy*, *20*, 163–77.

Money, J. & Ehrhardt, A.A. (1972). Man & woman boy & girl: Differentiation and dimorphism or gender identity from conception to maturity. Baltimore, MD: The John Hopkins University Press.

Murphy, G.H. (2003). Capacity to consent to sexual relationships in adults with learning disabilities. *Journal of Family Planning and Reproductive Health Care*, *28* (3), 148–9.

Murphy, W.D., Coleman, E.M. & Abel, G.G. (1983a). Human sexuality in the mentally retarded. In J.L. Matson & F. Andrasik (Eds), *Treatment issues and innovations in mental retardation*. New York: Plenum.

Murphy, W.D., Coleman, E.M. & Haynes, M. (1983b). Treatment and evaluation issues with the mentally retarded sex offender. In J. Greer & I. Stuart (Eds), *The sexual aggressor: Current perspectives on treatment*. New York: Van Nostrand Reinhold.

Neiderbuhl, J.M. & Morris, D.C. (1993). Sexual knowledge and the capability of persons with dual diagnoses to consent to sexual contact. *Sexuality and Disability*, *11* (4), 295–307.

Nezu, C.M., Nezu, A.M. & Dudeck, J. (1998). A cognitive behavioural model of assessment and treatment for intellectually disabled sexual offenders. *Cognitive and Behavioral Practice*, *5*, 25–64.

Phillips, N. (2000). Female sexual dysfunction: evaluation and treatment. *American Family Physician*, *62* (1). Retrieved on May 1, 2007 from www.aafp.org/afp/20000701/127.html.

Pithers, W. (1993). Treatment of rapists: Reinterpretation of early outcome data and explanatory constructs to enhance therapeutic efficiency. In G.G. Nagayama Hall, R. Hirrschman, J.R. Graham & M.S. Zaragoza (Eds), *Sexual aggression: Issues in etiology, assessment and treatment*. Washington, DC: Taylor & Francis.

Quinsey, V.L., Book, A. & Skilling, T.A. (2004). A follow-up of deinstitutionalised men with intellectual disabilities and histories of antisocial behaviour. *Journal of Applied Research in Intellectual Disabilities*, *17*, 243–53.

Richards, D., Miodrag, N. & Watson, S.L. (2006). Sexuality and developmental disability: Obstacles to healthy sexuality throughout the lifespan. *Developmental Disabilities Bulletin*, *34* (1), 137–55.

Richards, D., Miodrag, N., Watson, S.L., Feldman, M., Aunos, M., Cox-Lindenbaum, D. & Griffiths, D. (2008). Sexual rights and persons with intellectual disabilities. In D.M. Griffiths & F. Owen (Eds), *Rights of persons with intellectual disabilities: Historical, legal, policy and theoretical issues*. London: Jessica Kingsley.

Ruiter, I.D. (2000). *Allow me: A guide to promoting communication skills in adults with developmental delays*. Toronto: The Beacon Herald Fine Print Division.

Santamour, W. & West, B. (1978). *The mentally retarded offender and corrections*. Washington, DC: US Department of Justice.

Servais, L. (2006). Sexual Health Care in Persons with Intellectual Disabilities. Mental Retardation and Developmental Disabilities Research Reviews, *12*, 48–56.

Shapiro, S. (1986). Delinquent and disturbed behaviour within the field of mental deficiency. In A.V.S. deReuck & R. Porter (Eds), *The mentally abnormal offende*. New York: Grune & Stratton.

Sobsey, D. & Mansell, S. (1994). An international perspective on patterns of sexual assault and abuse of people with disabilities. *International Journal of Adolescent Medicine and Health*, *7* (2), 153–178.

Steiner, J. (1984). Group counselling with retarded offenders. *Social Work*, *29*, 181–82.

Torgrimson, B.N. & Minson, C.T. (2005). Sex and gender: What is the difference? *Journal of Applied Physiolology, 99* (3), 785–7.

Watson, S.L., Griffiths, D.M., Richards, D. & Dykstra, L. (2002). Sex education. In D.M. Griffiths, D. Richards, P. Fedoroff & S.L. Watson (Eds), *Ethical dilemmas: Sexuality and developmental disability*. Kingston, NY: NADD Press.

World Health Organization (1993). *International classification of mental and behaviour disorders: Diagnostic criteria for research*. Geneva: World Health Organization.

PART THREE

Risk Assessment

8

Assessing Recidivism Risk in Sex Offenders with Intellectual Disabilities

WILLIAM R. LINDSAY AND JOHN L. TAYLOR

INTRODUCTION

Since the early 1990s, a considerable amount of progress has been made in the assessment of long-term risk of future offending in criminal and forensic psychiatric populations (Lindsay and Beail 2004). This work arose out of dissatisfaction with predictions of risk for future offending made on the basis of clinical evaluations. At first, actuarial research was conducted on factors that might predict general recidivism and it was found that statistical prediction was more accurate than expert clinical judgement. Andrews (1989) reported that the predictive accuracy of a structured actuarial assessment in relation to general criminal recidivism was between 60 per cent and 80 per cent. Having demonstrated the possibility of predicting general recidivism, the next applied research task was to investigate the feasibility of improving the prediction of sexual and violent recidivism.

Harris, Rice and Quinsey (1993) conducted a large-scale study investigating a number of promising candidate variables that had emerged from previous research as possible predictors of future violent and sexual offences. In this study they grouped the variables into four categories: variables related to childhood, those relevant to adulthood, characteristics of the index offence and psychological/psychiatric assessment variables. Twelve childhood variables were included (e.g., elementary school maladjustment, parental crime, separation from parents under the age of 16), thirteen adult variables were included (e.g., longest employment, alcohol abuse, previous relationships, offence history), nine index offence variables (e.g., relationship to the victim, weapon use) and eight assessment variables (e.g., IQ, diagnosis of personality disorder). On each of the variables they then compared 191 recidivists and 427 non-recidivists in samples of men who had offended and who had been admitted for psychiatric assessment and

Assessment and Treatment of Sexual Offenders with Intellectual Disabilities: A Handbook
Edited by Leam A. Craig, William R. Lindsay and Kevin D. Browne
© 2010 John Wiley & Sons, Ltd.

treatment. Interestingly, from the point of view of the present chapter, there was no significant difference between recidivists and non-recidivists in IQ. However, a number of variables in each category did show highly significant differences between the two groups.

Inspection of these significant variables suggests that some of them are likely to be major markers for underlying psychological processes about which there is a considerable amount of theory and research. For example, parental alcoholism, parental crime and separation under the age of 16 from parents all significantly differentiated between the two groups. It is likely that these items represent a summary of the significant amount of research and theory on childhood development, family child-rearing style and attachment. These are highly important areas of research in the field of offenders. For example, one of the major developmental models for the onset of delinquency and criminal behaviour is that of Gerald Patterson (Patterson, 1986; Patterson & Yoerger, 1997). In an extensive series of studies based on learning and reinforcement theories, they found that from as early as 18 months, some families may promote a child's coercive behaviour, such as temper tantrums and hitting, because those behaviours have functional value in terminating conflict within the family. With repeated interactions, these behaviours are strengthened and firmly established in the child's repertoire. In other families, children learn interactions that are quite distinct from those learned in 'distressed families' (Patterson's terminology). In 'non-distressed' families, in which pro-social behaviours are reinforced, the child learns that interactions such as talking and negotiating are followed by a termination of conflict. In distressed families, not only are coercive behaviours promoted, but pro-social behaviours may not be particularly effective in terminating family conflict. Therefore, as these boys developed they failed to learn pro-social behaviours, problem solving and language skills but became highly skilled in antisocial behaviours.

Patterson and Yoerger (1997) related these findings to a theory concerning the development of early-onset and late-onset delinquency. In early-onset delinquency, the combination of the emergence of coercive behaviour and the high frequency of conflict within families accounted for almost half of the variance in the development of antisocial behaviour in boys as young as 6 or 7 (Snyder & Patterson, 1995). In late-onset delinquency, the ability and amount of time that parents devoted to monitoring their sons became a crucial variable in the movement of boys towards juvenile delinquency. They made the important point (Patterson & Yoerger, 1997) that almost all adolescents have some contact with deviant peers. The extent of parental monitoring played a significant role in the extent of contact and length of time period in contact with delinquent subcultures. While it is clearly not the only variable related to risk for future violent and sexual offending, the parenting items to emerge in the Harris, Rice and Quinsey (1993) study are likely to reflect this body of literature.

It is now becoming clear that family conflict is an equally important variable in the development of violent and criminal behaviour in individuals with intellectual disabilities (ID). Novaco and Taylor (2008) investigated the relationship between family volatility in childhood and anger and assault in 129 men with ID. Thirty-six percent of the men had previous convictions for violent behaviour and a further 38 per cent had a documented history of violence or aggression. Anger and aggression was assessed through self-report, staff ratings and archival records while family history of aggression was obtained in a set of 10 interview questions. They found a strong significant relationship between childhood exposure to parents' anger and aggression and current measures of self-reported anger, staff reported anger and physical assaults. They also found that those participants who had been physically abused by parents or caretakers had significantly higher levels of anger and assault on all measures.

Lindsay, Law, Quinn, Smart & Smith (2001) and Lindsay, Michie, Whitefield, Martin, Grieve & Carson (2006) examined characteristics of referrals to a forensic ID service and found that, when compared to other types of referrals such as sex offenders, violent offenders reported higher rates of physical abuse in childhood. In fact, while sexual offenders reported between 14 per cent and 16 per cent physical abuse, the violent offenders reported between 35 per cent and 38 per cent physical abuse in childhood. However, even when partialing out other significant variables such as childhood sexual abuse, Novaco and Taylor (2008) found that witnessing parental violence remained a significant predictor of future violence. This research would suggest that the major markers for parental problems found by Harris, Rice and Quinsey (1993) are relevant to the population of offenders with ID.

The results on separation from one parent in childhood may be even more significant in relation to sex offenders with ID. Harris, Rice and Quinsey (1993) found a highly significant difference in that recidivists had twice the rate of separation from parents in childhood when compared to the non-recidivists. If we ally this result to the results on parental problems (alcoholism and violence) then the item is likely to be a major marker for attachment difficulties in childhood development. Marshall (1989) had argued that one of the reasons some men commit sexual offences is that they may have failed to develop an ability to establish and maintain secure attachments in childhood. These developmental difficulties may lead to a lack of intimacy skills, failure to develop positive self-concept and a subsequent lack of skills to enter into intimate relationships with other adults. Despite the fact that these men may have poor heterosexual and social skills arising from attachment difficulties they continue to have a drive for sexual contact resulting in them gaining such contact through illegal means either with children or through force with other adults. Ward, Hudson and Marshall (1996) tested this hypothesis with 147 offenders with ID. They hypothesised the different types of attachment difficulty (dismissive, fearful and preoccupied) might be associated with different types of offending. They found that although the different types of attachment difficulty were not associated with particular types of offending, negative attachment was associated with all types of offending. Stirpe, Abracen, Stermac & Wilson (2006) reviewed the attachment style of 101 sexual and non-sexual offenders and found that all offenders tended towards insecure attachments. Therefore negative attachments through childhood are associated with a variety of types of offending (Marsa *et al.* 2004).

The literature and research on attachment has become increasingly complex and nuanced with disrupted attachments related to cognitive development which in turn drive the acquisition of implicit theories or 'world views' that develop in early childhood. These implicit theories then determine the way in which individuals relate to others. Ward and Keenan (1999) identified five distinct implicit theories among child molesters which determined cognitive distortions involved in their cycle of offending. However, there is now a wealth of research showing that offenders have a greater history of attachment difficulties than non-offenders and that these developmental disruptions may predict offending. In a comparison of 61 child molesters and 51 community controls, Wood and Riggs (2008) found that attachment anxiety contributed significantly in a logistic multiple regression to the odds that a participant would be a child molester.

In another study, specifically in the field of ID, Lindsay, Elliot and Astell (2004) reviewed a number of candidate variables in a comparison of recidivists and non-recidivists in 52 sex offenders and abusers with ID. Poor relationship with mother emerged as one of the variables significantly differentiating between groups and contributing significantly to the regression model predicting recidivism. Therefore, again, an item which indicates attachment difficulties is a significant predictor of recidivism in offenders with ID.

The significance of this body of research which reviews the family conflict and difficulties with childhood attachments is reflected in many risk assessment instruments. Several contain a major item on childhood maladjustment in which the assessor reviews precisely this body of work. Therefore, each of the items in a risk assessment instrument is likely to reflect a significant amount of depth in research and investigation. The available evidence, although it is not as extensive as that on mainstream offenders, is that these findings remain significant in relation to offenders with ID.

THE HISTORY AND DEVELOPMENT OF RISK ASSESSMENT INSTRUMENTS

The developmental research conducted by Harris, Rice and Quinsey (1993) progressed quickly to the establishment of the Violence Risk Appraisal Guide (VRAG) (Quinsey, Harris, Rice & Cormier, 1998, 2005). The VRAG employs the main variables to emerge from the developmental work and includes the four groupings of childhood, adult, index offence and assessment items. Because of its extensive empirical derivation, the VRAG and its sister risk assessment for sexual offences, the Sex Offender Risk Appraisal Guide (SORAG), have become a standard comparator against which other risk assessments have been compared for predictive accuracy. Both the VRAG and SORAG have been cross validated on a variety of forensic psychiatric populations and prisoner samples (Quinsey, Harris, Rice & Cormier 2005). In their original evaluation, Quinsey, Harris, Rice and Cormier (1998) found that the VRAG was as accurate with offenders who had intellectual limitations (IQ $<$ 80) as with offenders who did not.

As research on risk assessment developed over the subsequent 10 years, several groups of researchers compared the predictive accuracy of different risk assessment instruments on a range of databases. Barbaree, Seto, Langton and Peacock (2001) compared the VRAG, SORAG, Rapid Risk Assessment of Sexual Offence Recidivism (RRASOR: Hanson, 1997), Static-99 (Hanson & Thornton, 1999), the Minnesota Sex Offender Screening Tool – Revised (MmSOST-R: Epperson, Kaul, Huot, Hesselton, Alexander & Goldman, 1998) and the Multifactorial Assessment of Sex Offender Risk for Recidivism (MASORR). They employed a Canadian database of 215 sex offenders who had been released from prison for an average of 4.5 years. They found that the VRAG, SORAG, RRASOR and Static-99 successfully predicted general recidivism and sexual recidivism. Interestingly, the RRASOR, which included only four easily scored items, was superior to other instruments in predicting sexual recidivism.

Following on from the research of Barbaree, Seto, Langton and Peacock (2001), Langton, Barbaree, Seto, Peacock, Harkins and Hanson (2007) extended the study with 468 mainstream sex offenders followed up for an average of 5.9 years. They used the same assessments as previously with the addition of the updated Static-2002 (Hanson & Thornton, 2003). This study provides an indication of the extent to which research in the field should be treated with caution because with the addition of the extra 253 participants, the RRASOR was now the poorest predictor of future incidents, although all the instruments significantly predicted any offending. The VRAG and SORAG showed the largest effect sizes for any offending and those two assessments plus the Static-2002 showed the largest effect sizes for serious offending. For the prediction of future sexual offences, the SORAG and Static-2002 were significantly superior to the other instruments.

Other authors have compared the predictive accuracy of various instruments across a range of clients and cultures. Bartosh, Garby, Lewis and Gray (2003) compared the Static-99, RRASOR, MmSOST-R and SORAG in predicting recidivism in 251 sexual offenders in the USA. They categorised their participants in terms of index offence type and found that none of the four tests had consistent predictive validity across categories. However, the Static-99 and SORAG emerged as the instruments with the greatest consistency in terms of predictive accuracy for future sexual offences. Kroner and Mills (2001) compared the predictive accuracy of the Psychopathy Checklist – Revised (PCL-R: Hare, 1991), the VRAG and the HCR-20 (comprising the historical scale, the clinical scale and the risk management scale: Webster, Eaves, Douglas & Wintrup, 1995) with 97 mainstream offenders in Canada. The VRAG had the highest prediction correlations with minor and major incidents although there was no statistically significant differences between the instruments. In a follow-up of 51 mainstream offenders convicted of rape in Sweden, Sjostedt and Langstrom (2002) compared the accuracy of several instruments including the VRAG, RRASOR, PCL-R and Sexual Violence Risk – 20 (SVR-20: Boer, Hart, Kropp & Webster, 1997). Follow-ups were for an average of 92 months and only the RRASOR showed predictive accuracy for sexual recidivism while the other instruments showed some predictive accuracy with violent non-sexual recidivism.

Finally, in a further follow-up to their original series of studies, Harris, Rice, Quinsey, Lalumiere, Boer and Lang (2003) compared the VRAG, SORAG, RRASOR and Static-99 in the prediction of recidivism for 396 sexual offenders in Canada. All four instruments predicted recidivism with significantly greater accuracy than chance. Prediction of violent recidivism was consistently higher for the VRAG and SORAG with the effect sizes large for violence recidivism and moderate for sexual recidivism.

Given these various studies, there is little doubt that prediction of future sexual and violent offending based on actuarial/historical variables can be conducted with a reasonable degree of accuracy. It should be remembered that, generally, the prediction of risk is based on statistics borrowed from signal detection theory which accumulate predictive accuracy based on individual successes and failures rather than group data. There has been a recent debate on the confidence with which individual predictions can be made based on these studies. However, as Quinsey (2007) amusingly illustrates with reference to buying a new car, predictions about the reliability of individual cars can be made based on the statistics used (Receiver Operator Characteristics) which accumulate information on the basis of the reliability of previous cars in this category (Hart, Michie & Cook, 2007).

ACTUARIAL ASSESSMENT AND OFFENDERS WITH INTELLECTUAL DISABILITY

Given that the VRAG and SORAG have often been included as comparators in risk assessment evaluations, it is gratifying that the first form of evaluation of a standardised risk assessment was completed using the VRAG. Quinsey, Book and Skilling (2004) investigated the predictive validity of the VRAG in men with ID. Their study employed 58 men with serious histories of antisocial and aggressive behaviour who were followed up for an average of 16 months. Eighty per cent of the participants had at least one additional diagnosis, 56 per cent had a diagnosis of some type of personality disorder, 36 per cent had been diagnosed with some type of paraphilia, 11 per cent had a diagnosis of psychosis and 9 per cent were diagnosed with affective disorder. Around 70 per cent of the clients had documented incidents or arrests for sexual offences of various kinds. Almost all of the sexual offences constituted physical contact made with the victim. More than half of the clients presented chronic management problems involving sexual and physical aggressiveness within their community placement and there were over 500 incidents reported during the follow-up period. Thirty-nine of the 58 participants had at least one incident over the follow-up period. They found that the VRAG showed significant predictive value with medium effect sizes (auc = 0.69). They also found that monthly staff ratings of client behaviour were significantly related to antisocial incidents. One of the interesting developments in this study was that they substituted the PCL-R (Hare, 1991), a somewhat technical item on the VRAG, with the Child and Adolescent Taxon (CAT), which is a much simpler measure of antisociality. The CAT is based on interview and file material regarding childhood behavioural difficulties. Quinsey, Harris, Rice and Cormier (2005), in their revision of the VRAG, found that the CAT could replace the PCL-R with no significant reduction in accuracy.

Two subsequent studies have compared the relative predictive accuracy of a number of risk assessment instruments including the VRAG. The first was by Gray, Fitzgerald, Taylor, MacCulloch and Snowden (2007) in an evaluation of the VRAG, the PCL – Screening Version (Hart, Cox & Hare, 1995) and the HCR-20. They compared the instruments on a group of 145 offenders with ID and 996 mainstream offenders all discharged from four independent sector hospitals and followed up for a minimum of two years. For the ID group, all the assessments predicted future incidents with a medium-to-large effect size for both violent and general recidivism. Indeed, all the risk predictors showed greater accuracy with the ID group than with the mainstream, non-ID offenders.

Lindsay *et al.* (2008) completed a further evaluation of a number of risk assessments on a sample of 212 offenders with ID from a range of community and secure settings. They followed participants up for a period of one year and compared the VRAG, HCR-20, Static-99 and Risk Matrix 2000 (Thornton *et al.*, 2003). They also used two measures of dynamic risk assessment which shall be dealt with later in this chapter. The VRAG and HCR-20 showed significant predictive accuracy with Areas Under the Curve (AUCs) of 0.71 and 0.72 respectively. The RM2000 had poorer predictive accuracy with a small effect size but the authors noted that the assessment was promising since the scoring criteria were relatively straightforward. Therefore, the results from these various studies suggest that the predictive validity of actuarial risk assessment with offenders with ID is at least as good as that on mainstream offenders. Furthermore, it is interesting that despite differing lengths of follow-up in the three studies discussed, the predictive results for the VRAG were broadly similar.

STRUCTURED CLINICAL JUDGEMENT AND THE PSYCHOPATHY CHECKLIST – REVISED

The most commonly employed structured clinical judgement is the HCR-20. This has been mentioned above in the section on studies comparing the predictive accuracy of different risk assessments and it is also explained extensively later in this book, in Chapter 10. However, since it is perhaps the most frequently used risk assessment, combining actuarial approaches and clinical judgement to consider risk levels and risk management needs in offenders, it should be reviewed at least briefly in the present chapter. The HCR-20 has three sections – historical, which includes 10 items; clinical, including five items; and risk, including five items. Each item is rated on a three-point scale from 0, no evidence of the variable, through 1, some evidence of the variable, to 2, clear evidence of the variable. All research studies employ this manner of scoring in order to compare the predictive ability with other instruments. However, the authors do not recommend making decisions on the basis of total score. Rather, they recommend that the items are structured in order to help the consideration of a comprehensive range of variables with a view to arriving at a final judgement. In this way, actuarial, historical variables are combined with an assessment of current clinical status and consideration of future risk variables.

As mentioned in Chapter 10, a great deal of research work has been conducted on the HCR-20 in different settings and with different populations. These studies have found that the HCR-20 predicts future violent incidents with a medium-to-large effect. Chapter 10 also describes more recent research on the HCR-20 and offenders with ID. Gray, Fitzgerald, Taylor, MacCulloch and Snowden (2007) found that the historical scale had the highest predictive value for future offending of the various assessments they employed. Lindsay *et al.* (2008) found that when the HCR-20 was judged against other similar actuarial predictors it had a medium effect size which was comparable to the VRAG and better than the RM2000.

Taylor *et al.* (2008) conducted a more extensive analysis on the HCR-20 data which were reported in summary fashion in Lindsay *et al.* (2008). Taylor *et al.* (2008) used the information from 212 adult male offenders with ID who had been drawn from three different settings. These included 73 participants from a high secure setting, 70 participants from medium and low secure settings and 69 participants from a community forensic ID service. The three settings represented mature services for forensic referrals with ID and they have been described and compared in detail on referral information, personal characteristics, criminal history, psychiatric history and index crimes in separate publications (Hogue *et al.*, 2006). In summary, the cohorts differed significantly in age with the community referrals younger than both other cohorts; rates of mental illness with medium/low secure referrals having lower rates than the other cohorts; violent offences with maximum secure referrals having a significantly higher frequency than the other two cohorts. There were no differences between the groups on IQ or the number of participants with a history of sexual offences. Parallel datasets were collected across all three sites and all historical information was available from the clinical files. Violent and sexual incidents were recorded over a period of one year. A significant incident was defined as recorded verbal aggression, physical aggression, destruction of property and inappropriate sexual behaviour. There were no incidents of absconding. Therefore, the HCR-20 was assessed for predictive accuracy across a range of community and secure settings.

In this study, there were significant differences between the groups on the H scale and total score with the community group having lower scores than the other two sites. This relatively orderly, predictable result was not mirrored with the risk and clinical items which are more dynamic risk assessments (see later). There were no significant differences between the groups on the clinical scale and on the risk management scale, the medium/low secure had significantly lower scores than the other two sites. One might expect those in medium and low secure services to have higher risk management scores than those in the community. However, on reflection, the community forensic service catered for individuals who lived at home with their families, in their own supported accommodation and in group homes. Most had constant unsupervised access to the community and so would present a constant risk as judged by the services. Therefore, it is perhaps less surprising that they were judged as having higher risk scores. In comparisons between individuals who did and did not perpetrate a violent incident in the subsequent year, there were significant differences between the groups on all three scales with those who committed further incidents having higher scores. When they calculated the predictive accuracy of the HCR-20 for those who did and did not perpetrate a further incident, they found an AUC = 0.68 for the H scale, AUC = 0.67 for the C scale, AUC = 0.62 for the R scale and for the total score, they found an AUC = 0.72. It seems, then, that the HCR-20 has reasonable predictive accuracy for offenders with ID across this range of settings.

Work on the PCL-R and offenders with ID is discussed in detail in Chapter 9. Morrissey and colleagues (Morrissey *et al.*, 2005, 2007; Morrissey, Mooney, Hogue, Lindsay & Taylor, 2007) have conducted a series of analyses investigating the usability, applicability and psychometric properties of the PCL-R in this population. Firstly, Morrissey *et al.* (2005) reported good internal consistency for total score and factor one of the PCL-R. Internal consistency for factor two was lower but remained acceptable. Inter-rater reliability between trained raters was also good with intra-class correlations of greater than 0.8. They then compared participants in high secure, medium/low secure and community settings. Mean results for each group were orderly with the high secure participants having a significantly higher average PCL-R total than the other two groups. Full-scale IQ did not correlate with either the total score or any of the factor scores. In separate publications, these authors found that while PCL-R scores predicted treatment progress with higher scoring individuals showing poorer progression (Morrissey, Mooney, Hogue, Lindsay & Taylor 2007), the instrument did not predict aggressive behaviour over the subsequent 12 months (Morrissey *et al.*, 2007). Therefore, while the PCL-R showed some clinical utility in terms of predicting progress through treatment, it was less successful in predicting future violent incidents.

DYNAMIC/PROXIMAL RISK ASSESSMENT

As with static/historical risk assessment, there have been a considerable number of developments with dynamic/immediate risk assessment variables and their predictive validity. In their evaluation of the predictive utility of a range of candidate variables, Lindsay, Elliot and Astell (2004) included both historical and proximal variables. This study was specifically on sexual offenders with ID and sexual offence recidivism and it included 15 historical variables and 35 proximal/dynamic variables drawn from previous research. They found that a number of dynamic variables were significantly correlated with re-offending, including antisocial attitude, low self-esteem, lack of assertiveness, allowances made by staff, staff complacency, poor response to treatment, attitudes tolerant of sexual crimes and erratic attendance. In a subsequent regression analysis which investigated the variables which predicted sexual recidivism, the variables with the strongest predictive power were allowances made by staff, antisocial attitude and poor relationship with mother. As can be seen, two of these variables are dynamic, related to staff supervision and the offenders antisocial attitudes.

Antisocial attitudes emerged again as an important dynamic predictor of recidivism in the study by Quinsey, Book and Skilling (2004). They investigated the predictive value of a number of dynamic risk indicators using an experimental design employed previously by Quinsey, Coleman, Jones and Altrows (1997). In this, they gathered monthly ratings of client behaviours on antisociality, psychotic symptoms, poor compliance, mood problems, antisocial behaviour, medication compliance and denial of problems. Because they had monthly ratings of behaviour and also recorded incidents, they could correlate each month's ratings with problem incidence. They argued that the ratings taken on the month of the incident might be influenced by the fact that an incident was occurring or had occurred but that this would be impossible for ratings taken in the month prior to the incident. They found that client's risk scores increased in the month before incidents occurred. They found that for any incident (including sexual incidents) there were significant increases in the month prior to the incident for ratings of psychotic behaviour, inappropriate and antisocial behaviour, mood problems, social withdrawal, dynamic antisociality and denial. The most significant of these was antisocial behaviour which had predictive validity even when other variables were controlled in the statistical analysis. Therefore, antisocial behaviour and antisocial attitude appear to have significant predictive value as dynamic variables in relation to future sexual incidents.

Boer, Tough and Haaven (2004) outlined a number of variables which they considered to be important in the structured assessment of future recidivism for sex offenders with ID. These fall into four categories: stable dynamic (staff and environment), acute dynamic (staff and environment), stable dynamic (offenders) and acute dynamic (offenders). In total, they reviewed 30 dynamic variables including such items as communication among supervisory staff, client specific knowledge of staff, new staff entering the clinical team, monitoring of the offender by staff, attitudes towards compliance of the offender, mental health problems, relationship skills, impulsiveness, changes in social support, changes in substance abuse and coping strategies of the offender. They did not provide any empirical support for the model and it is likely that with 30 dynamic variables there would be a significant amount colinearity among the variables with some redundancy. However, as a theoretical framework it is a useful beginning to the consideration of the important aspects for current management of sexual offenders with ID.

In another development on dynamic risk assessment for offenders with ID, Lindsay, Elliot and Astell (2004) used the same experimental design as Quinsey, Book and Skilling (2004) but shortened the time periods to days rather than months. They developed the Dynamic Risk Assessment and Management System (DRAMS), which employed a similar set of variables to previous studies, including mood, antisocial behaviour, aberrant thoughts, psychotic symptoms, self-regulation, therapeutic alliance, substance abuse, compliance, emotional relationships and victim access. Since their participants were drawn from a high secure setting, there were no opportunities for substance abuse or victim access. By gathering daily ratings of participant behaviour they were able to relate them to independently collected incident data. They found that for individual participants ratings taken on the day before an incident were significantly higher than ratings taken at least seven days distant from any incident. The significant variables were mood, antisocial behaviour, aberrant thoughts and total score. In a subsequent, larger scale study, Steptoe, Lindsay, Murphy and Young (2008) found that sections of mood, antisocial behaviour and intolerance/agreeableness had significant predictive values with future incidents (auc > 0.70) and there were highly significant differences with large effect sizes between assessments taken one or two days prior to an incident and the control assessments conducted at least seven days from an incident. While this study was conducted on the prediction of violent incidents, it reinforces the importance of dynamic variables and in particular dynamic antisociality in relation to future incidents for offenders with ID.

A final recent development has been related to another finding from the Harris, Rice and Quinsey (1993) original work. In addition to examining the predictive value of the historical/ actuarial variables, in their study they also found that both 'attitudes unfavourable to convention' and 'pro-criminal values' showed highly significant differences between recidivists and non-recidivists. Thornton (2002) has also incorporated antisocial attitudes into his framework for assessing dynamic risk in sex offenders and has shown the difference between sex offenders and non-sex offenders on attitudes supportive of sexual offending. Several measures have been developed to asses such attitudes in this client group, and Kolton, Boer and Boer (2001) have shown that an adapted version of the Abel and Becker Cognitions Scale, a scale for measuring attitudes towards sexual relationships with children, could be used reliably with offenders with ID. Lindsay, Whitefield and Carson (2007) reported on the Questionnaire on Attitudes Consistent with Sex Offending (QACSO), which is an instrument designed to be used with offenders with ID. The QACSO has seven scales and assesses attitudes in the areas of rape, exhibitionism, voyeurism, dating abuse, stalking, homosexual assault and offences against children. They demonstrated that it had an appropriate reading age (although all items are read to clients), good reliability, good internal consistency and discriminated between sexual offenders and non-offenders. Several treatment studies have found that it is sensitive to change after treatment (Rose, Anderson, Hawkins & Rose, 2007, Lindsay & Smith, 1998) and its specific scales have been found to differentiate between offenders against adults and offenders against children (Lindsay, Steele, Smith, Quinn & Allan, 2006). Therefore there are assessments which are sensitive and appropriate for this aspect of risk in sex offenders with ID.

CONCLUSIONS

There have been a significant number of developments in the evaluation of risk assessment for sex offenders and general offenders with ID. The available studies suggest that risk assessments based on actuarial variables predict violent and sexual incidents at least as well as they do in mainstream offender groups. The study by Gray, Fitzgerald, Taylor, MacCulloch and Snowden (2007) found that the HCR-20 historical items showed superior predictive accuracy on offenders with ID when compared to mainstream offenders. These results were for general and violent offending rather than sexual offending but suggest that risk assessments are likely to be as valid for this client group as they are for mainstream criminal populations. For the PCL-R, Morrissey *et al.* (2007) and Morrissey, Mooney, Hogue, Lindsay and Taylor (2007) found that the instrument was less successful in predicting future violence over a period of one year but was related to treatment progress.

Dynamic variables are important considerations for the population of offenders with ID. A number of studies have found that dynamic risk assessment provides additional predictive value and that dynamic variables may be as useful as distal variables in predicting future incidents. Therefore, while the research on risk assessment for sex offenders with ID is at an early stage there have already been significant advances adding to knowledge which can be used in a most practical fashion.

REFERENCES

Andrews, D.A. (1989). Recidivism is predictable and can be influenced: Using risk assessments to reduce recidivism. *Forum on Corrections Research, 1,* 11–18.

Barbaree, H.E., Seto, M.C., Langton, C.M. & Peacock, E.J. (2001). Evaluating the predictive accuracy of six risk assessment instruments for adult sex offenders. *Criminal Justice & Behaviour, 28,* 490–521.

Bartosh, D.L., Garby, T., Lewis, D. & Gray, S. (2003). Differences in the predictive validity of actuarial risk assessments in relation to sex offender type. *International Journal of Offender Therapy & Comparative Criminology, 47,* 422–38.

Boer, D.P., Hart, S.D., Kropp, P.R. & Webster, C.D. (1997). *Manual for the sexual violence risk – 20: Professional guidelines for assessing risk of sexual violence.* Vancouver, British Columbia: British Columbia Institute on Family Violence & Mental Health, Law & Policy Institute, Simon Fraser University.

Boer, D.P., Tough, S. & Haaven, J. (2004). Assessment of risk manageability of developmentally disabled sex offenders. *Journal of Applied Research in Intellectual Disabilities, 17,* 275–84.

Epperson, D.L., Kaul, J.D., Huot, S.J., Hesselton, D., Alexander, W. & Goldman, R. (1998). *Minnesota sex offender screening tool–revised (MnSOST-R).* St Paul: Minnesota Department of Corrections.

Gray, N.S., Fitzgerald, S., Taylor, J., MacCulloch, M.J. & Snowden, R.J. (2007). Predicting future reconviction in offenders with intellectual disabilities: The predictive efficacy of VRAG, PCL-SV and the HCR-20. *Psychological Assessment, 19,* 474–9.

Hanson, R.K. (1997). *The development of a brief actuarial risk scale for sexual offence recidivism.* (User report 1997-04). Ottawa: Department of the Solicitor General of Canada.

Hanson, R.K. & Thornton, D. (1999). *Static-99: Improving actuarial risk assessments for sex offenders.* (User report 1999-02). Ottawa: Department of the Solicitor General of Canada.

Hanson, R.K. & Thornton, D. (2003). *Notes on the development of the Static-2002.* (User report 2003-01). Ottowa: Department of the Solicitor General of Canada.

Hare, R.D. (1991). *The Hare Psychopathy Checklist – revised.* Toronto, Ontario: Multi-Health Systems.

Harris, G.T., Rice, M.E. & Quinsey, V.L. (1993). Violent recidivism of mentally disordered offenders: The development of a statistical prediction instrument. *Criminal Justice & Behaviour, 20,* 315–35.

Harris, G.T., Rice, M.E., Quinsey, V.L., Lalumiere, M.L., Boer, D. & Lang, C. (2003). A multi-site comparison of actuarial risk instruments for sex offenders. *Psychological Assessment, 15,* 413–25.

Hart, S.D., Cox, D.N. & Hare, R.D. (1995). *The Hare PCL:SV.* Toronto, Ontario: Multi-Health Systems.

Hart, S., Michie, S. & Cooke D. (2007). Precision of actuarial risk assessment instruments. *The British Journal of Psychiatry 190,* s60–s65.

Hogue, T.E., Steptoe, L., Taylor, J.L., Lindsay, W.R., Mooney, P., Pinkney, L., Johnston, S., Smith, A.H.W. & O'Brian, G. (2006). A comparison of offenders with intellectual disability across three levels of security. *Criminal Behaviour & Mental Health, 16,* 13–28.

Kolton, D.J. C., Boer, A. & Boer, D.P. (2001). A revision of the Abel and Becker cognition scale for intellectually disabled sexual offenders. *Sexual Abuse: A Journal of Research & Treatment, 13,* 217–19.

Kroner, D.G. & Mills, J.F. (2001). The accuracy of five risk appraisal instruments in predicting institutional misconduct and new convictions. *Criminal Justice & Behaviour, 28,* 471–89.

Langton, C.M., Barbaree, H.E., Seto, M.C., Peacock, E.J., Harkins, L. & Hanson, K.T. (2007). Actuarial assessment of risk for re-offence amongst adult sex offenders: Evaluating the predictive accuracy of the Static-2002 and five other instruments. *Criminal Justice & Behaviour, 24,* 37–59.

Lindsay, W.R. & Beail, N. (2004). Risk assessment: Actuarial prediction and clinical judgement of offending incidents and behaviour for intellectual disability services. *Journal of Applied Research in Intellectual Disabilities, 17,* 229–34.

Lindsay, W.R., Elliot, S.F. & Astell, A. (2004). Predictors of sexual offence recidivism in offenders with intellectual disabilities. *Journal of Applied Research in Intellectual Disabilities, 17,* 299–305.

Lindsay, W.R., Hogue, T., Taylor, J.L., Steptoe, L., Mooney, P., Johnston, S., O'Brien, G. & Smith, A.H. W. (2008). Risk assessment in offenders with intellectual disabilities: A comparison across three levels of security. *International Journal of Offender Therapy & Comparative Criminology, 52*, 90–111.

Lindsay, W.R., Law, J., Quinn, K., Smart, N. & Smith, A.H. W. (2001). A comparison of physical and sexual abuse histories: Sexual and non-sexual offenders with intellectual disability. *Child Abuse & Neglect, 25*, 989–95.

Lindsay, W.R., Michie, A.M., Whitefield, E., Martin, V., Grieve, A. & Carson, D. (2006). Response patterns on the questionnaire on attitudes consistent with sexual offending in groups of sex offenders with intellectual disability. *Journal of Applied Research in Intellectual Disabilities, 19*, 47–54.

Lindsay, W.R., Murphy, L., Smith, G., Murphy, D., Edwards, Z., Grieve, A., Chettock, C. & Young, S.J. (2004). The dynamic risk assessment and management system: An assessment of immediate risk of violence for individuals with intellectual disabilities, and offending and challenging behaviour.

Lindsay, W.R. & Smith, A.H.W. (1998). Responses to treatment for sex offenders with intellectual disability: A comparison of men with 1 and 2 year probation sentences. *Journal of Intellectual Disability Research, 42*, 346–53.

Lindsay, W.R., Steele, L., Smith, A.H.W., Quinn, K. & Allan, R. (2006). A community forensic intellectual disability service: Twelve year follow-up of referrals, *analysis of referral patterns and assessment of harm reduction. Legal & Criminological Psychology, 11*, 113–30.

Lindsay, W.R., Whitefield, E. & Carson, D. (2007). The development of a questionnaire to measure cognitive distortions in sex offenders with intellectual disability. *Legal & Criminological Psychology, 12*, 55–68.

Marsa, F., O'Reilly, G., Carr, A., Murphy, P., O'Sullivan, M., Cotter, A. & Hevey, D. (2004). Attachment styles and psychological profiles of sex offenders in Ireland. *Journal of Interpersonal Violence, 19* (2), 228–51.

Marshall, W.L. (1989). *Pornography and sex offenders*. In D. Zillmann & J. Bryant (Eds), *Pornography: Recent research, interpretations and policy considerations* (pp. 185–214). Hillsdale, NJ: Lawrence Erlbaum.

Morrissey, C., Hogue, T., Mooney, P., Allen, C., Johnston, S., Hollin, C., Lindsay, W.R. & Taylor, J. (2007). Predictive validity of the PCL-R in offenders with intellectual disabilities in a high secure setting: Institutional aggression. *Journal of Forensic Psychology & Psychiatry, 18*, 1–15.

Morrissey, C., Hogue, T., Mooney, P., Lindsay, W.R., Steptoe, L., Taylor, J.L. & Johnston, S. (2005). Applicability, reliability and validity of the Psychopathy Checklist – Revised in offenders with intellectual disabilities: Some initial findings. *International Journal of Forensic Mental Health, 4*, 207–20.

Morrissey, C., Mooney, P., Hogue, T., Lindsay, W.R. & Taylor, J.L. (2007). Predictive validity of psychopathy in offenders with intellectual disabilities in a high security hospital: Treatment progress. *Journal of Intellectual & Developmental Disabilities, 32*, 125–33.

Novaco, R.W. & Taylor, J.L. (2008). Anger and assaultiveness of male forensic patients with developmental disabilities: Links to volatile parents. *Aggressive Behaviour, 34*, 380–93.

Patterson, G.R. (1986). Performance models for antisocial boys. *American Psychologist, 41*, 432–44.

Patterson, G.R. & Yoerger, K. (1997). A developmental model for late onset delinquency. In D.W. Osgood (ed.), *Motivation and delinquency* (pp. 119–77). Lincoln: University of Nebrasca Press.

Quinsey, V. (2007). Old saws and modern instances: On not making inferences based on 'group data'. *Crime Scene, 14* (2), 3.

Quinsey, V.L., Book, A. & Skilling, T.A. (2004). A follow-up of deinstitutionalised men with intellectual disabilities and histories of antisocial behaviour. *Journal of Applied Research in Intellectual Disabilities, 17*, 243–54.

Quinsey, V.L., Coleman, G., Jones, B. & Altrows, I. (1997). Proximal antecedents of eloping and re-offending among supervised mentally disordered offenders. *Journal of Interpersonal Violence, 12*, 794–813.

Quinsey, V.L., Harris, G.T., Rice, M.E. & Cormier, C.A. (1998). *Violent offenders: Appraising and managing risk*. Washington, DC: American Psychological Association.

Quinsey, V.L., Harris, G.T., Rice, M.E. & Cormier, C.A. (2005). *Violent offenders, appraisal and managing risk: Second edition*. Washington, DC: American Psychological Association.

Rose, J., Anderson, C., Hawkins, C. & Rose, D. (2007). A community based sex offender treatment group for adults with intellectual disabilities. Paper presented to the World Congress of Behavioural and Cognitive Psychotherapy, Barcelona.

Sjostedt, G. & Langstrom, N. (2002). Assessment of risk for criminal recidivism among rapists: A comparison of four different measures. *Psychology, Crime & Law, 8*, 25–40.

Snyder, J.J. & Patterson, G.R. (1995). Individual differences in social aggression: A test of a reinforcement model of socialisation in the natural environment. *Behaviour Therapy, 26*, 371–91.

Steptoe, L., Lindsay, W.R., Murphy, L. & Young, S.J. (2008). Construct validity, reliability and predictive validity of the Dynamic Risk Assessment and Management System (DRAMS) in offenders with intellectual disability. *Legal & Criminological Psychology*.

Stirpe, T., Abracen, J., Stermac, L. & Wilson, R. (2006). Sexual offenders' state-of-mind regarding childhood attachment: A controlled investigation. *Sexual Abuse: A Journal of Research and Treatment, 18*, 289–302.

Taylor, J.L., Lindsay, W.R., Hogue, T.E., Mooney, P., Steptoe, L., Johnston, S. & O'Brien, G. (2008). Use of the HCR-20 in offenders with intellectual disability. Paper presented to the Annual Conference of the Forensic Division of the British Psychological Society, Edinburgh.

Thornton, D. (2002). Constructing and testing a framework for dynamic risk assessment. *Sexual Abuse: A Journal of Research & Treatment, 14*, 139–53.

Thornton, D., Mann, R., Webster, S., Blud, L., Travers, R., Friendship, C. & Erikson, M. (2003). Distinguishing and combining risks for sexual and violent recidivism. *Annals of the New York Academy of Sciences, 989*, 225–35.

Ward, T., Hudson, S.M. & Marshall, W.L. (1996). Attachment style in sex offenders: A preliminary study. *Journal of Sex Research, 33*, 17–26.

Ward, T. & Keenan, T. (1999). Child molesters implicit theories. *Journal of Interpersonal Violence, 14*, 821–38.

Webster, C.D., Eaves, D., Douglas, K.S. & Wintrup, A. (1995). *The HCR-20: The assessment of dangerousness and risk*. Vancouver, Canada: Simon Fraser University and British Colombia Forensic Psychiatric Services Commission.

Wood, E. & Riggs, S. (2008). Predictors of child molestation. *Journal of Interpersonal Violence, 23*, 259–75.

9

Psychopathy and other Personality Disorders in Sexual Offenders with Intellectual Disabilities

CATRIN MORRISSEY

INTRODUCTION

The presence of personality disorder can be an important factor when intervening with sexual offenders and may have an impact on case formulation, treatment approaches and on risk assessment. This chapter aims to provide an overview of the relevant literature related to personality disorder, and psychopathy in particular, both for forensic populations in general and for those with intellectual disabilities (ID). The assessment and treatment considerations for those individuals with ID who sexually offend and who may also have personality disorder will be outlined.

What is Personality Disorder?

According to DSM-IV-TR (American Psychiatric Association, 2000), personality disorder is 'an enduring pattern of inner experience and behaviour that deviates markedly from the expectations of the individual's culture' (p. 685). Such patterns are inflexible and pervasive across a broad range of personal and social situations, with symptoms usually evident from childhood or adolescence, and significantly affect the individual's lifetime functioning.

A personality disorder can be manifested in an individual's cognition, affective response, interpersonal functioning and impulse control. DSM-IV-TR classifies 10 specific personality disorders in three clusters: those characterised as primarily odd and eccentric (Cluster A: Paranoid, Schizoid and Schizotypal); those classified as dramatic or erratic (Cluster B:

Assessment and Treatment of Sexual Offenders with Intellectual Disabilities: A Handbook
Edited by Leam A. Craig, William R. Lindsay and Kevin D. Browne
© 2010 John Wiley & Sons, Ltd.

Antisocial, Borderline, Histrionic and Narcissistic) and those which are principally anxious or fearful in nature (Cluster C: Avoidant, Dependent and Obsessive).

DSM-IV also includes a category Personality Disorder (Not Otherwise Specified), in which there are features of more than one disorder but the features do not meet the full criteria for any specific personality disorder. It should be acknowledged that concerns have nevertheless been raised about the reliability and validity of these categorical personality disorder classifications (e.g., Alwin, Blackburn, Davidson, Hilton, Logan & Shine, 2006; Costa & McRae, 1999; Livesley, 2001), as well as those of other nosological systems such as ICD-10 (World Health Organization, 1992), with arguments being made for a dimensional approach.

Closely related to DSM-IV Antisocial Personality Disorder (APD) (and Dissocial Personality Disorder, a parallel disorder in ICD-10) is the clinical construct of *psychopathy*. This construct extends the primarily behavioural concepts in APD to include further aspects of affective and interpersonal functioning. As defined by Cleckley (1941), 'psychopaths' are emotionally defective and shallow, lacking characteristics such as anxiety, empathy, guilt and remorse. Interpersonally, they are grandiose, deceitful, manipulative and egocentric, but also superficially charming. Their behaviour is irresponsible and impulsive and they fail to profit from experience or to respond to punishment. Psychopathy has a long history in clinical psychopathology (Millon, Simonsen, Morton Birket-Smith & Davis, 1998), but despite its apparent significance it does not appear as a separate disorder in either of the main diagnostic systems. There has been considerable debate concerning exactly how the psychopathy construct fits with that of DSM-IV APD (e.g., Blair, Mitchell & Blair, 2005; Hare, 2003; Lykken, 1995; Skilling, Harris, Rice & Quinsey, 2002). However, there is broad agreement that psychopathy describes a much smaller subset (probably less than 25 per cent) of those who meet APD criteria (Blair, Mitchell & Blair, 2005; Hare, 2003). The modern conceptualisation of psychopathy is, therefore, as a specific and severe type of personality disorder (Hart & Hemphill, 2002; Cooke, Michie, Hart & Clarke, 2005). Since the early 1990s, the psychopathy construct has become synonymous with the Psychopathy Checklist – Revised (PCL-R) (Hare, 1991, 2003), a widely validated measure of psychopathy. The PCL-R is a 20-item checklist, which reflects a superordinate construct of psychopathy underpinned by two factors and four facets of the disorder: interpersonal and affective traits contribute to Factor 1; and lifestyle manifestations, such as impulsivity and irresponsibility, and persistent antisocial behaviour, contribute to Factor 2 (see Figure 9.1).

Personality Disorders in Forensic Populations

Unsurprisingly, personality disorders with antisocial and psychopathic features are strongly associated with criminal behaviour. Fazel and Danesh (2002) reviewed 62 studies of prison inmates and concluded that around 46 per cent of prisoners have APD. In high security psychiatric hospitals in the UK an even higher incidence of APD is reported (Blackburn, Logan, Donnelly & Renwick, 2003). Where psychopathy is concerned, around 15–20 per cent of male prisoners in the USA, and around 5–15 per cent of those in the UK are classified as psychopathic using the PCL-R (Hare, 2003). Among forensic psychiatric patients in North America, again around 15 per cent are classified as psychopathic, and as many as a third of a sample of high security psychiatric hospital patients in

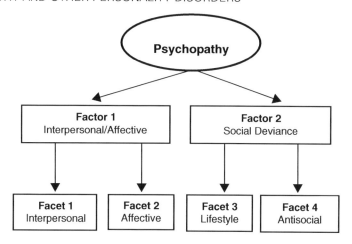

Figure 9.1 The scale structure of the PCL-R, 2nd edn (from Hare, 2003)

the UK have been reported to have elevated PCL-R scores (Blackburn, Logan, Donnelly & Renwick, 2003).

There is known to be a very robust relationship between future violence and APDs, psychopathy in particular. There have been several meta-analytic reviews of this relationship (e.g., Salekin, Rogers & Sewell, 1996; Hemphill, Hare & Wong, 1998; Walters, 2003), all of which have established clearly that psychopathy significantly increases the risk of both general and violent re-offending, in prisoners, forensic psychiatric and civil psychiatric populations. As a result of this body of evidence, psychopathy is a heavily weighted item in a number of violence risk prediction instruments, These include the Violence Risk Appraisal Guide (VRAG) (Quinsey, Rice, Harris & Cormier, 1998) and the Historical Clinical Risk – 20 (HCR-20) (Webster, Douglas, Eaves & Hart, 1997), as well as in some assessments of sexual violence risk (e.g., the Sexual Violence Risk – 20 (SVR-20) (Boer, Hart & Kropp, 1997) and the Sexual Offending Risk Appraisal Guide (SORAG) (Quinsey, Rice, Harris & Cormier, 1998)F. see earlier question on order). Notably, evidence of any personality disorder is also weighted in these assessments.

Sexual Offending

The relationship between personality disorder and sexual offending is less clear than that between personality disorder and violence. The literature is again focussed on psychopathy as opposed to other personality disorders. The PCL-R measure tends to be only weakly or inconsistently related to the number of convictions or charges for sexual offences (Cooke, 1995; Quinsey, Rice & Harris, 1995), and Hare (2003) acknowledges that psychopathy is more strongly associated with general and violent re-offending than with sexual offending. Nevertheless, several pieces of research have indicated that there is an important sub-group of sexual offenders who are psychopathic and who present a particularly high risk. These are typically generalised offenders whose sexual offences are part of a wider repertoire of offending which involves instrumental violence and violating the rights of others. It has been consistently found that rapists of adult females have significantly higher PCL-R scores than sex offenders who solely offend against children (e.g., Forth & Kroner, 1994; Olver & Wong, 2006; Porter, Fairweather, Drugge, Herve, Birt & Boer, 2000). Such psychopathic rapists are generally opportunistic offenders with criminally versatile histories. Interestingly, in the study by Porter and colleagues of a diverse sample of imprisoned sex offenders it was found that a particularly high proportion (64 per cent) of offenders who had victimised *both* children and adults were psychopaths, suggesting that psychopaths tend to cross boundaries between victim groups. Furthermore, those convicted of sexual homicides have also been found to have high levels of psychopathic traits (Firestone, Bradford, Greenberg & Larose, 1998; Porter, Woodworth, Earle, Drugge & Boer, 2003).

There is a further body of research which indicates that sex offenders with a combination of a deviant sexual arousal pattern and a high level of psychopathic traits are at particularly high risk of sexual recidivism. Rice and Harris (1997) investigated the interaction of deviant sexual arousal (as measured by a preference for inappropriate sexual stimuli using the penile plethysmograph (PPG)) and psychopathy when following up a sample of 288 sex offenders. They found that 70 per cent of those who were both defined as psychopathic and had deviant sexual arousal committed a new sexual offence within five years in comparison with around 40 per cent in other groups. Similarly, Serin, Mailloux and Malcolm (2001) followed 68 sexual offenders for seven years, and found that those higher on psychopathic traits and with sexual deviance offended at more than four times the rate of those low on psychopathy and without sexual deviance. Measuring sexual deviance on a rating scale, as opposed to physiologically, Olver and Wong (2006) and Hildebrand, de Ruiter and Vogel (2004) also found that the combination of psychopathy and higher ratings of deviant arousal was associated with a significantly higher rate of sexual recidivism. It therefore seems that the presence of deviant sexual arousal combined with the thrill seeking, interpersonal manipulation and lack of empathy characteristic of psychopathy is particularly likely to lead to repeated sexual offending.

Personality Disorder and Treatment

Given its lifelong nature, personality disorder is generally believed to be very resistant to change, and therefore difficult to treat successfully. Less severe personality disorders may, however, respond to certain types of theoretically coherent, intensive and longer term treatment (Alwin, Blackburn, Davidson, Hilton, Logan & Shine, 2006; Bateman & Fonagy, 2006; Bateman & Tyrer, 2004; Blackburn, 2000), although there are few well controlled studies. Psychopathy in particular has long been associated with clinical pessimism regarding treatment outcome (Cleckley, 1941; McCord & McCord, 1964). In fact, a relatively small number of studies have explicitly examined the predictive power of psychopathy diagnoses in relation to response to treatment, and few studies have been methodologically rigorous (for reviews see D'Silva, Duggan & McCarthy, 2004; Harris & Rice, 2006; Salekin, 2002). On the whole, however, the studies that have been done indicate that psychopaths perform more poorly on outcome measures such as motivation (Hildebrand, 2004), reported improvement (e.g., Ogloff, Wong & Greenwood, 1990) and behaviour in treatment (Hobson, Shine & Roberts, 2000) as well as in terms of re-offending post treatment (e.g., Rice, Harris & Cormier, 1992; Hare, Clark, Thornton & Grann, 2000; Seto & Barbaree, 1999). The latter three studies even suggest that re-offending may be at *higher* rates among those psychopaths who have undergone treatment than among those who have not. In the Seto and Barbaree study, those psychopaths who were perceived to have had 'successful' treatment offended at the highest rate, although follow-up studies have cast doubt on the validity of such findings (Barbaree, 2005).

As with other psychopathic offenders, sex offenders with psychopathy appear to be difficult to treat successfully. Following sex offender treatment they recidivate more seriously and more quickly than other sex offenders (Barbaree, Seto & Langton, 2001; Hildebrand, de Ruiter & Vogel, 2004; Looman, Abracen, Serin & Marquis, 2005), although this recidivism may not necessarily be sexual in nature. Sex offenders high in psychopathy also commit institutional misdemeanours more frequently than non-psychopathic sex offenders and are therefore more difficult to manage in treatment contexts (Buffington-Vollum, Edens, Johnston & Johnston (2002)). Despite this, Langevin (2006) found that those with higher PCL-R scores were more likely to enter treatment than other sex offenders.

Notwithstanding the more positive outlook for treatment of psychopathic offenders expressed by Salekin (2002), it can be reasonably concluded that there is as yet no firm evidence that there are treatments which are effective for psychopaths, and there are some strong indications that they are more difficult to treat effectively than other offenders.

PERSONALITY DISORDER AND INTELLECTUAL DISABILITY

General Issues

It could be argued that understanding of personality disorder is as important for people with ID as for any other clinical population (Reid, Lindsay, Law & Sturmey, 2004). However, in common with other psychiatric disorders, diagnosis of personality disorders in ID populations has suffered from 'diagnostic overshadowing' (Reiss, Levitan & Syszko, 1983; Mason & Scior, 2004), a process whereby the disability 'masks' the recognition of other disorders. It is only since the mid 1990s that detailed consideration has been given to assessment and diagnosis of personality disorders in this group (e.g., Flynn, Matthews & Hollis, 2002; Goldberg, Gitta & Puddephatt, 1995; Khan, Cowan & Roy, 1997; Lindsay *et al.*, 2006; Lindsay, 2007; Naik, Gangadharan & Alexander, 2002; Torr, 2003). Alexander and Cooray (2003) have reviewed the evidence in this field and have concluded that the diagnosis of personality disorders in ID is a complex and difficult area, particularly for those with more severe disability. They observed, from studies using a variety of instruments, that prevalence estimates of personality disorder vary widely, and they judged this variation in estimates to be too great to be explained by real differences. Instead they attributed the variation to a range of difficulties with assessment of personality disorder in this group. Firstly, methodological problems were identified which relate both to the reliability of the assessment instruments and to the validity of the diagnostic criteria in this population. Secondly, it was argued that the communication, physical and sensory difficulties of some people with ID affect the ease with which a personality disorder can be assessed and diagnosed. Lastly, the reviewers observed that there is a problem with the overlap of behaviour commonly occurring in ID (e.g., self-harm; impulsivity; affective lability) and key features of certain personality disorders, and that in particular there is lack of clarity about the boundaries between personality disorders, Pervasive Developmental Disorders (PDD) and behaviour disorders. Fundamentally, as Lindsay (2007) has noted, the delayed development of people with ID will result in less completely developed personalities, and it is therefore debatable whether personality disorder can be accurately diagnosed in some cases.

In response to these diagnostic problems, the early 2000s have seen the production of supplements and guidelines to the main diagnostic systems for psychiatric criteria in ID, including for personality disorder. The Diagnostic Criteria in Learning Disability (DC-LD; Royal College of Psychiatrists, 2001) supplements ICD-10. A parallel set of guidelines for DSM-IV-TR, the *Diagnostic manual – ID* (DM-ID) (Fletcher, Luschen, Stavrakaki & First, 2007), has a chapter on personality disorders (Lindsay, Gabriel, Dana, Young & Dosen, 2007). DC-LD is explicit that a diagnosis of personality disorder should be precluded if the disturbance is a direct consequence of the severity of the ID, and that diagnosis should only be made when personality characteristics seem to be the most important factor driving the behaviour. A diagnosis of personality disorder in severe/ profound ID is considered inadvisable, and in both DC-LD and DM-ID, the minimum age of diagnosis is increased to 21 years to take into account the fact that the developmental phase for lasting personality characteristics is longer in people with ID. Slight changes to specific criteria are made: for example, in DM-ID the pre-15 criteria for conduct disorder within APD is increased to 18 years. As of 2010, however, no substantial studies have been published using DC-LD or DM-ID criteria, and their reliability and validity has not as yet been established.

While diagnosis of any kind of personality disorder in people with ID continues to be problematic, the general consensus in this developing area is that work furthering understanding of personality disorder in this population is important, with development of valid and reliable assessment instruments being a priority.

Antisocial Personality Disorders in Offenders with Intellectual Disabilities

The literature certainly suggests that an understanding of APDs and psychopathy may have relevance to some offenders who also have ID. Since 2000, a number of groups of researchers, primarily in the UK, have begun to examine these aspects of functioning in this population. For example, Lindsay *et al.*, (2006) assessed personality disorder in a sample of 164 males in ID forensic health settings in the UK (mean full scale IQ = 66), covering community-based, low, medium and high security services. This important study, assessed personality disorder using a DSM-IV criteria checklist conducted from three perspectives using a file review, clinician ratings and nurse observations and also the Structured Assessment of Personality (Pilgrim & Mann 1990), completed by care staff. A 'consensus' rating was used to diagnose personality disorder. Total prevalence of personality disorder in this forensic sample was 39.5 per cent, with the high security sample predictably having a significantly higher level of such diagnoses (57 per cent). Inter-rater reliability between file and clinician derived ratings was reported to be good. APD was by far the largest category of personality disorder, followed by Personality Disorder (Not Otherwise Specified). Formal existing diagnoses of personality disorder on clinical files were evident in only 22.6 per cent of cases (Morrissey, 2006a), suggesting that, even in this forensic population, under-diagnosis of personality disorder was prevalent. As part of the same study the authors also examined the relationship between degree of personality disorder and several risk assessment instruments. They grouped participants according to the extent to which they met the criteria for 'severe personality disorder' as defined by high PCL-R scores (over 25) and/or number of personality disorder diagnoses.[1] Fourteen percent of the sample met at least one of the criteria for severe personality disorder. Those with severe personality disorder had higher scores on the VRAG risk assessment although, as personality disorder and psychopathy are items weighted heavily in the VRAG, this particular relationship is unsurprising. There was also a strong relationship with the Risk Matrix 2000-Violence (Thornton, Mann, R., Webster, Blud, Travers & Friendship, 2003) (which is not weighted by personality disorder diagnoses) and to a lesser extent with the sex offence risk measures the STATIC-99 (Hanson & Thornton, 2000) and Risk Matrix 2000-Sex. Although it is important to point out that this study does not establish a relationship between personality disorder and actual recidivism in people with ID but only with risk prediction *measures*, these findings nevertheless provide some initial validation for the construct of severe personality disorder in this client group.

Alexander, Crouch, Halstead and Pichaud (2006), however, provided some evidence that a diagnosis of personality disorder does indeed increase risk in this population. They examined two cohorts of patients discharged over a 12-year period from a UK medium-secure service for people with ID. In the first 33 per cent (n = 27) and in the second 21 per cent (n = 40) had an ICD-10 diagnosis of personality disorder. Dissocial Personality Disorder (similar to DSM-IV APD) was again the most common diagnosis in these groups. Importantly, diagnosis of personality disorder was one of the factors that significantly increased the risk of reconviction in this ID sample, suggesting that among such offenders in mainstream populations personality disorder is predictor of re-offending risk.

Psychopathy

In his classic early work on psychopathy, Cleckley (1941) specified that *superficial charm and good intelligence* were among the key characteristics of the condition, and explicitly distinguished between a patient who was 'mentally defective' and one who was psychopathic. Nevertheless, the findings of most studies that have investigated the relationship between global intelligence and the PCL-R measure (e.g., Hart & Hare, 1989; Hart, Forth & Hare, 1990; Shine & Hobson, 1997) have led Hare (2003) to conclude that the total score is essentially uncorrelated with standard measures of intelligence. This said, more recent worked has uncovered a differential relationship between intelligence and the various facets of psychopathy (Vitacco, Neumann & Jackson, 2005; Vitacco, Neumann & Wodusheck, 2008), so the relationship may be more complex than was previously thought.

In contrast to Cleckley's position, since the development of the PCL-R there has been widespead acknowledgement of the co-morbidity of psychopathy with other disorders (Brinkley, Newman, Widiger & Lynam, 2004) and there therefore seems to be no valid argument for excluding those with ID from psychopathy assessment. Accordingly, the three-site study described above also examined psychopathy using the PCL-R, rated from file review and an

---

[1] 'Severe personality disorder' is an administrative concept used in the UK in relation to management of people who are dangerous and have severe personality disorder (DSPD) (Home Office & Department of Health, 1999).

interview with the responsible clinician, for 203 cases (see Morrissey *et al.*, 2005; Morrissey, 2006a). It was acknowledged by this study that there were both conceptual and practical difficulties with using the PCL-R in this population, which reflect the problems identified by Alexander and Cooray in relation to personality disorder more generally. These problems include differences in the presentation of the core characteristics of the disorder as a result of communication and adaptive deficits; confusion between symptoms arising from intellectual limitations and those arising from psychopathy; restricted opportunities to manifest all the characteristics of psychopathy as a result of lower levels of adaptive functioning; and problems with the client interview as a methodology with this population. In response to these practical and theoretical difficulties, Morrissey (2003, 2006b) developed practice guidelines for using the PCL-R with offenders with ID which were employed in the three-site study and subsequently revised following a series of validation studies (see Morrissey, 2006a; Morrissey *et al.*, 2007; Morrissey, Mooney, Hogue, Lindsay & Taylor 2007).

Internal consistency for the PCL-R total score was reported to be reasonable (alpha = 0.82), and inter-rater reliability for the total score using this methodology was also good (ICC = 0.89). Although adequate, internal reliability coefficients were lower for the sub-scales representing antisocial behaviour and lifestyle facets of psychopathy (alpha = 0.62-0.64), a finding which may be explained by the interpretation of the items in the context of restricted occupational and social functioning of people with ID. Convergent and discriminant validity of the PCL-R was found to be broadly similar to that observed in other male offender populations and, overall, PCL-R scores were associated in expected ways with most of the available criterion variables. Moreover, it was found that the PCL-R score was not associated with IQ, suggesting that the scale is not measuring an aspect of global cognitive functioning within this lower ability group. As expected, the scale was positively associated with prior antisocial behaviour and with recent externalising behaviour problems, and those with high PCL-R scores were also more likely to be rated as dominant, coercive and hostile in their interpersonal behaviour as measured by the interpersonal circle (Blackburn & Renwick, 1996). Around 12 per cent of the total sample had a PCL-R total score of over 25, a score usually denoting a high level of psychopathic traits, with higher scores being evident in the high security setting (18 per cent over 25). Multi-group confirmatory factor analysis comparing the ID sample and a UK prison sample found that the three-factor model of psychopathy (proposed by Cooke & Michie, 2001) fitted the ID data and that there was structural equivalence for the PCL-R between offenders with and without ID. This finding suggests that the same 'latent trait' is being measured in those with and without ID, which in turn provides evidence that the psychopathy construct can be generalised to people with ID. However, more sophisticated item response theory analyses conducted in his series of studies provided evidence for 'metric differences' in the ratings of psychopathy symptoms between the group and the comparison UK prison group. This suggested that, for a variety of reasons, the PCL-R appears to *underestimate* psychopathy when used to assess people with ID. The same scores obtained on the PCL-R in the two groups cannot, therefore, be considered equivalent, which has implications for the interpretation of scores obtained with people with ID and for applying the cut-off scores commonly used for clinical decision making (Morrissey, 2006a; Morrissey Cooke, Michie, Hollin, Lindsay & Hogue, 2010). Consequently, it is currently reasonable to suggest that PCL assessments on those with ID are used for formulation and treatment planning, but that total scores and subscale scores are not used.

To date, there are few studies on the predictive validity of psychopathy in populations with ID. Gray, Fitzgerald, Taylor, MacCulloch and Snowden, (2007), in a retrospective case file study, found that the PCL: SV had reasonable predictive validity for an outcome of reconviction in an ID sample (auc = 0.76). The predictive power was as good, if not better, than in comparable sample without ID. There is less evidence for the predictive validity of the PCL-R, which has been explored only in two small prospective studies relating to the high secure sample described above (Morrissey *et al.*, 2007; Morrissey, Mooney, Hogue, Lindsay & Taylor 2007). Unexpectedly, where institutional aggression was concerned, neither the PCL-R nor its main factors were found to predict institutional aggression, whereas a number of other risk assessment measures, including the HCR-20, did. However, PCL-R scores were found to be significantly negatively associated with the outcome of positive progress from the high security hospital, a relationship which was independent of the seriousness of the offence, length of stay in the hospital and previous convictions. The mechanisms by which psychopathy mediates such progress, therefore, remain to be explored.

Further exploratory work has found that the different item descriptions employed in alternative measures of psychopathy (PCL – Youth Version (PCL-YV) (Forth, Kosson & Hare, 2003) and PCL – Screening Version (PCL: SV) (Hart, Cox & Hare, 1995) resulted in better content validity and improved psychometric properties for these scales as compared to the PCL-R (Morrissey, 2006a). In particular, an external validity criterion of concurrent antisocial behaviour was more strongly related to both these alternative scales than to the PCL-R. The findings provide preliminary evidence that the PCL-YV and PCL: SV may have promise as more 'ID appropriate' measures of psychopathy. In conclusion, while the psychometric properties of the PCL-R can be considered to be adequate, certain problems in its applicability to people with ID have been identified. At present, therefore, some caution is advised in the use of the PCL-R in offenders with ID, particularly where clinical decision-making is likely to be influenced. This measure, and guidelines for its use in ID groups, is discussed further below.

There is a paucity of studies relating to treatment of those with ID and psychopathic traits. In reviewing the recent literature on personality disorder in ID, Torr (2003) noted the dearth of intervention studies in this area and, at present, there is no definitive evidence that those with ID and personality disorder do less well in treatment. However, the finding of Morrissey, Mooney *et al.*, 2007 suggests that treatment may need to be lengthier in personality disordered patients with ID, which is consistent with the evidence for mainstream groups.

Sexual Offenders with Intellectual Disabilities

No studies have thus far specifically examined the relationship between personality disorder and sexual offending in those who have ID. It is, nevertheless, interesting to note that of six cases in an early descriptive study of APD and 'mental retardation' by Hurley and Sovner (1995), five had sex offence histories. There seems little doubt that examination of personality disorder is likely to be relevant to some sexual offenders with ID.

In the large UK study of personality disorder and ID referred to above (Lindsay *et al.*, 2006) over 50 per cent of the sample had histories which included sexual offending.

The incidence of personality disorder was found to be almost identical in the sex offender group (38.6 per cent) as compared to the non-sex offender group (38.7 per cent). It was also observed that sex offenders with personality disorder scored higher on risk measurements (HCR-20; VRAG; Static-99; and RM-2000/Sex) than did those without personality disorder. This study also found that those sex offenders who were personality disordered exhibited higher levels of internalising and externalising behaviour problems than those without personality disorder (Morrissey, 2006a), which suggests that the treatment and management needs of those with personality disorder may be different during, and subsequent to, sex offender treatment.

How Should Personality Disorder and Psychopathy be Assessed in Clients with Intellectual Disabilities?

Initial Screening

Assessment of personality disorder or psychopathy is time-consuming and requires specialist expertise; in many settings it will therefore be unlikely that all referral cases can have a full assessment. In such circumstances it is preferable that screening assessment is conducted in order to identify cases suitable for more comprehensive assessment. Where personality disorder is concerned, it may be preferable to complete a DSM-IV checklist of criteria (such as that prepared by D'Silva & Hogue, 2003) using file review and observational data, with referral for further investigation if necessary. In the case of psychopathy, the P-SCAN (Hare and Hervé, 1999) can be completed by a relatively inexperienced mental health or criminal justice practitioner. The P-SCAN is a checklist of items relevant to psychopathic features that can indicate whether further, more in-depth assessment is required by someone trained in the use of the PCL-R or PCL – Screening Version. The P-SCAN cannot, however, be used to make a formal assessment of psychopathy.

Measures of Personality Disorder

Assessment of personality disorder should be undertaken using a structured assessment format relating to either ICD-10 or DSM-IV criteria, although none have yet been devised or modified specifically for assessment of people with ID. One widely used assessment is the International Personality Disorder Examination (IPDE) (Loranger, Janca & Sartorius, 1997), a semi-structured interview which can be adapted to the needs of a person with ID and does allow for informant information to be incorporated. The Structured Assessment of Personality (Pilgrim & Mann, 1990) has been used to assess individuals with ID in a number of studies (e.g. Lindsay *et al.*, 2006; Reid & Ballinger, 1987), typically using informant report methodology. However, it is known to be over inclusive in identifying personality disorder (see Alexander & Cooray, 2003). For higher functioning clients with mild ID self-report instruments may additionally be used, particularly if administered by interview (e.g., Personality Assessment Inventory (Morey, 1991); PDQ-4 (Hyler, Skodol, Oldham, Kellman & Doidge 1992)).

Guidance for Assessment of General Personality Disorder

The following guidance outlines appropriate considerations when assessing personality disorder in clients with ID:

1. If ICD-10 classification is employed, the Diagnostic Criteria for Learning Disability (DC:LD) (Royal College of Psychiatrists, 2001) should be referred to. For DSM-IV, DM-ID should be consulted.
2. Personality disorder should not be diagnosed in those with severe or profound disabilities, and diagnoses should not be made below the age of 21 years.
3. Particular care should be taken to differentiate between aspects of functioning which are driven by the ID and those attributable to the personality disorder. This is not always straightforward, and efforts should be made to gather evidence from a range of perspectives: for example, client interview; carer interview; file information and behavioural observation.
4. The cultural norm for people with similar levels of ID should be kept in mind when determining what is and is not a deviation from 'the expectations of an individual's culture' as described in DSM-IV.
5. It is crucial that the traits observed are enduring across time and different environments, and are not a function of adaptation to a particular setting.
6. Attention should also be paid to differentiation between PDD and personality disorders as in the former group the general diagnostic criteria for personality disorder are quite likely to be met. If the diagnosis of PDD is better able to account for the symptoms then this diagnosis should be used. Nevertheless, in some cases an Axis 2 diagnosis can be necessary and useful in addition to a PDD diagnosis.

Measures of Psychopathy

As noted above, the most widely used measure of psychopathy is currently the PCL-R (see Table 9.1 and Figure 9.1), along with a shorter 12-item version, the Psychopathy Checklist – Screening Version (PCL- SV) (Hart, Cox & Hare, 1995). For those under 21 the PCL-R Youth Version (PCL-YV) (Forth, Kosson & Hare, 2003) can be applied, although assessment at below age 21 is not recommended for individuals with ID (see below). In the PCL-R, the 20 items are scored 0-2, giving a total possible score of 40. In the United States, a high level of psychopathic traits are typically represented by a score of 30 or more, whereas in the United Kingdom and Europe, a score of 25 or more is commonly applied (Cooke, Michie, Hart & Clark, 2005). (However, caution should be applied in using such cut-offs in ID populations; see below.) Factor 1 represents the interpersonal and affective aspects of the disorder and Factor 2, the lifestyle and antisocial disorder manifestations. As noted above, adequate reliability and validity for the PCL-R has been demonstrated in a relatively large sample with ID. On balance, it has been considered that development of new or revised measures of psychopathy specifically for ID populations is not appropriate, not least because it would not allow comparison with groups without ID. Instead, evidence-based guidelines for the assessment of psychopathy using these instruments in people with ID have recently been developed (Morrissey, 2006b) based on the studies described earlier

Table 9.1 PCL-R items and their location in the factor structure (Hare, 2003)

	Psychopathy (superordinate factor)				
Factor 1 *Affective/Interpersonal*		Factor 2 *Lifestyle/Antisocial*			
Facet 1 *Interpersonal*	Facet 2 *Affective*	Facet 3 *Lifestyle*	Facet 4 *Antisocial*		*No Factor Loading*
1. Glibness/superficial charm	6. Lack of remorse/guilt	3. Need for stimulation	10. Poor behavioural controls		11. Promiscuous sexual behaviour
2. Grandiose sense of self worth	7. Shallow affect	9. Parasitic lifestyle	12. Early behavioural problems		17. Many marital relationships
4. Pathological lying	8. Callous/lack empathy	13. Lack realistic goals	18. Juvenile delinquency		
5. Conning - manipulative	16. Failure to take responsibility	14. Impulsivity	19. Revocation conditional release		
		15. Irresponsibility	20. Criminal versatility		

Table 9.2 PCL-R Total, factor and facet scores by level of security: Data from a study in three forensic ID settings (from Morrissey *et al.*, 2005)

	All	High	Medium–Low	Community
		Level of Security		
N	203	66	68	69
	M (*SD*)	M (*SD*)	M (*SD*)	M (*SD*)
PCL-R Total	16.02 (7.3)	18.25 (7.2)	15.39 (6.2)	14.50 (7.9)
Factor 1	6.38 (3.8)	6.99 (4.1)	5.75 (3.4)	6.43 (3.9)
Factor 2	8.18 (4.2)	9.69 (4.5)	8.31 (3.3)	6.78 (4.3)
Total 13	10.10 (5.4)	11.67 (6.0)	9.19 (4.4)	9.75 (5.6)
Facet 1	2.31 (2.1)	2.49 (2.2)	1.67 (1.9)	2.77 (2.1)
Facet 2	4.10 (2.3)	4.70 (2.3)	4.00 (2.1)	3.64 (2.4)
Facet 3	3.87 (2.5)	–	3.41 (2.0)	3.32 (2.4)
Facet 4	4.49 (2.5)	5.00 (2.4)	5.05 (2.3)	3.51 (2.6)

Note: Total 13 is the 13 item total using the items described by Cooke & Michie, 2001. There were insufficient valid cases in the high secure sample where Facet 3 could be calculated because of the number of omitted items.

in the chapter. The main principles of these guidelines are summarised below. Although the guidelines cover both instruments, on balance the evidence is in favour of using the PCL: SV as opposed to the PCL-R for a number of reasons. Firstly, the PCL: SV does not include some of the items which were found to be problematic for application to people with ID in the validation study (e.g., many marital relationships; sexual promiscuity; parasitic lifestyle). Secondly, the PCL: SV items associated with antisocial behaviour depend less than the PCL-R on formal charges and convictions and on a versatile range of offending behaviour being exhibited. This approach is more appropriate for people with ID, whose offending behaviour tends to be narrower in scope and is often not processed through the criminal justice system. Moreover, there are indications that the predictive validity of the PCL: SV in relation to aggressive institutional behaviour and recidivism is better than the PCL-R. Unfortunately, however, ID comparative data is available only on the PCL-R at the present time (see Table 9.2). An alternative to using the PCL: SV is to use Cooke and Michie's (2001) 13 selected items from the PCL-R, which contribute to their three-factor model of psychopathy (deficient affective experience; arrogant and deceitful interpersonal style and impulsive and irresponsible behavioural style). This model excludes all items from the antisocial behaviour facet of the PCL-R, which, in particular, was found to have low reliability, and poorer ability to discriminate in the ID sample described in Morrissey *et al.*, 2005. Moreover, confirmatory factor analysis has indicated that the three-factor model fits the available ID data.

Guidance for Assessment of Psychopathy using the PCL-R/PCL: SV

The following is a summary of the guidelines reproduced in Morrissey (2006b) in relation to assessment of psychopathy using the PCL-R and PCL: SV:

1. Appropriate PCL-R/SV training is required for assessors, as is established inter-rater reliability, preferably with both an ID and non-ID population. Appropriate clinical

experience with both ID and offenders with psychopathic characteristics is essential for raters so that clinical judgement may be used in individual cases to determine whether a particular score on an item is indeed reflective of psychopathic traits. As a general principle, two raters should be used.

2. The evidence thus far cannot support use of the measure with those with IQ below 55 as there were insufficient numbers of participants in the validation study functioning at below this intellectual level. Furthermore, there is evidence of the disorder having poorer validity at lower levels of functioning. While there are validation studies of the scales with females (e.g., Vitale, Smith, Brinkley & Newman 2002), it has not been validated on females with ID.

3. In line with DC-LD, because of developmental delays, and particularly the fact that the developmental phase for personality characteristics in people with ID should be viewed as longer than that for a person of average ability, the PCL-R/SV should not be used on adults under 21 years.

4. As with personality disorder more generally, care should be taken to differentiate between aspects of functioning that are driven by the ID and those attributable to psychopathy. As a benchmark for some items (e.g., Item 15; *Irresponsibility*), it is relevant to use the expected behavioural norm for people at the same level of intellectual and adaptive functioning who are non-offenders living in community settings.

5. When scoring the PCL-R, it is often useful to consider the underlying *function* of the behaviour to ensure that the behaviour observed in the person with ID is consistent with the intent of the item (e.g., *Pathological lying*; *Conning/manipulative*).

6. Efforts should be made to gather evidence from a range of perspectives. The use of informants should be routine and, if possible, more than one informant should be used. These informants would include direct care staff and family where possible. It is advisable wherever possible to obtain school reports, social-work reports and direct reports as descriptive evidence of behaviour. Observation of interpersonal behaviour is also advisable.

7. If an interview with the client is possible this should also be carried out. However, it should be recognised that such interview evidence may be less reliable with people with ID. Raters should be aware that inconsistent historical accounts (usually interpreted as deceitfulness in the PCL-R) may be a result of cognitive/memory deficits rather than deliberate distortion. For people with more significant levels of ID the interview evidence may be very limited. The PCL-R interview guide has also been revised to be more applicable to people with ID (Morrissey, 2006b).

8. The guidelines for ID are not intended to change the flavour or intent of the items, and the manual for the PCL-R second edition (Hare, 2003) (or in the PCL: SV manual: Hart, Cox & Hare, 1995) should be adhered to, as with any other case. The characteristics identified must be chronic and pervasive, reflect lifetime functioning and be identifiable in a range of personal and social situations, even if it is not the full range (e.g., employment; marital etc.) specified in the manual. They should in most cases have been apparent by adolescence.

9. For the PCL-R, there are no exclusion criteria on the grounds of other disorders; for example, diagnosis of an autistic spectrum disorder should not preclude a high score. Typically, however, the validation research found that people with such disorders may score positively on the affective items but do not typically score positively on the

interpersonal and lifestyle items of the PCL-R. There are, nevertheless, individuals who meet the criteria for both autistic spectrum disorders and psychopathic disorders.

10. The guidelines expand the item descriptions, where appropriate, to include what are considered to be ID relevant behaviour or examples, and in some cases add different possible sources of information. Because of many parallels between youth and people with ID, some of the examples are derived from the PCL-YV manual (Forth, Kosson & Hare, 2003) where this is considered appropriate. For certain items, it is recommended that the criteria for evidence for the behaviour are broadened (for example, for Item 20 *Criminal Versatility*, that all behaviour which would constitute offending in a mainstream population should be considered, not only charges and convictions).

11. Because of the typically restricted social, occupational and life opportunities for people with ID, it is recommended that if there has been insufficient opportunity to exhibit evidence for an item (e.g., *Parasitic lifestyle*; *Many marital relationships*), the item should be omitted.

12. The PCL-R total and factor scores should not be compared directly with those for samples without disabilities, nor should commonly employed cut-offs be used. This is because using item response theory analyses, PCL-R scores in the ID samples investigated in Morrissey *et al.* (2005) were found not to be metrically equivalent to those without such disabilities. Nevertheless, use of means and standard deviations of scores from the ID study referred to above may be useful for comparative purposes (Table 9.2). The standard error of measurement for the total scale for this group is 3.0 points, which is comparable to that in mainstream populations.

13. The evidence base for the utility of psychopathy as a construct in ID is at an early stage; because of this, caution should be applied in use of the scores. There is, for example, not yet strong empirical evidence that psychopathy is a significant risk factor for aggression in this group of people, and therefore until such evidence becomes more available the scores should be used with caution to influence risk assessments either alone or as a weight in instruments such as the HCR-20 or VRAG. Use of the measure for other types of clinical decision-making should also be cautious. By and large, qualitative descriptions (e.g., 'high number of psychopathic traits') can be used to describe PCL-R scores.

14. Since there is some evidence that high PCL-R scorers with ID may make poorer progress in treatment, attention may need to be paid to the treatment strategies applied to this subgroup of ID offenders, and specific intervention programmes for those with ID who are high scorers may be appropriate. Item scores and facet profiles can be useful for the purposes of formulation and for identifying specific treatment needs. High PCL-R scores should not be used as a reason to exclude individuals from treatment.

ASSESSMENT OF PERSONALITY DISORDER IN SEXUAL OFFENDERS WITH INTELLECTUAL DISABILITIES

Intervention and Management Issues

There are a number of intervention and management issues on which a diagnosis of personality disorder in a person with ID who offends sexually may have a bearing, and these will be briefly reviewed in turn.

Firstly, if a personality disorder is diagnosed, awareness of the constellation of traits evident in the individual's presentation can be very important in developing a formulation of their sexual offending behaviour prior to treatment. This formulation may identify dysfunctional schemas (or belief systems) underlying these traits and specific skills deficits which need to be addressed through treatment. Because of the more complex set of problems likely to be encountered in personality disordered sex offenders with ID it is usually necessary to provide treatment which is targeted more broadly than standard sex offender treatment approaches. Particularly in longer term treatment settings, it may be appropriate that broader aspects of the personality disorder itself are treated before addressing the sexual offending. This may be achieved through either group or individual intervention aiming to modify the schema or 'world view' underlying the emotional and behavioural symptoms. In sexual offenders, this 'world view' can include mistrust of others; belief about self-defectiveness; and beliefs about entitlement. Examples of appropriate therapies might include: Schema Focussed Therapy (Young, 1994); Cognitive-Analytic Therapy (Ryle, 1995); and other forms of Cognitive Behaviour Therapy for personality disorder (Linehan, 1991; Davidson, 2008), all of which have been modified in various clinical settings to increase applicability to people with ID. In addition, specific skills training may be warranted in order to address skills deficits such as lack of means–ends problem solving, lack of emotional regulation, poor recognition of others' needs and feelings and lack of impulse control. If these areas have first been addressed, there is some anecdotal evidence that subsequent treatment for the sexual offending behaviour may be more successful.

A second important consideration is that potential clients with personality disorders are frequently poorly motivated to change (Beck & Freeman, 1990), and this is a particular challenge of working with this group. Therapist skills in motivational interviewing (Miller & Rollnick, 2002) are therefore likely to be useful, and clients referred for treatment may require a significant period of motivational and engagement work prior to a sex offence focussed intervention.

The interpersonal difficulties associated with a personality disorder diagnosis can also have an impact on response to and behaviour within sex offender treatment. For example, those with a hostile-dominant interpersonal style characteristic of psychopathy tend to have a poorer therapeutic alliance (Muran, Segal, Samstag & Crawford, 1994) and to be disruptive or dominating in group-based treatment (Hobson, Shine & Roberts, 2000). Alternatively, those individuals with characteristics related to borderline personality disorder may find aspects of sex offender treatment lead to periods of emotional dysregulation, which may provoke urges to self-harm or lead to treatment drop out. It is important that behaviours which interfere with therapy are addressed in a consistent and structured fashion. In line with research evidence on fluctuating engagement in personality disordered individuals, particular efforts have to be made first to form an adequate therapeutic alliance and to maintain engagement in treatment. This task can be all the more difficult as clients with personality disorder are known to provoke strong, even negative and hostile, reactions in therapists and care staff (Beck & Freeman, 1990; Rotgers & Maniacci, 2006), and 'splitting' of teams is a common consequence of working with personality disordered clients. A final note of caution is that although clients with antisocial and psychopathic disorders may see no need to change they may nevertheless master the 'language' of treatment in order to convince therapists that they have changed: skilful assessment of genuine shifts in attitudes is therefore necessary.

Awareness of the impact of personality disorder on the above therapeutic processes is crucial, particularly in the context of supervision of staff conducting work with this client group. However, if anticipated, these difficulties can be planned for and worked with constructively. For example, appropriate selection and combination of clients for group work can be considered in the light of any expected difficulties with those with personality disorder diagnoses. Another approach that has had some clinical success for preventing treatment drop out in this client group is concurrent individual support sessions for some or all sex offender treatment group members (Terry, Willows & Rose, 2005).

A final important reason for assessing personality disorder in sexual offenders with ID referred for treatment is the determination of risk of further offending, given the evidence base described earlier in this chapter. It has been noted that diagnosis of personality disorder and psychopathy lead to increased risk scores on several structured assessments. Level of risk has a bearing on duration and intensity of treatment (Beech & Mann, 2002) and on appropriate management following treatment. Thus, consideration may need to be given to longer term intervention and follow-up; and a highly structured relapse prevention plan with a high level of monitoring and support of the client with ID may be more important in an individual with concurrent personality disorder.

The preceding discussion emphasises the importance of assessing for personality disorder in those referred to sex offender treatment in ID settings and, indeed, that failing to recognise such disorder may result in a failure to provide appropriate treatment and management for the client. The fictional case example (Mr J) described below provides some pointers to ways that personality disorder can influence the presentation of a sex offender with ID and examples of how such understanding might be incorporated into both formulation and a comprehensive treatment approach.

Case Example

Diagnosis

- DSMIV diagnosis of APD and borderline personality disorder
- PCL-R score in the top 2 per cent of the distribution of scores for offenders with ID (see Table 9.1)

Background

- aged 24: full scale IQ = 66
- chaotic family with few sexual boundaries; father abused male and female children within family including Mr J
- taken into care at age 12
- several incidents of sexually inappropriate behaviour in children's home: not charged
- previous offences of burglary and theft
- index offence: conviction for rape of adult female with ID in residential home when Mr J aged 21
- detained under Mental Health Act (1983) classification of Psychopathic Disorder and Mental Impairment in a low security unit

Personality disorder assessment (DSM-IV Checklist; PCL: SV)

- Combination of personality disorder traits: failure to conform to social norms; impulsivity; irritability; intense uncontrolled anger and aggressiveness; lack of remorse

for actions; identity disturbance; affective instability; transient paranoid ideation; some self-harm.
- Psychopathy: high level of affective symptoms (deficient affective experience, poor empathy); interpersonal symptoms (deceitfulness; manipulation of others).
- Self-reported deviant arousal to rape.
- Maladaptive schemas relating to entitlement, mistrust/abuse and lack of self-control underpin offending and have led to deficiencies in abilities to maintain internal limits, assume responsibility to others and orient Mr J to long-term goals.
- Offences typically occur when Mr J is in an unstable, angry mode.

Risk
Identified as 'high' risk of sexual re-offending on SORAG and RSVP assessments

Treatment issues

- Maladaptive schemas relating to entitlement, mistrust and abuse by others; *Schema Therapy (30 sessions) undertaken by psychologist prior to SOTP with focus on maintaining motivation and on the therapeutic relationship. Attention paid to the effect of sexual abuse on schema development.*
- Reluctant to engage in sex offender treatment, particularly group treatment: *lengthy motivational work undertaken prior to SOTP.*
- In SOTP group considers self superior to other participants; dominates group; occasionally disruptive; tutors have considered removal from group: *appropriate management of consistent boundaries within group and consideration of personality disorder issues raised in supervision.*
- Unreliable attendance: *allocated tutor for individual follow up and support.*
- Idealises one tutor and devalues other. Devalued tutor appears covertly hostile to client: *appropriate supervision of team with exploration of counter-transference issues.*
- High risk: *allocate to longer term treatment group with concurrent additional individual support; longer follow-up and robust relapse management and supervision plan devised; Multi Agency Public Protection Arrangements to be involved on discharge.*

CONCLUSIONS

Personality disorder and psychopathy are important considerations in the assessment and treatment of sex offenders with ID. The characteristics associated with these disorders may have a bearing on formulation, risk assessment, risk management and aspects of treatment. Careful assessment of such personality disorders must be conducted using guidelines specific to this group and awareness needs to be increased with respect to the ways ID interacts with such disorders. Finally, it is important to recognise that a label of personality disorder has negative connotations and can have diverse implications for an individual. For those already living with the stigma of ID, such a diagnosis should therefore be used with caution unless it has clear clinical utility.

REFERENCES

Alexander, R. & Cooray, S. (2003). Diagnosis of personality disorders in learning disability. *British Journal of Psychiatry, 44* (Suppl.), 528–31.

Alexander, R.T., Crouch, K., Halstead, S. & Pichaud, J. (2006). Long-term outcome from a medium secure service for people with ID. *Journal of ID Research, 50,* 305–15.

Alwin, N., Blackburn, R., Davidson, K., Hilton, M., Logan, C. & Shine, J. (2006). *Understanding personality disorder.* BPS: Lecicester.

American Psychiatric Association. (2000). *Diagnostic and statistical manual of mental disorders,* 4th edn., text revision. Washington DC.

Barbaree, H.E. (2005). Psychopathy, treatment behaviour and recidivism in a follow-up of Seto and Barbaree. *Journal of Interpersonal Violence, 20* (9), 1115–31.

Barbaree, H.E., Seto, M.C., Langton, C.M. & Peacock, E.J. (2001). Evaluating the predictive accuracy of assessment instruments for adult sex offenders. *Criminal Justice and Behaviour,* Vol. *28,* No. 4, 490–521.

Bateman, A. & Fonagy, P. (2006). Progress in the treatment of borderline personality disorder. *The British Journal of Psychiatry, 188,* 1–3.

Bateman, A.W. & Tyrer, P. (2004). Psychological treatment for personality disorders. *Advances in Psychiatric Treatment, 10,* 378–88.

Beck, A.T. & Freeman, A. (1990). *Cognitive therapy of personality disorders.* New York: Guilford Press.

Beech, A. & Mann, R (2002). Recent developments in the treatment of sexual offenders. In J. McGuire (Ed.), *Offender rehabilitation and treatment* (pp. 259–89). Chichester: Wiley.

Blackburn, R. (2000). Treatment or incapacitation? Implications of research on personality disorders for the management and diagnosis of offenders. *Legal and Criminological Psychology, 5,* 1–21.

Blackburn, R., Logan, C., Donnelly, J. & Renwick, S. (2003). Personality disorders, psychopathy and other mental disorders: Co-morbidity among patients at English and Scottish high-security hospitals. *Journal of Forensic Psychiatry and Psychology, 14,* 111–37.

Blackburn, R. & Renwick, S.J. (1996). Rating scales for measuring the interpersonal circle in forensic psychiatric patients. *Psychological Assessment, 8,* 76–84.

Blair, J. (2005). Responding to the emotions of others: dissociating forms of empathy through the study of typical and psychiatric populations. *Consciousness and Cognition, 14* (4), 698–718.

Blair, J., Mitchell, D. & Blair, K. (2005). *The psychopath: Emotion and the brain.* Blackwell: Oxford.

Boer, D.P., Hart, S.D. & Kropp, P.R. (1997). *Manual for the sexual violence risk – 20.* British Columbia: SFU.

Brinkley, C.A., Newman, J., Widiger, T.A. & Lynam, D.R. (2004). Two approaches to parsing the heterogeneity of psychopathy. *Clinical Psychology: Science and Practice, 11,* 69–94.

Buffington-Vollum, J., Edens, J.F., Johnston, D.W. & Johnston, J.K. (2002). Psychopathy as a predictor of institutional misbehaviour among sex offenders: A prospective replication. *Criminal Justice and Behaviour, 29* (5), 497–511.

Cleckley, H. (1941). *The Mask of Sanity.* St Louis, MO: Mosby.

Cooke, D.J. (1995). Psychopathic disturbance in the Scottish prison population: Cross cultural generalisability of the Hare Psychopathy Checklist. *Psychology, Crime and the Law, 2,* 101–18.

Cooke, D.J. & Michie, C. (2001). Refining the construct of psychopathy: Towards a hierarchical model. *Psychological Assessment, 13,* 171–88.

Cooke, D.J., Michie, C., Hart, S.D. & Clark, D. (2005). Searching for the pan-cultural core of psychopathic personality disorder. *Personality and Individual Differences, 39,* 283–95.

Costa, R.R. & McRae, P.T. (1999). *A five factor theory of personality: Theory and research.* Guilford Press.

Davidson, K. (2008). *Cognitive therapy for personality disorders: A guide for clinicians.* London: Routledge.

D'Silva, K., Duggan, C. & McCarthy, L. (2004). Does treatment really make psychopaths worse? A review of the evidence. *Journal of Personality Disorders, 18,* 163–77.

D'Silva, K. & Hogue, T.E. (2003). DSM-IV personality disorder assessment procedure. (Unpublished.)

Fazel, S. & Danesh, J. (2002). Serious mental disorder in 23,000 prisoners: A systematic review of 62 surveys. *Lancet, 359,* 545–50.

Firestone, P., Bradford, J.M., Greenberg, D.M. & Larose, M.R. (1998). Homicidal sex offenders: Psychological phallometric and diagnostic features. *Journal of American Academic Psychiatry and Law, 26,* 537–52.

Fletcher, R., Loschen, E., Stavrakaki, C. & First, M. (Eds). (2007). *Diagnostic manual ID (DM-ID): A textbook of diagnosis of mental disorders in persons with ID.* Kingston, NY: NADD Press.

Flynn, A., Matthews, H. & Hollis, S. (2002). Validity of the diagnosis of personality disorder in adults with learning disability and severe behavioural problems: Preliminary study. *British Journal of Psychiatry, 180,* 543–6.

Forth, A.E., Kosson, D. & Hare, R.D. (2003). *Hare psychopathy checklist: Youth version (PCL:YV).* Toronto, Ontario: Multi Health Systems.

Forth, A.E. & Kroner, D. (1994). The factor structure of the Hare psychopathy checklist – revised in sex offenders. Department of Psychology, Corkton University, Ottowa, Ontario. (Unpublished.)

Goldberg, B., Gitta, M.Z. & Puddephatt, A. (1995). Personality and trait disturbances in an adult mental retardation population: Significance for psychiatric management. *Journal of ID Research, 39,* 284–94.

Gray, N., Fitzgerald, S., Taylor, J., MacCulloch, M.J. & Snowden, R.J. (2007). Predicting future reconviction in offenders with intellectual disabilities: The predictive efficacy of VRAG, PCL: SV, and the HCR-20. *Psychological Assessment, 19* (4), 474–9.

Hanson, R.K. & Thornton, D. (2000). Improving risk assessment for sex offenders: A comparison of three actuarial scales. *Law and Human Behavior, 24,* 119–36.

Hare, R.D. (1991). *The Hare psychopathy checklist – Revised.* Toronto, Ontario: Multi-Health Systems.

Hare, R.D. (2003). *The Hare psychopathy checklist – Revised.* 2nd edn. Toronto, Ontario: Multi-Health Systems.

Hare, R.D., Clark, D., Thornton, D. & Grann, M. (2000). Psychopathy and the predictive validity of the PCL-R: An international perspective. *Behavioral Sciences and the Law, 18* (5), 623–45.

Hare, R.D. & Hervé, H. (1999). *Hare P-SCAN: Research version.* Toronto, Ontario: Multi-Health Systems.

Harris, G.T. & Rice, M.E. (2006). Treatment of psychopathy: A review of empirical findings. In C. J. Patrick (Ed.), *Handbook of psychopathy.* New York: Guilford Press.

Hart, S.D., Cox, D.N. & Hare, R.D. (1995). *The Hare PCL: SV.* Toronto, Ontario: Multi-Health Systems.

Hart, S.D., Forth, A.E. & Hare, R.D. (1990). Performance of criminal psychopaths on selected neuropsychological tests. *Journal of Abnormal Psychology, 99,* 374–9.

Hart, S.D. & Hare, R.D. (1989). Discriminant validity of the Psychopathy Checklist in a forensic psychiatric population. *Psychological Assessment, 1,* 211–18.

Hart, S.D. & Hemphill, J.F. (2002). Psychopathic personality disorder: Assessment and management. In E. Blaauw & L. Sheridan (Eds), *Psychopaths: Current International Perspectives.* The Hague: Elsevier.

Hemphill, J.F., Hare, R.D. & Wong, S. (1998). Psychopathy and recidivism: A review. *Legal and Criminological Psychology, 3,* 139–70.

Hildebrand, H. (2004). *Psychopathy in the treatment of forensic psychiatric patients.* Amsterdam: Dutch University Press.

Hildebrand, M., de Ruiter, C. & Vogel, V. (2004). Psychopathy and sexual deviance in treated rapists: Association with sexual and non-sexual recidivism. *Sexual Abuse: A Journal of Research and Treatment, 16*, 1–24.

Hobson, J., Shine, J. & Roberts, R. (2000). How do psychopaths behave in a prison therapeutic community? *Psychology, Crime, and Law, 6* (2), 139–54.

Home Office & Department of Health (1999). *Managing people with a severe personality disorder: Proposals for policy development.* London, Home Office.

Hurley, S. & Sovner, R. (1995). Six cases of patients with mental retardation who have antisocial personality disorder. *Psychiatric Services, 46* (8), 828–31.

Hyler, S., Skodol, A., Oldham, J., Kellman, H. & Doidge, N. (1992). Validity of the Personality Diagnostic Questionnaire – revised: A replication in an outpatient sample. *Comparative Psychiatry, 33*, 73–7.

Khan, A., Cowan, C. & Roy, A. (1997). Personality disorders in people with learning disabilities, a community survey. *Journal of ID Research, 41*, 324–30.

Langevin, R. (2006). Acceptance and completion of treatment among sex offenders. *Journal of Offender Therapy and Comparative Criminology, 150*, 402–17.

Lindsay, W.R., Gabriel, S., Dana, L., Young, S. & Dosen, A. (2007). *Personality disorders.* In R. Fletcher, E. Loschen & P. Sturmey (Eds), *Diagnostic manual of psychiatric disorders for individuals with mental retardation.* Kingston, NY: National Association for Dual Diagnosis.

Lindsay, W.R., Hogue, T., Taylor, J.L., Mooney, P., Steptoe, L., Johnston, S.O., Brien, G. & Smith, A.H.W. (2006). Two studies of the prevalence and validity of personality disorder in three forensic ID samples. *Journal of Forensic Psychiatry and Psychology, 17*, 485–506.

Lindsay, W.R. (2007). Personality Disorders. In: N. Bouras & G. Holt (Eds), *Psychiatric and behavioral disorders in developmental disabilities.* 2nd edn. Cambridge: CUP.

Linehan, M. (1991). *Cognitive-behavioural treatment of borderline personality disorder.* New York: Guilford Press.

Livesley, W.J. (2001). Conceptual and taxonomic issues. In: W.J. Livesley (Ed.), *Handbook of personality disorders: Theory, research and treatment.* New York: Guilford Press.

Looman, J., Abracen, J., Serin, R. & Marquis, P. (2005). Psychopathy, treatment change and recidivism in high risk, high need sexual offenders. *Journal of Interpersonal Violence, 20*, 549–68.

Loranger, A.W., Janca, A. & Sartorius, N. (1997). *Assessment and diagnosis of personality disorders: The ICD-10 international personality disorder examination.* CUP: Cambridge.

Lykken, D.T. (1995). *The antisocial personalities.* Hillsdale, NJ: Lawrence Earlbaum Associates.

McCord, W. & Mc Cord, J. (1964). *The psychopath: An essay on the criminal mind.* Princeton, NJ: Van Nostrand.

Mason, J. & Scior, K. (2004). Diagnostic overshadowing amongst clinicians working with people with intellectual disabilities in the UK. *Journal of Applied Research in Intellectual Disabilities, 17* (2), 85–90.

Millon, T., Simonsen, E., Birket-Smith, M. & Davis, R.D. (1998). *Psychopathy: antisocial, criminal, and violent behavior.* NY: Guilford Press.

Miller, W.R. & Rollnick, S. (Eds). (2002). *Motivational interviewing. Preparing people for change,* 2nd edn. New York: Guilford Press.

Morey, L.C. (1991). *Personality assessment inventory manual.* Psychological Assessment Resources: Florida.

Morrissey, C. (2003). The use of the PCL-R in forensic populations with learning disability. *British Journal of Forensic Practice, 5*, 20–4.

Morrissey, C. (2006a). Assessment of offenders with intellectual disabilities. PhD thesis, University of Leicester.

Morrissey, C., (2006b). Guidelines for assessment of psychopathy in offenders with intellectual disabilities. Available at: http://institutemh.org.uk.

Morrissey, C., Cooke, D., Michie, C., Hollin, C., Lindsay, W.R. & Hogue, T.E. (n.d.). Test item and structural generalisability of the PCL-R for offenders with intellectual disabilities.

Morrissey, C., Hogue, T., Mooney, P., Allen, C., Johnston, S., Hollin, C., Lindsay, W.R. & Taylor, J.L. (2007). The predictive validity of the PCL-R in offenders with ID in a high secure hospital setting: Institutional aggression. *Journal of Forensic Psychiatry and Psychology, 18*, 1–15.

Morrissey, C., Hogue, T., Mooney, P., Lindsay, W.R., Steptoe, L., Taylor, J. & Johnston, S. (2005). Applicability, reliability, and validity of the psychopathy checklist-revised in offenders with intellectual disabilities: Some initial findings. *International Journal of Forensic Mental Health, 4*, 207–20.

Morrissey, C., Mooney, P., Hogue, T., Lindsay, W.R. & Taylor, J. (2007). Predictive validity of psychopathy in offenders with ID in high security: Treatment progress. *Journal of Intellectual and Developmental Disability, 32* (2) 125–33.

Muran, J.C., Segal, Z.V., Samstag, L.W. & Crawford, C.E. (1994). Patient pre-treatment interpersonal problems and therapeutic alliance in short-term cognitive therapy. *Journal of Consulting and Clinical Psychology, 62*, 85–90.

Naik, B.I., Gangadharan, S.K., & Alexander, R.T. (2002). Personality disorders in learning disability – the clinical experience. *British Journal of Developmental Disabilities, 48*, 95–100.

Ogloff, J., Wong, S. & Greenwood, A. (1990). Treating criminal psychopaths in a therapeutic community program. *Behavioral Sciences and the Law, 8* (2), 181–90.

Olver, M.E. & Wong, S.C. (2006). Psychopathy, sexual deviance and recidivism among sex offenders. *Sexual abuse: A Journal of Research and Treatment, 18*, 65–82.

Pilgrim, J. & Mann, A. (1990). Use of the ICD–10 version of the standardized assessment of personality to determine the prevalence of personality disorder in psychiatric inpatients. *Psychological Medicine, 20*, 985–92.

Porter, S., Fairweather, D., Drugge, J., Herve, H., Birt, A. & Boer, D.P. (2000). Profiles of psychopathy in incarcerated sexual offenders. *Criminal Justice and Behaviour, 27*, 2, 216–34.

Porter, S., Woodworth, M., Earle, J., Drugge, J. & Boer, D. (2003). Characteristics of violent behaviour exhibited during sexual homicides by psychopathic and non-psychopathic murderers. *Law and Human Behavior, 27*, 459–70.

Quinsey, V.L., Rice, M.E., Harris, G.T. & Cormier, C. (1998). *Violent offenders: Appraising and managing risk*. Washington, DC: American Psychological Association.

Quinsey, V.L., Rice, M.E. & Harris, G.T. (1995). Actuarial prediction of sexual recidivism. *Journal of Interpersonal Violence, 10*, 85–105.

Reid, A.H. & Ballinger, B.R. (1987). Personality disorder in mental handicap. *Psychological Medicine, 17* (4), 983–7.

Reid, A.H., Lindsay, W.R., Law, J. & Sturmey, P. (2004). The relationship of offending behaviour and personality disorder in people with developmental disabilities. In: W.R. Lindsay, J. Taylor & P. Sturmey (Eds), *Offenders with developmental disabilities*. Chichester: Wiley.

Reiss, S., Levitan, G.W. & Syszko, J. (1983). Emotional disturbance and mental retardation: Diagnostic overshadowing. *American Journal of Mental Deficiency, 86*, 567–74.

Rice, M.E. & Harris, G.T. (1997). Cross validation and extension of the violence risk appraisal guide for child molesters and rapists. *Law and Human Behaviour, 21*, 231–41.

Rice, M.E., Harris, G.T. & Cormier, C.A. (1992). An evaluation of a maximum security therapeutic community for psychopaths and other mentally disordered offenders. *Law and Human Behavior, 16* (4), 399–412.

Rotgers, F. & Maniacci, M. (2006). *Antisocial personality disorder: A practitioners guide to comparative treatments*. New York: Springer.

Royal College of Psychiatrists. (2001). *Diagnostic criteria for learning disability (DC-LD)*. London: Gaskell.

Ryle, A. (1995). *Cognitive analytic therapy: Developments in theory and practice*. Chichester: Wiley.

Salekin, R.T. (2002). Psychopathy and therapeutic pessimism: Clinical lore or clinical reality? *Clinical Psychology Review*, *22* (1), 79–112.

Salekin, R., Rogers, R. & Sewell, K.W. (1996). A review and meta-analysis of the Psychopathy checklist and psychopathy checklist-revised: Predictive validity of dangerousness. *Clinical Psychology: Science and Practice*, *3*, 203–215.

Serin, R., Mailloux, D. & Malcolm, P. (2001). Psychopathy, deviant sexual arousal and recidivism among sexual offenders. *Journal of Interpersonal Violence*, *16* (3), 234–46.

Seto, M.C. & Barbaree, H.E. (1999). Psychopathy, treatment behavior, and sex offender recidivism. *Journal of Interpersonal Violence*, *14* (12), 1235–48.

Shine, J.H. & Hobson, J.A. (1997). Construct validation of the Hare psychopathy checklist – Revised on a UK prison population. *Journal of Forensic Psychiatry*, *8*, 546–64.

Skilling, T.A., Harris, G.T., Rice, M.E. & Quinsey, V.L. (2002). Identifying persistently antisocial offenders using the Hare psychopathy checklist and DSM antisocial personality disorder criteria. *Psychological Assessment.*, *14* (1), 27–38.

Terry, S., Willows, D. & Rose, S. (2005). A sex offender treatment programme for sexual offenders in a high security hospital. Paper presented at IAFMHS Conference (June), Melbourne, Australia.

Thornton, D., Mann, R., Webster, S., Blud, L., Travers, R., Friendship, C., *et al.* (2003). Distinguishing and combining risks for sexual and violent recidivism. *Annals of the New York Academy of Sciences*, *989*, 225–35.

Torr, J. (2003). Personality disorder in ID. *Current Opinion in Psychiatry*, *16* (5), 517–21.

Vitacco, M.J., Neumann, C.S. & Jackson, R.L. (2005). Testing a four-factor model of psychopathy and its association with ethnicity, gender, intelligence, and violence. *Journal of Consulting and Clinical Psychology*, *73* (3), 466–76.

Vitacco, M.J., Neumann, C.S. & Wodushek, T. (2008). Differential relationships between the dimensions of psychopathy and intelligence: Replication with adult jail inmates. *Criminal Justice and Behavior*, *35*, 48–55.

Vitale, J.E., Smith, S.S., Brinkley, C.A. & Newman, J.R. (2002). The reliability and validity of the psychopathy checklist–revised in a sample of female offenders. *Criminal Justice and Behaviour*, *29*, 202–31.

Walters, G.D. (2003). Predicting institutional adjustment and recidivism with the psychopathy checklist factor scores: A meta analysis. *Law and Human Behavior*, *27*, 541–58.

Webster, C.D., Douglas, K.S., Eaves, D. & Hart, S.D. (1997). *The HCR-20 scheme (version 2): The assessment of risk for violence*. Burnaby, BC: Mental Health, Law, and Policy Institute, Simon Fraser University.

World Health Organization. (1992). *The ICD-10 classification of mental and behavioural disorders: Clinical descriptions and diagnostic guidelines*. Geneva: WHO.

Young, J. (1994). *Schema focussed therapy: A practitioner's guide*. Guilford Publications: New York.

10

Suggested Adaptations to the HCR-20 for Offenders with Intellectual Disabilities

DOUGLAS P. BOER, MATTHEW FRIZE, RUTH PAPPAS, CATRIN MORRISSEY AND WILLIAM R. LINDSAY

INTRODUCTION

Although there are a number of well-researched structured professional judgement (SPJ) instruments available for purposes of risk assessment of violent offenders none of these instruments provide explicit rules for the differential assessment of intellectually disabled (ID) offenders.[1] That is, there are no generally accepted guidelines for the application of the standard items in commonly used SPJ instruments to ID clients. As a result, researchers and clinicians who have found evidence that SPJ instruments are valid with ID offenders have adapted the items in these instruments in idiosyncratic ways and, to date, have not always been clear as to how this was done for the purposes of their research. For example, there is evidence that the Historical-Clinical-Risk – 20 (HCR-20) (Webster, Douglas, Eaves & Hart, 1997) is valid for violent offenders with ID (e.g., Lindsay *et al.* 2008), but these authors do not explicitly explain how they adapted the HCR-20 in their study.

The present chapter aims to provide some guidelines for the use of the HCR-20 primarily with ID individuals who have been charged with non-sexual violent crimes. Furthermore, we

---

[1] In this chapter ID individuals are seen as those individuals with a full scale IQ of less than 75 and those individuals with a measured IQ of less than 80 but with significant adaptive behaviour deficits. An IQ cut-off of 75 takes into account the standard error of measurement of most of the commonly used intelligence tests. It is noted that Morrissey (2006) suggested that her PCL-R guidelines be applied to offenders with intellectual disabilities and that intellectual disability is to be inclusive of individuals with diagnosed intellectual disability (i.e., those with an IQ of less than 70) and also those individuals with borderline intellectual disability (i.e., those with an IQ of less than 80) who also have significant adaptive behaviour deficits.

Assessment and Treatment of Sexual Offenders with Intellectual Disabilities: A Handbook
Edited by Leam A. Craig, William R. Lindsay and Kevin D. Browne
© 2010 John Wiley & Sons, Ltd.

would also propose that the principles and strategies elucidated in this chapter applied in risk assessment of offenders with intellectual disabilities could potentially be adapted to provide an assessment framework for people with intellectual disabilities who, though not ever (or at least not currently) involved in the criminal justice system, exhibit behaviours labelled as *challenging*. That is, 'culturally abnormal behaviours of such an intensity, frequency or duration that the physical safety of the person or others is likely to be placed in serious jeopardy, or behaviour which is likely to seriously limit the use of, or result in the person being denied access to ordinary community facilities' (Emerson, 2001, p. 3). While some ID individuals may commit violent behaviour, such behaviours are not always legally consequenced owing to issues regarding mental capacity and intent – both of which are somewhat beyond the scope of this chapter – although both are addressed briefly under item 'H1' of the HCR-20 (see below).

APPLICATION TO ID OFFENDERS

A recent set of studies by Morrissey and colleagues on the applicability of the Psychopathy Checklist – Revised (PCL-R) (Hare, 2003) to ID offenders (e.g., Morissey *et al.*, 2007) was based on a set of guidelines produced by Morrissey in 2003, evaluated by Morrissey *et al.* in 2005, and then revised in 2006. The latter guidelines are available from the author (see Chapter 9).[2] These guidelines formed the basis of a systematic study of a reasonably large sample of ID offenders in several settings in the UK. The present chapter attempts to emulate Morrissey's guidelines for assessing ID offenders with the HCR-20. However, unlike Morrissey's guidelines, those which follow do not have empirical support – these are suggested alterations only, and these suggestions require empirical validation before adoption as anything but research suggestions or clinical guidelines.

In keeping with Morrissey (2006), we are suggesting that the present guidelines be applied only to offenders with intellectual disabilities and that intellectual disability is to be inclusive of individuals with diagnosed intellectual disability (i.e., those with an IQ of less than 70) and also those individuals with borderline intellectual disability who also have significant adaptive behaviour deficits. Most of the general principles listed below are modelled on those elucidated by Morrissey in her 2006 edition of guidelines for assessing psychopathy in ID offenders.

GENERAL PRINCIPLES

Although these guidelines change the content of the items to varying degrees, no change to the flavour or intent of the items of the original HCR-20 manual was intended.

- We acknowledge that the current research findings are more supportive of the validity of these instruments with males with mild ID. There is some evidence of validity of the HCR-20 with females with ID. Of course, the fact that Morrissey (2006) did not evaluate the

[2] Please contact Catrin Morrissey at catrin.morrissey@nottshc.nhs.uk for a copy of the PCL-R and PCL:SV ID guidelines.

PCL-R with female offenders with an ID limits the applicability of the HCR-20 to such female offenders.

- As with the diagnostic criteria for personality disorder for patients with ID in the Diagnostic Criteria – Learning Disability from the United Kingdom (DC-LD) (Royal College of Psychiatrists, 2001), we suggest that the HCR-20 not be used with adults under 21 years. This is based on the delayed development of individuals with ID.
- The current version of the HCR-20 incorporates the PCL-R or PCL-SV. Thus, it is recommended that prior to giving an ID offender a personality disorder diagnosis, including that of psychopathy (arguably an extreme form of antisocial personality disorder), assessors need to consider other possible reasons for an offender's presentation and behaviour. With ID individuals this would include the influence of conditions such as autistic spectrum disorder and foetal alcohol spectrum disorder (FASD) among others. Of course, the presence of any particular disorder may not necessarily preclude a high risk finding on any of these instruments, but certain items may reflect one syndrome more than another and therefore need to be considered carefully. For example, impulsivity is a key characteristic of FASD as well as a risk issue for SPJ instruments and the PCL-R, and the role of impulsivity may be functionally quite different in such cases.
- We do not suggest the use of these guidelines with individuals with an IQ of less than 55 because of limitations in the assessment of psychopathy (i.e., poor inter-rater reliability and low numbers in Morrissey's samples) with ID offenders.
- We endorse the general guidelines in the HCR-20 manual – the use of a good clinical interview, a thorough collateral file review (that is, all reports, such as care and support worker reports, school reports, and any relevant agency reports should be obtained), as well as consultation with significant others whenever possible.

Finally, we note that the authors of the HCR-20 have not granted their official approval for these replacement items for use with ID offenders, nor are we suggesting that these items are any better or more useful than any the reader could derive themselves. However, there is a trade-off in not having some standard suggested items for ID usage. If all users of the HCR-20 were to derive their own item applications then, logically, there would be greater variability and lack of precision in ID offender assessment – the very problem we are seeking to help reduce. The HCR-20 manual itself indicates that some flexibility is required in that 'any overly complicated scheme would stand little chance of success', and therefore its 'main value at this point may lie in the general principles it espouses rather than in its detail' (p. 5). However, we would strongly suggest that researching similar items for use with ID increases our ability to do good work for our ID clients and further our ability to increase effective reintegration and increase public safety.

HCR-20

The HCR-20 (Webster, Douglas, Eaves and Hart, 1997) has been the most widely used and well-researched SPJ with ID offenders. It is organised into three sections – Historical (10 items), Clinical (5 items) and Risk (5 items), with each item rated on a three-point scale from 0, no evidence of the variable, through 1, some evidence of the variable, to 2, clear evidence of the variable. The total score is the sum of the items, although the authors do not generally recommend making decisions on the basis of the total score. Rather, they recommend that the items are structured in order to help the consideration of a comprehensive range of variables with a view to arriving at a final judgement. In this way, historical variables are combined with an assessment of current clinical status and consideration of future risk variables.

The HCR-20 has been the subject of a considerable quantity of research work in a range of settings for mainstream offenders in both correctional and mental health facilities. Since it has a range of clinical variables it is unsurprising that much of the research has been carried out in forensic psychiatric settings or with mentally disordered offenders. A number of reports have now appeared reviewing the predictive accuracy and value of the HCR-20 in clinical practice and the prediction of re-offending with ID forensic clients.

Gray, Fitzgerald, Taylor and Snowden (2007) reviewed the predictive accuracy of the HCR-20 in relation to the Violence Risk Appraisal Guide (VRAG) (Quinsey, Harris, Rice & Cormier, 2003) and Psychopathy Checklist – Screening Version (PCL-SV) (Hart, Cox & Hare, 1995). They employed 118 men and 27 women with ID who had all been discharged from hospital following admission for conviction of a criminal offence or exhibiting behaviour that might have led to a conviction in different circumstances. This ID group were compared with a similar control group of 843 men and 153 women who were mainstream, mentally disordered offenders without ID. Following up these individuals for a period of five years, they found that all three instruments predicted violent recidivism with large effect sizes. For violent offending, the HCR historical items predicted recidivism with an AUC of 0.81, the clinical items with an AUC of 0.71 and the risk management items with an AUC of 0.64. These predictive values were considerably better than those found for the non-ID group, which were 0.69, 0.55 and 0.63 respectively. Generally, the HCR-20 had predictive values which were at least as good as those found for the VRAG and PCL-SV, although there were no significant differences in the predictive accuracy between assessments.

In related research, Morissey et al. (2005) investigated the relationship between the Psychopathy Checklist – Revised (Hare, 2003), the VRAG and the HCR-20, in addition to measures of personality disorder and emotional problems. This was an exploratory study primarily aimed at investigating the usability of the PCL-R but these authors reported convergence between the HCR-20 total score (with the PCL-R item removed), the three subscales of the HCR-20 and the PCL-R. This study was conducted on 212 offenders with ID drawn from a range of community, low secure, medium secure and maximum secure settings, and Morissey et al. (2007) went on to investigate the predictive value of these instruments in relation to institutional aggression. They found that the HCR-20 total score was significantly correlated with aggression in contrast to the PCL-R item totals, which were not significantly correlated with any type of institutional aggression. The HCR-20 was also significantly more accurate in predicting violence than the PCL-R (AUC = 0.68–0.77). In a final report on this population of offenders with ID, Morissey et al. (ibid.) showed that the HCR-20 total score significantly predicted positive treatment progress but that the PCL-R total demonstrated incremental predictive power over the HCR-20.

Lindsay et al. (2008) employed the same population in a comparison of the predictive validity of a number of risk assessments including the HCR-20. Participants were followed up for a period of one year for the recording of violent and sexual incidents. They found that the VRAG and HCR-20 had similar predictive validity with AUCs of 0.71 and 0.72 respectively. Therefore, there is some evidence from these two research groups (Gray, Fitzgerald, Taylor &

Snowden, 2007 and Morissey *et al.*, 2007) that the predictive accuracy of the HCR-20 is reasonable in offenders with ID.

Adapted HCR-20 Items – 'Qualifiers'

Please note that the following suggestions are to be used in parallel sequence with, not in replacement of, the original HCR-20 item. In other words, you should read the manual item and then the ID item 'qualifier' – the additional information that may influence your item rating. Then rate the item using the existing coding from the manual, unless new coding is indicated by research on the suggested parallel items. We have used the male pronoun throughout the following items; although we endorse the use of these items with female ID clients as well (there are simply more of the former).

H1. Previous Violence

- This item encapsulates one of the main differences between ID and non-ID clients: the issue of intent. The HCR-20 manual definition of violent behaviour implies that that there is intent on the part of the person to cause harm to others. The issue of intent subsumes, to some degree, the issue of challenging behaviour versus offending behaviour. Doyle (2004) appeared to view offending behaviour (albeit in his article this is specifically sexual offending the argument clearly applies to non-sexual behaviour) as 'challenging' when the perpetrator committing the behaviour is doing so without intent to harm another person. Challenging behaviour can still be criminal in that the victim of the unintentional behaviour may be injured or even killed, in such circumstances the behaviour was obviously illegal. Further, lack of intent does not necessarily reduce the person's potential to cause harm in the future.
- As a result, when this item is applied to ID clients, the assessor should examine intent of previous violence and the extent of previous violence as well as frequency and severity of violence. As a matter of course, assessors need to examine the client's file. Is there a history of violence in the file? Who are the targets of the violence? Is he the victim who fights back, or the perpetrator?
- It is quite possible that ID clients may have a high baseline frequency of low–moderate severity violent actions (e.g., throwing plates at staff, biting other residents) as opposed to non-ID offenders (e.g., assaulting others with weapons). We have assumed a very simple operational definition of a violent act: any behaviour of a violent or threatening nature that has been recorded in any of the client's files and as a result constitutes a problematic issue for the client. The more the behaviour is repeated, and the more serious the consequences, the more problematic the issue becomes, as reflected in the escalation of the consequences it provokes (for example, perhaps less serious behaviour is initially ignored, but more serious behaviour could result in loss of privileges or relocation to a more secure environment). This sort of simple definition obviates the question of whether the violent action is considered a 'challenging' behaviour or one that is considered serious enough to be reported to the authorities. That is a separate decision – both sorts of behaviours are considered 'previous violence', albeit probably of differing degrees of severity and intent.
- The operational definition here also allows for the same scoring as described in the manual but utilising a client's file information.

H2. Young Age at First Violent Incident

- The authors of the HCR-20 note that their prescribed age divisions were 'admittedly arbitrary', and we are quite sure that these age divisions would be somewhat different for ID clients depending on level of ID or adaptive behaviour deficits. For example, there would be developmental differences, with some of the older ID clients having significant lower mental ages than their non-ID chronologically similar peers.
- We are mainly concerned here with the earliest appearance of violent behaviour in the client's records. It is quite possible that ID clients begin showing recordable incidents of violent much earlier than non-ID clients, in which case the recommended HCR-20 coding categories will be useless in differentiating between risk levels. This is an empirical issue to be resolved but means the scoring as it applies in the manual should be retained. If the assessor has serious concerns about the mental age of the client (and feels this should allow some moderation of scoring), then this should be described in the report.

H3. Relationship Instability

- The HCR-20 manual confines this item to romantic and intimate relationships and explicitly excludes relationships with friends and family. In a study of a community forensic ID service, Lindsay, Smith, Law, Quinn, Anderson, Smith and Allan (2004) reported that only around 2 per cent of male ID offenders had been in a stable intimate relationship.
- If the item is based on the importance of stable social support, the ability of an individual to take advantage of such support and the protective effect of stable social support against further violence then this item needs to be expanded for ID application. For individuals with ID, it is appropriate to consider their general attachment ability and style with individuals in their life irrespective of whether or not these relationships are romantic. In this way, prior relationships with peers, siblings and caseworkers are all likely to be important in considering this item.
- For ID clients who have not had the opportunity (or do not have the skill or functioning level) to develop any sort of intimate relationship, we should look at their ability to initiate/maintain any sort of close relationship, (friendships, family, carers, support workers, housemates). We should contrast appropriate relationship-seeking with attempts to develop inappropriate relationships.
- The basic point here is that stable, supportive social relationships mitigate the classification of the individual as violent by showing that the person can maintain a stable relationship (thereby suggesting the importance of reasonable interpersonal skills and the converse – violent interactions reduce the likelihood of support people remaining supportive).
- If the person engages in stable but inappropriate relationships (e.g., is violent in the context of friendships or intimate relationships) then these stable social relationships may be indicative of increased risk.
- When scoring this item, a person who is able to maintain stable and positive relationships but has had limited opportunity to develop intimate relationships should score 0. A score of 1 would be appropriate where the client shows some difficulty maintaining their relationships (e.g., reports from contacts indicate that the client is difficult to get along with) but has not lost supports because of behaviour or personality or that they have had some opportunity but have failed to engage in intimate relationships. A score of 2 is used where the person has a history

of difficulty in maintaining supports or where the person has not had their autonomy limited and by definition should have been able to develop intimate relationships but appears to not have been able to do this.

H4. Employment Problems

- Lindsay and Taylor (2008) opined that most individuals with ID have the opportunity to engage in supported activities through ID services, such as attendance at voluntary or paid employment placements, attendance at special needs college courses, attendance at social work resource centres, day programmes and so on. The ID individual's ability to engage with these occupation centres should be reviewed in a similar light to open employment for mainstream offenders. Therefore, the person's record of ability to engage with occupation, education and recreation services throughout their adult life is relevant to this item and should be considered in the scoring.
- Employment problems should be extended to meet the broadened definition of employment. Regular lateness or failure to attend (differentiated, of course, from such difficulties as transport problems or staffing issues) should score a 1, and refusing to attend or being dismissed from programmes because of behaviour or attitude would count as a 2 for this item.

H5. Substance Use Problems

- The HCR-20 manual includes misuse of prescription drugs as substance abuse. The ability to misuse drugs implies the ability to access drugs and/or self-administer medication, activities for which ID clients may not have the opportunity in many situations. Also, inappropriate administration of medication by staff or family would not count. And, if given the opportunity to access medication, sometimes the misuse would be unintentional for ID clients.
- It is worth noting that studies of offenders with ID that include one significant item on alcohol abuse have consistently produced significant predictive results for recidivism (e.g., Lindsay & Taylor, 2008). As a result, if the drug or alcohol usage is clearly intentional and related to offending behaviour it seems appropriate to consider this item in the same way as for mainstream offenders.

H6. Major Mental Illness

- We note that the diagnosis of mental illness with ID clients is problematic. White, Chant, Edwards, Townsend and Waghorn (2005) found evidence of a high level of dual diagnoses of ID clients in a large Australian sample. In fact, 8 per cent of the ID sample had been diagnosed as depressed and another 14 per cent with an anxiety disorder (although according to the HCR-20 an anxiety disorder does not count). In 2004, Kerker, Owens, Zigler and Horwitz found that some mental illnesses were more prevalent in the ID than in the non-ID population. These authors reflected on the problems in making accurate diagnoses with ID patients in their excellent article.
- The HCR-20 manual indicates that a person with an ID would score a 2 automatically. However, in the present context we suggest that a person with a diagnosed ID (i.e., IQ below 70 or significant adaptive behaviour deficits) only be given a 1 and be given a 2 only if the

client has an Axis I disorder in addition to ID, or clear symptomology warranting a referral for diagnosis and treatment. A client with a borderline ID would be scored as a 0 and only be given a 1 or a 2 if diagnosed with an Axis I disorder.

- Of course, for the sake of manageability it is also critical that the assessor identify symptoms and histories of other major mental illness and how these symptoms present or complicate the clinical picture in the ID or borderline ID client.

H7. Psychopathy

- This item is valid for ID, and there is a substantial literature in this regard (e.g., Gray, Fitzgerald, Taylor & Snowden, 2007; Gray, Hill, McGleish, Timmons, MacCulloch & Snowden, 2003; Morissey et al., 2007). The reader is referred to Morrissey's ID guidelines (2006) for practical direction. Given Gray's research using the PCL-SV, it may be the case that the PCL-SV is generally used in preference to the full PCL-R, but if psychopathy is a possible issue (that is, a diagnosis thereof is important to the case or to the management of the case), then it is probably better practice to administer the full test (using the Morrissey items). Any user of the PCL-R is cautioned to ensure that they have met at least the minimum training standards for the use of that instrument and are aware of local validation samples (if any) for the use of the test in their jurisdiction. The PCL-R is not a SPJ instrument in the pure sense – the scores are validated for use within certain populations and therefore it cannot be assumed that the test is valid in a new setting or with an unusual population of clients.

H8. Early Maladjustment

- Maladjustment during childhood may disrupt appropriate socialisation. With ID individuals, disruptions with appropriate bonding may occur because of factors outside the child's control, such as a service's inability to provide adequate support so the person is 'shuffled' around. This sort of socialisation disruption would be unusual for non-ID children.
- In addition, ID children would appear to be at greater risk of victimisation because of their vulnerability owing to greater levels of family psychopathology, psychosocial deprivation, behavioural disturbances at school, psychiatric illness, social naivety and poor ability to form normal sexual and personal relationships, (e.g., Winter, Holland & Collins, 1997).
- We suggest some caution in assigning a high score when there is a high rate of out-of-home placement – this is not uncommon for ID clients. In such cases it is important to consider why this occurred. Maladjustment should only be considered where the out-of-home placement was for reasons of behaviour (parent or client) as opposed to medical requirement.
- Therefore, in scoring this item, while the same scoring criteria should apply, the assessor should be careful to ascertain the reason for maladjustment.

H9. Personality Disorder

- It can be difficult to distinguish characteristics of ID from personality disorder, including impulsivity, emotional dysregulation, attachment difficulties, self-injury and attention-seeking behaviour among other characteristics. In addition to behavioural disorders, communication problems and physical or sensory disorders often associated with ID adversely affect the accuracy of diagnosis of personality disorder in the ID person (Khan, Cowan & Roy, 1997). Khan and colleagues noted that the issue of accuracy is further complicated by their finding that personality disorders are sometimes diagnosed as behavioural disorders in the person with severe ID as personality diagnosis requires subjective reports of thoughts and feelings which may be difficult to elicit from the severely ID (or for the neophyte clinician to identify). The opposite was found with those with a mild or moderate level of ID; that is, particular patterns of behaviour were more often diagnosed as a personality disorder than a behavioural disorder in higher functioning clients.

- It is well known that the development of personality characteristics takes longer in people with ID than in non-ID people (Royal College of Psychiatrists, 2001).
- The difficulty in accurate diagnosis is exemplified by a review conducted by Alexander and Cooray (2003) in which they found a range of less than 1 per cent to over 90 per cent in community samples and a range of 22 per cent to 92 per cent in hospital settings. Clearly such variability is too large to be explained by real differences between such settings. Alexander and Cooray (ibid.) concluded that specific criteria be developed for the diagnosis of personality disorders in ID for various developmental levels and suggested that objective proxy measures such as behavioural observations be used particularly for those with severe disabilities.
- Further, the criteria for some of the personality disorders (e.g., dissocial and paranoid) seem to assume a level of cognitive ability which may be absent in those with an ID (Goldberg, Gitta & Puddephatt, 1995).
- When scoring this item, a 1 should be provided when the person is under the age of 25 (to account for the longer development of personality) unless it is very evident that the cognitions underlying the personality disorder are present and very stable. A 1 should be scored where there is no diagnosis but file information has noted traits of a personality disorder – for example, severe and persistent fears of abandonment.

H10. Prior Supervision Failure

- With ID clients, this item should include any sort of imposed supervision, not necessarily just those imposed for criminal activity. This would then include supervision or imposed restrictions because of challenging or offensive behaviour.
- The scoring of this item should vary with the client's level of understanding of his restrictions, including not just what the restrictions are but why they were imposed. With non-ID clients, supervision failure may be more often for nefarious reasons than for ID clients, for whom the supervision failure may be because the person did not understand or know what or why there was a restriction.
- The HCR-20 manual says to score 0 if the person has never had a period of institutional or community supervision – legally imposed restrictions. Many ID clients with violent behaviour do not end up having contact with the criminal justice system because of tolerance of violence by staff in support services (Lyall, Holland & Collins, 1995). This means that many people with an ID would not have had legally-imposed restrictions if their violent behaviour was classified as challenging as opposed to being an offence. Furthermore, many courts might redirect a client to treatment services rather than impose a court order. However, if restrictions were placed on a person to limit his opportunity to commit violent behaviour

and he disregarded the restriction (regardless of understanding) we would suggest scoring a 1; more serious failures (e.g., new violence or other illegal activity) we suggest should score a 2.

- We emphasise that the supervision issues in this item have to do with issues related to violent behaviour. We emphasise that the supervision issues in this item have to do with issues related to violent behaviour. We would not consider other forms of non-compliance, such as absconding from a house to buy cigarettes or simply not following the direction of staff to turn off a TV, say, worth scoring for this item. A qualifier to this would be if the person going unsupervised to obtain their cigarettes has a history of committing sexually violent or sexually offensive challenging acts when unsupervised. In this situation a 2 would be warranted.

- Finally, in almost all jurisdictions, community service orders and treatment plans are meted out to ID clients. Most of the items in such orders are, in essence, to do with housekeeping and time structuring for the client. There may be explicit issues related to mitigating the risk for violence in such orders, and the in-house consequence of this may be loss of privileges. This should be recognised as a supervision failure (e.g., 1 point), or some assessors might forget or ignore these types of supervision.

C1. Lack of Insight

- ID clients vary dramatically in their ability to formulate insight, and also the way that insight is revealed is sometimes even more subtle than in non-ID persons. We caution that, as the client's insight may be undetectable without experience and time, it is very inappropriate to simply score a 1 or 2 simply on the basis of the nature of a client's ID. Of course, if there is lack of insight it remains a risk factor, and one which is not necessarily lessened because it is the result of cognitive deficits.

- Therefore it is important to ascertain the client's insight with specific reference to their offences and not to make assumptions based on their cognitive ability. It remains the case that, regardless of reason, a lack of insight linked to violence propensity is scored.

C2. Negative Attitudes

- Clients with ID may be more susceptible to holding, or at least appearing to hold, negative attitudes due to their desire for inclusion with other ID and non-ID peers. They may not really support or even understand the negative attitudes they appear to display. However, there is no reason to believe that this would reduce the potency of this risk factor if that were the case, which indicates that the scoring in the manual would equally apply to those with an ID.

- At the same time, there is evidence to suggest that people with an intellectual disability have higher levels of suggestibility. This requires that an assessor use open-ended questions when interviewing a client to obtain attitudes related to offending.

C3. Active Symptoms of Major Mental Illness

- This item applies fully to the ID client, but the assessor is reminded of the cautions of the H6 (Major Mental Illness) item. Symptoms of mental illness must be clearly the result of a

mental illness as described in H6 and not ID (or any other mental health problem such as acquired brain injury, as per any diagnostic scheme).
- In this item, active symptoms do not include the ongoing symptomology of ID.

C4. Impulsivity

- Parry and Lindsay (2003) reported that ID non-sexual violent offenders were more impulsive than ID sexual offenders. But it is not necessarily the case that ID clients are always impulsive. In fact, a perusal of the relevant literature suggests that this is a common but perhaps unfounded assumption warranting more investigation. Regardless of the dynamics of the issue and whether impulsivity is actually more problematic in the ID client, this factor is still relevant in terms of its role in affecting a client's risk of violent offending.
- In the HCR-20, the issue seems to be strongly related to emotional lability, whereas with ID clients this item could also relate to motor impulsivity, and emotional lability may or not be an issue. Regardless of the type of impulsivity, this item needs particular knowledge regarding how impulsivity manifests itself with ID clients and how the client's level and type of impulsivity impacts on their risk for violence. Therefore a client who has a high level of motor impulsivity might still only score a 1 if it appears this impulsivity has little relationship with their aggression.

C5. Unresponsive to Treatment

- The HCR-20 manual seems more focussed on non-compliance with any sort of medical, clinical or vocational intervention, that is, intentional unresponsiveness. For some ID clients, this could be an issue, but we assume that a client's facility for intentional non-compliance will vary with level of ID.
- We also note that the range of interventions will be generally much broader for ID clients – particularly those related to their disabilities (e.g., skill building or management of other challenging behaviours).
- For ID clients, we are unsure if intentionality necessarily affects risk (culpability certainly, not necessarily risk), none the less, we would suggest, in general, that a 2 be scored when it is clear that there is intentional non-compliance and a 1 when it is unclear that the non-compliance is intentional. However, we would add the rider clause that if the non-compliance is clearly related to risk that a 2 be scored as per the manual, regardless of intentionality.
- Finally, the scoring of the item should also vary if the assessor is unclear whether the person is unresponsive to treatment or whether the treatment was appropriate for the level of cognitive ability of the person or appropriately implemented. If there is doubt, we recommend scoring a 1; describing the scoring issue as failure in a cognitive therapy does not mean other interventions like medication or environmental management would not be unsuccessful.

R1. Plans Lack Feasibility

- This item is very similar to that of the PCL-R Item 13 or PCL-SV Item 9. As Morrissey (2006) suggested, this item should take into account what is appropriate for persons according to their 'level of ability and adaptive skills, and in terms of the person's comprehension of what is ... attainable for them' (p. 8).

- We would add that the HCR-20 and PCL items seem to be related mainly to post-release plans and this ignores the fact that many ID clients are not in custody and many of those in the community are actually in long-term placement.
- Further, it may also be more difficult for people to judge what is realistic for an ID client, in that people often underestimate their abilities or ability to learn.
- As a result, we encourage assessors to focus not only on feasibility but ability and willingness. If a client is willing and able to discuss and engage in planning goals; and if they are able to formulate good plans or adjust plans to make them realistic with a bit of support, then a 0 is warranted.
- Higher scores should be given when the goals are unrealistic, unattainable and this lack of realism and ability to either achieve the goal or realise the inherent infeasibility of the goal actually contributes to the risk the client presents to the community.

R2. Exposure to Destabilisers

- In principle, this item applies fully to ID clients. The nature of the destabilisers may be a little different (in general, less exposure to antisocial peers, less exposure to drugs and alcohol), but also the nature of the professional supervision will be different. For example, instead of weekly or intermittent appointments with parole officers for the non-ID client, ID clients could be living in a residential care setting or have specially trained caseworkers assigned to them on an individual or small-group basis. Hopefully, the specialised training of ID care or support workers would result in many ID clients scoring lower on this item than non-ID clients.
- While a person with an ID might have less exposure to factors that are significantly criminogenic (thus warranting a 2), a person with an ID might have greater exposure to additional stressors (see R5) that may be destabilising and require scoring a 1 on this item.

R3. Lack of Personal Support

- This item has some unique ID considerations. For example, depending on level of ID, a person could be living in a residential care setting, have 24-hour active case management and automatically score a 0 with the current HCR-20 scoring guidelines. However, we would suggest that the quality of the staff support and care be factored in to reach a score. Inattentive staff, or staff with poor attitudes, poorly-integrated services, and inconsistent, absentee or neglectful parents all may reflect a lack of personal support relative to that needed to manage the level of risk present.
- We doubt that many ID clients would decide against accepting support from family, but this is possible. Further, we would contend that more ID clients would have immediate family support (as well as support for the supportive family) for years in comparison with non-ID clients.
- When scoring this item, a 0 should reflect a level and quality of support required to address the behaviour. A 1 would be appropriate where the level of support is sufficient but the lack of quality is likely to lead to violent behaviour. A 2 would be given where necessary supports are not available or where supports appear to promote violent behaviour.

R4. Noncompliance with Remediation Attempts

- In most circumstances, remediation attempts in disability services refer to behaviour intervention plans implemented by support services and the administration of medication. When considering compliance with such plans, it is important that it is compliance with those aspects related to reducing violent behaviour.
- Although this item is concerned with the individual's predicted level of future non-compliance, the item assumes that there are plans for the future, or that there have been previous attempts at remediation on which to assess the future. Services supporting those with ID will often have neither any remediation plans in place nor plans for any such in the future. Reasons include lack of recognition that the client actually requires this or the fact the ID services often operate in crisis mode and future planning is not always a high priority or reality.
- In terms of intent, when scoring this item for ID comments relating to intent in precious items (H1, H5 and C5) should be taken into consideration. Obviously, where the non-compliance is clearly intentional it should be scored in the same way as for mainstream offenders. Whether present or future intent is assumed, the focus should be on the outcome of noncompliance, that is, an increase of risk. The level of ID will also impact on the on the level of intentional non-compliance.
- The type of remediation or intervention and its relationship to offending should be taken into consideration in terms of intent when scoring this item. It is suggested that the probability of non-compliance to planned future interventions not directly related to offending behaviour be scored as a 1 (e.g., daily routine) and those directly related to offending (e.g., line of sight supervision) a 2.
- This item specifically mentions medication as a remediation. Individuals with an ID are more likely to be on medication than are members of the mainstream population. In scoring this item it is suggested that if the medication compliance is not related to offending and predicted non-compliance may be for a valid reason, (e.g., not wanting to take the medication because of the side effects), then a 0 is given. If the medication is not related to offending & the reason for non-compliance relates to attitudes or personality factors that are consistent with re-offending (e.g., being disagreeable) a 1 is scored. If the medication being refused is directly related to offending then a score of 2 is given regardless of the reason for refusal.

R5. Stress

- Individuals with ID are likely to be vulnerable to similar types of stressors as are the mainstream population. The three general areas family, peer and employment (day occupation) would be valid for the ID population.
- Individuals with ID are likely to have additional stressors because of their cognitive and functional (including communication) deficits. They have an increased need to rely on others and are often living in congregate care not necessarily with others who are compatible. In addition, they often have fewer resources and less capacity and opportunity to escape from stressors, and they are often forced to remain in highly stress-provoking situations. Coupled with their cognitive and functional deficits (e.g., decreased coping, problem solving and

communication skills) it would be expected that individuals with ID would potentially score higher on this item than mainstream individuals.

- Given probable communication deficits the assessor should take into account the possibility that the individual with ID may display offence-unrelated challenging behaviours as a way of expressing their level of stress.
- Because of their vulnerability individuals with an ID are often themselves victims of violence so Felson's (1992) point that persons who were under stress were only more likely to be violent than those who were not under stress if they also had been victims of violence, is particularly relevant.
- The definition of 'serious stressors' is open to a broader interpretation for this group given the points above. In scoring, though, the item does take into consideration the individual's ability to cope with them.

CONCLUSIONS

There are several studies indicating that the HCR-20 has predictive validity for non-sexually violent ID offenders (e.g., Morissey *et al.*, 2007). However, the elaboration of test items or the validation of such tests with ID offenders does not help in all cases because many individuals with ID are not charged for their offending (or challenging) behaviour and hence these instruments (indeed all commonly used risk assessment instruments, including all the actuarial tests) would be inapplicable. For the assessment of risk for individuals with ID with actual charges or convictions for non-sexual violent offences we suggest that the literature supports the use of the HCR-20 and a relevant actuarial instrument for the risk assessment of non-sexually violent ID individuals.

In order to use the HCR-20 more appropriately with ID clients who either offend or show violent challenging behaviour, we have offered some suggestions to conceptualise or expand the current SPJ items within an ID context. We suggest that the convergence of the risk posed by the original and parallel sets of items will help to provide an overall picture of the level of risk posed by the individual in the context of the environmental variables that comprise the individual's current circumstances. It is our opinion that only by contextualising the individual's risk within an ecological framework can an accurate portrayal of current dynamic risk (and hence the management of that risk) be construed.

REFERENCES

Alexander, R. & Cooray, S. (2003). Diagnosis of personality disorders in learning disability. *The British Journal of Psychiatry*, *182*, 28–31.

Doyle, D.M. (2004). The differences between sex offending and challenging behaviour in people with an intellectual disability. *Journal of Intellectual and Developmental Disability*, *29* (2), 107–18.

Emerson, E. (2001). *Challenging behaviour: Analysis and intervention in people with severe intellectual disabilities*, 2nd edn. Cambridge, UK: Cambridge University Press.

Felson, R.B. (1992). 'Kick 'em when they're down': Explanations of the relationship between stress and interpersonal aggression and violence. *Sociological Quarterly*, *33*, 1–16.

Goldberg, B., Gitta, M.Z. & Puddephatt, A. (1995). Personality and trait disturbances in an adult mental retardation population: Significance for psychiatric management. *Journal of Intellectual Disability Research, 39*, 284–94.

Gray, N.S., Fitzgerald, S., Taylor, J., MacCulloch, M.J., & Snowden, R.J. (2007). Predicting future reconviction in offenders with intellectual disabilities: The predictive efficacy of VRAG, PCL-SV and the HCR-20. *Psychological Assessment, 19*, 474–9.

Gray, N.S., Hill, C., McGleish, A., Timmons, D., MacCulloch, M.J. & Snowden, R.J. (2003). Prediction of violence and self-harm in mentally disordered offenders: A prospective study of the efficacy of HCR-20, PCL-R, and psychiatric symptomatology. *Journal of Consulting and Clinical Psychology, 71* (3), 443–51.

Hare, R.D. (2003). *The Hare psychopathy checklist - revised*, 2nd edn. Toronto, Ontario: Multi-Health Systems.

Hart, S.D., Cox, D.N. & Hare, R.D. (1995). *The Hare PCL:SV*. Toronto, Ontario: Multi-Health Systems.

Kerker, B.D., Owens, P.L., Zigler, E. & Horwitz, S.M. (2004). Mental health disorders among individuals with mental retardation: Challenges to accurate prevalence estimates. *Public Health Reports, 119*, 409–17.

Khan, A., Cowan, C. & Roy, A. (1997). Personality disorders in people with learning disabilities, a community survey. *Journal of Intellectual Disability Research, 41*, 324–30.

Lindsay, W.R., Hogue, T.E., Taylor, J.L., Steptoe, L., Mooney, P., O'Brien, G., Johnston, S. & Smith, A.H.W. (2008). Risk assessment in offenders with intellectual disability. *International Journal of Offender Therapy and Comparative Criminology, 52* (1), 90–111.

Lindsay, W.R., Smith, A.H.W., Law, J., Quinn, K., Anderson, A., Smith, A. & Allan, R. (2004). Sexual and non-sexual offenders with intellectual and learning disabilities: A comparison of characteristics, referral patterns and outcome. *Journal of Interpersonal Violence, 19*, 875–90.

Lindsay, W.R. & Taylor, J.L. (2008). Assessment and treatment of offenders with intellectual and developmental disabilities. In K. Soothill, P. Rogers, and M. Dolan (Eds), *Handbook of forensic mental health*, UK: Willan Press.

Lyall, I., Holland, A.J., Collins, S. (1995). Offending by adults with learning disabilities and the attitudes of staff to offending behaviour: Implications for service development. *Journal of Intellectual Disability Research, 39* (6), 501–8.

Morrissey, C. (2003). Guidelines for use of the PCL-R in offenders with intellectual disabilities. Unpublished manuscript.

Morrissey, C. (2006). Guidelines for assessing psychopathy in offenders with intellectual disabilities using the PCL-R and PCL: SV. Unpublished manuscript.

Morissey, C., Hogue, T., Mooney, P., Lindsay, W.R., Steptoe, L., Taylor, J.L. & Johnston, S. (2005). Applicability, reliability and validity of the Psychopathy Checklist-Revised in offenders with intellectual disabilities: Some initial findings. *International Journal of Forensic Mental Health, 4* (2), 207–20.

Morissey, C., Hogue, T., Mooney, P., Allen, C., Johnston, S., Hollin, C., Lindsay, W.R. & Taylor, J.L. (2007). Predictive validity of the PCL-R in offenders with intellectual disability in a high secure hospital setting: Institutional aggression. *Journal of Forensic Psychiatry and Psychology, 18*, 1–15.

Parry, C.J. & Lindsay, W.R. (2003). Impulsiveness as a factor in sexual offending by people with mild intellectual disability. *Journal of Intellectual Disability Research, 47* (6), 483–7.

Quinsey, V.L., Harris, G.T., Rice, M.E. & Cormier, C.A. (2003). *Violent offenders: Appraising and managing risk* (2nd edn). Washington, DC: American Psychological Association.

Royal College of Psychiatrists (2001). *Diagnostic criteria for learning disability (DC-LD)*. London: Gaskell.

Webster, C.D., Douglas, K.S., Eaves, D. & Hart, S.D. (1997). *HCR-20: Assessing risk for violence (version 2)*. Burnaby, British Columbia, Canada: The Mental Health, Law, and Policy Institute of Simon Fraser University.

White, P., Chant, D., Edwards, N., Townsend, C. & Waghorn, G. (2005). Prevalence of intellectual disability and comorbid mental illness in an Australian community sample. *Australian and New Zealand Journal of Psychiatry*, *39* (5), 395–400.

Winter, N., Holland, A.J. & Collins S. (1997). Factors predisposing to suspected offending by adults with self-reported learning disabilities. *Psychological Medicine*, *27*, 595–607.

11

Suggested Adaptations to the SVR-20 for Offenders with Intellectual Disabilities

DOUGLAS P. BOER, MATTHEW FRIZE, RUTH PAPPAS, CATRIN MORRISSEY AND WILLIAM R. LINDSAY

INTRODUCTION

As noted in the previous chapter,[1] while there are a number of well-researched structured professional judgement (SPJ) instruments available for risk assessment purposes of violent and sexual offenders, none of these instruments provide explicit rules for the differential assessment of intellectually disabled (ID) offenders.[2] That is, there are no generally accepted guidelines for the application of the standard items in commonly used SPJ instruments to ID clients. As a result, researchers and clinicians who have found evidence that SPJ instruments are valid with ID offenders have adapted the items in these instruments in idiosyncratic ways and, to date, have not always been clear as to how this was done for the purposes of their research. For example, while there is some evidence that certain SPJ instruments, such as the Sexual Violence Risk – 20 (SVR-20) (Boer, Hart, Kropp & Webster, 1997) appears valid with

---

[1] The usefulness of the present chapter hinges on the assumption that the reader will also read the Chapter 10 of this book on the adaptation of the HCR-20 (Webster, Douglas, Eaves & Hart, 1997) items for use with ID offenders. Certain basic sections were not repeated in this chapter (for example, the sections entitled 'application to ID offenders' and 'general principles') but are clearly relevant to the use of the SVR-20 with ID offenders.

[2] Here and in Chapter 10, individuals with ID are seen as those individuals with a full scale IQ of less than 75 and those individuals with a measured IQ of less than 80 but with significant adaptive behaviour deficits. An IQ cut-off of 75 takes into account the standard error of measurement of most of the commonly used intelligence tests. It is noted that Morrissey (2006) suggested that her PCL-R guidelines be applied to offenders with ID and that ID is to be inclusive of individuals with diagnosed intellectual disability (that is, those with an IQ of less than 70) and also those individuals with borderline intellectual disability (that is, those with an IQ of less than 80) who also have significant adaptive behaviour deficits.

Assessment and Treatment of Sexual Offenders with Intellectual Disabilities: A Handbook
Edited by Leam A. Craig, William R. Lindsay and Kevin D. Browne
© 2010 John Wiley & Sons, Ltd.

ID sexual offenders (e.g., Lambrick, 2003), these same authors note that some of the factors have to be interpreted with caution. But Lambrick did not explain how the SVR-20 was adapted in practice.

The present chapter aims to provide some guidelines for the use of the SVR-20 with ID individuals who have been charged with, or convicted of, sexually violent crimes. Furthermore, we would also propose that the principles and strategies elucidated in this chapter applied in risk assessment of offenders with ID could potentially be adapted to provide an assessment framework for people with ID who, though not ever (or at least not to date) involved in the criminal justice system, exhibit sexual behaviours labelled as *challenging*; viz., 'culturally abnormal behaviours of such an intensity, frequency or duration that the physical safety of the person or others is likely to be placed in serious jeopardy, or behaviour which is likely to seriously limit the use of, or result in the person being denied access to, ordinary community facilities' (Emerson, 2001, p. 3).

While some ID individuals may commit sexually violent behaviour, such behaviours are not always legally consequenced because of issues regarding mental capacity and intent – a substantive discussion of which is beyond the scope of this chapter. However, in brief, Doyle (2004) viewed sexual offending as 'challenging' behaviour when the perpetrator committing the behaviour is doing so without intent to harm another person. Challenging sexual behaviour can still be criminal, particularly if the victim of the unintentional behaviour feels offended against or legal consequences ensue. Further, lack of intent does not reduce the person's potential to cause harm in the future.

In the preceding chapter, we noted that research by Morrissey *et al.* (2007) demonstrated the applicability of the Psychopathy Checklist – Revised (PCL-R) (Hare, 2003) to ID offenders. This research was based on a set of guidelines produced by Morrissey in 2003 and revised in 2006 that are available from the author. The present chapter follows Morrissey's guidelines for the use of the PCL-R when assessing ID offenders with the SVR-20. However, unlike Morrissey's guidelines, the following guidelines do not have empirical support – these are suggested alterations only, and these suggestions require empirical validation before adoption as anything but research suggestions.

In keeping with Morrissey (2006), we are suggesting that the present guidelines be applied to offenders with ID and that ID is to be inclusive of individuals with diagnosed ID (that is, those with an IQ of less than 70) and also those individuals with borderline ID who also have significant adaptive behaviour deficits. Also, Morrissey (ibid.) listed a number of general principles for assessing psychopathy in ID offenders. In the preceding chapter, we paraphrased these general principles to apply them to the use of the HCR-20 with ID offenders. These same principles hold true for the application of the SVR-20 with ID offenders.

Most importantly, we acknowledge that the following guidelines do change the content of the original items to some degree, but we have striven to maintain the original intent of the SVR-20 items. We also want to stress that these guidelines should only be used on ID individuals who are 21 years of age or older (Royal College of Psychiatrists, 2001), and not with ID individuals with IQs of less than 55 based on the findings by Morrissey *et al.* (2006) of poor inter-rater reliability with this group. It would seem reasonable to pay attention to the general principles elucidated by Morrissey *et al.* (2006) in the use of any SPJ with ID an individual which, like the SVR-20, utilises psychopathy as an item.

Finally, the other authors of the SVR-20 have not granted their approval for these replacement items for use with ID sexual offenders, nor are we suggesting that these items are any better or more useful than any the reader could derive themselves. However, if all users of the SVR-20 were to derive their own ID items, then logically there would be greater variability and lack of precision in ID offender assessment – the very problem we are seeking to help reduce. In closing, we suggest that researching similar items for use with ID increases our ability to do good work for our clients and further our ability to increase effective reintegration and increase public safety.

SVR-20

The current version of the SVR-20 (Boer, Hart, Kropp & Webster, 1997) was constructed using a subset of the HCR-20 (Webster, Douglas, Eaves & Hart, 1997) historical items with a number of items related specifically to sexual offending. Like the HCR-20, it is organised into three sections – Psychosocial Adjustment or history (11 items), Sexual Offences (7 items) and Future Plans (2 items) – each broadly related to historical, current clinical (offence-related) and future risk issues. Each of the items may be rated on a three-point scale from 0, no evidence of the variable, through 1, some evidence of the variable, to 2, clear evidence of the variable. The total score is the sum of the items, although the authors do not generally recommend making decisions on the basis of the total score. Rather, it is recommended that the items are structured in order to help the consideration of a comprehensive range of variables with a view to arriving at a final judgement based on supervision and treatment needs of the individual offender.

  The SVR-20 has been the subject of a considerable quantity of research work in a range of settings for mainstream sexual offenders in both correctional (e.g., Dempster, 1998) and forensic psychiatric treatment facilities (e.g., de Vogel, de Ruiter, van Beek & Mead, 2004) and has regularly shown increased predictive validity over that of actuarial scales designed specifically for sexual offender risk assessment such as the Static-99 (Hanson & Thornton, 1999). The latter fact, coupled with the fact that the Static-99 and other actuarial measures do have adequate predictive validity with ID sexual offenders (all of which have poorer predictive validity than the SVR-20 according to some meta-analyses – e.g., Hanson & Morton-Bourgon, 2004), suggests that the SVR-20 would likely also be a valid risk instrument with this population. However, to our knowledge, there are no published reports reviewing the predictive accuracy and value of the SVR-20 in clinical practice and the prediction of re-offending with ID forensic clients at the present time. None the less, there are a number of studies (under the supervision of some of the authors of this chapter among others) nearing completion that will hopefully show that the SVR-20 works validly with ID sexual offenders. The reader is encouraged to contact the first author of this chapter for such information.[3]

ADAPTED SVR-20 ITEMS – 'QUALIFIERS'

Please note that for all items, the standard item from the SVR-20 manual should be read first. The following suggestions are to be used in parallel with, not in replacement of, the original

---

[3] Please contact Dr Douglas P. Boer at drdoug@waikato.ac.nz for up-to-date research findings or inquiries regarding collaborative research on the SVR-20 or related instruments for ID offenders.

item. In other words, read the manual item, then the ID item 'qualifier' – the additional information that may influence your item rating. Then rate the item using the existing coding from the manual unless new coding is indicated by research on the suggested parallel items. Although we endorse the use of these items with both female and male ID clients we have used the male pronoun throughout the following items as there are simply more of the latter. The items are provided in the same order as in the manual, beginning with the Psychosocial Adjustment (PA) items, the Sexual Offences (SO) items and the Future Plans (FP) items. In general, the PA and FP items have more differences from the standard items for ID application than the SO items, most of which seem quite applicable as they stand in the the SCR-20 manual (with a few caveats).

Psychosocial Adjustment Items

PA1. Sexual Deviation

- The manual describes deviant sexual preference or paraphilia as a relatively stable pattern of sexual arousal to inappropriate sexual stimuli that causes distress or social dysfunction. However, as Lambrick (2003) noted, sex offenders with an ID may be exposed to unusual sexual circumstances compared to other individuals. For example, they often lack privacy through living in supervised settings. Thus, being found masturbating by staff (sometimes in their own rooms or in the toilets) could be mistakenly considered to be exhibitionism. Or, wearing the wrong clothing could be mistakenly considered to be cross-dressing or fetishism.
- On the other hand, some research (e.g., Day, 1994; Langevin & Pope, 1993; and Thompson, 1997) suggests that ID sexual offenders may have multiple markers of sexual deviancy, including attraction to a wide range of potential victims (non-specific to age and gender) coupled with a more marked level of sexual impulsivity.
- In scoring this item, assessors should be sensitive to the client's limited access to opportunities for sexual interaction or for masturbation (including any sexual behaviour being 'against the rules'), low levels of sexual knowledge, different fantasies, different preoccupations – all of which may result in odd challenging behaviour as opposed to intentional 'deviant' sexual behaviour, but which may still result in the victimisation of others.

PA2. Victim of Child Abuse

- All forms of child abuse, unfortunately, are linked with youth and adult criminality, non-sexual violence, and sexual violence (e.g., Hanson & Bussière, 1996). Lindsay, Law, Quinn, Smart, and Smith (2001) found a significant relationship between abuse type and adult offending behaviour. In this study, 38 per cent of the ID sex offenders had experienced sexual abuse as children, while 13 per cent of the non-sexual offenders had similar abuse experiences. However, 33 per cent of the non-sexual (violent) ID offenders had experienced physical abuse as children in contrast to 13 per cent of the sexual offenders. Thus, it appears that there is some evidence that experiences of sexual abuse may influence the development of deviant sexual preference with ID clients. Also, refusal of naive therapists to address this issue results in poor therapeutic alliance. It is certainly a barrier to treatment if not addressed adequately.

- ID considerations would include being a victim of abuse – not just as a child, but as a young adult as well – all forms of abuse by family, direct care staff, and others (including other persons with an ID). Transitions to care because of challenging behaviour by the client may be made in an indifferent or possibly vindictive fashion (sometimes moving is very upsetting to the client and this may or may not be known to parents or care staff).
- The agent of abuse need not be the family. In the case of ID clients, abusers can also be direct care and support workers (in both group homes and institutions), but may also have been at school or day placements. Abusers could also include other ID clients.
- The spectrum of abuse is detailed in the SVR-20 manual. But for ID clients, the spectrum can be enlarged to include a large number of early transitions or transfer of care by disability services because of challenging behaviour. Some may think that a transition to care may be sufficient to consider abuse when it is because of the client's behaviour. ID clients may lack the understanding of the rationale for transfer, find it upsetting and feel abused.

PA3. Psychopathy

- In the SVR-20 manual we defined 'psychopathic personality disorder' as 'psychopathy as defined by the characteristics of the PCL-R (Hare, 2003) or PCL-SV (Hart, Cox & Hare, 1995). In sexual offenders, psychopathy is related to opportunistic and sadistic offending.
- This item is the same for the SVR-20 and the HCR-20. There is a substantial literature validating the PCL-R and PCL-SV with ID violent offenders (e.g., Gray, Fitzgerald, Taylor & Snowden, 2007; Gray, Hill, McGleish, Timmons, MacCulloch & Snowden, 2003; Morrissey *et al.*, 2007). The reader is referred to Morrissey's ID guidelines (2006) for practical direction. Given Gray's research using the PCL-SV, it may be the case that the PCL-SV is generally used in preference to the full PCL-R, but if psychopathy is a possible issue (that is, a diagnosis thereof is important to the case or to the management of the case), then it is probably better practice to administer the full test (using the Morrissey items). Any user of the PCL-R is cautioned to ensure that they have met at least the minimum training standards for the use of that instrument and are aware of local validation samples (if any) for the use of the test in their jurisdiction. The PCL-R is not a SPJ instrument in the pure sense – the scores are validated for use within certain populations and therefore it cannot be assumed that the test is valid in a new setting or with an unusual population of clients.
- We do have one caveat – while there is ample research supporting the use of the PCL-R and PCL-SV with ID violent offenders, there is less for ID sexually violent offenders.

PA4. Major Mental Illness

- For the inexperienced clinician, the diagnosis of major mental illness (MMI) with ID clients is problematic, particularly since the diagnosis of ID itself may cloud or impede the accuracy of any further diagnostic issues. None the less, White, Chant, Edwards, Townsend and Waghorn (2005) found evidence of a high level of dual diagnoses with ID clients in a large Australian sample. In fact, 8 per cent of the ID sample had been diagnosed as depressed and another 14 per cent with an anxiety disorder (although according to the HCR-20 and SVR-20 anxiety disorders do not count as major mental illnesses). Kerker, Owens, Zigler and Horwitz (2004) found that some mental illnesses were more prevalent in the ID than in the non-ID population. These authors provided some valuable insights on the problems in making accurate diagnoses with ID patients.

- We would add that dual diagnosis issues (ID plus an MMI) may potentiate risk as a result of the ID client experiencing difficulty or inability in the management of his MMI (for example, not taking medications) or being unable to notice symptoms prior to being compromised or incapacitated by the illness. Further, in some cases, acquired brain injury (ABI) has resulted in ID in a previously undisabled person. In any complex case, the responsible assessor should know his or her diagnostic limitations and refer appropriately.
- As with our suggestion for the ID application of this item for non-sexual violent offenders (regarding the HCR-20 manual), we suggest, contrary to the SVR-20 manual, that a person with an ID would not score a 2 automatically. Rather, a client with an ID would score a 1, and only if the ID client had an Axis I diagnosis or clear symptomology warranting a referral for diagnosis and treatment would he receive a 2 on this item. Similarly, a client with a borderline ID would score 0, and only 1 or 2 if the client had Axis I mental health problems.

PA5. Substance Use Problems

- Alcohol and substance use have long been associated with crime, and the variable has been shown to be significantly related to recidivism by a number of studies (Harris, Rice & Quinsey, 1993; Swanson, 1994). Studies on offenders with ID which include one significant item on alcohol abuse have consistently produced significant predictive results. However, Lindsay, Elliot and Astell (2004) in their review of variables related to offending in sex offenders found that increases in alcohol use did not have a significant relationship with re-offending. Apart from this one study, we are not aware of any work relating alcohol use to offending in the population of individuals with ID, and until such evidence is accumulated it seems appropriate to consider this item in the same way that one would for mainstream offenders.
- It is worth noting that studies on offenders with ID that include one significant item on alcohol abuse have consistently produced significant predictive results for recidivism (e.g., Lindsay & Taylor, 2008). As a result, if the drug or alcohol usage is clearly intentional and related to offending behaviour it seems appropriate to consider this item as one would for mainstream offenders.
- The SVR-20 manual includes misuse of prescription drugs as substance abuse. The ability to misuse drugs implies the ability to access drugs and/or self-administer medication, activities for which ID clients may not have the opportunity in many situations. Also, inappropriate administration of medication by staff or family should not count as a substance-use problem. And, if given the opportunity to access medication, sometimes the misuse would be unintentional for ID clients.
- Other ID considerations: access to drugs and alcohol may be more limited than for a non-ID client, resulting in abuse of unusual substances such as petrol or solvents; sometimes a person with ID is used by others to gain access to alcohol or prescription drugs; there is potential for unusual drug interactions (prescription drugs plus alcohol or other substances).

PA6. Suicidal/Homicidal Ideation

- While suicidal or homicidal ideation may be considered, by definition, indicators of elevated risk, as suggested by the SVR-20 manual, this is not necessarily the case for ID sex offenders. There are some additional considerations with this item for ID clients. For example, self-injurious behaviour (SIB) is a common feature of ID clients, whether sex offenders or otherwise (e.g., Collacott, Cooper, Branford & McGrother, 1998), sometimes with devastating results (e.g., Martin & Guth, 2005). Further, as Collacott, Cooper, Branford and McGrother (1998) suggest, SIB may have very different causes and functions in ID (e.g., self-stimulation).
- In our opinion, suicidal or homicidal ideation may have more to do with violence and deviance than SIB, which, though it may seem similar to suicidal behaviour possibly has more to do with the reduced ability of the person with ID to impact on their environment (a result of frustration or anger) or his inability to communicate his needs/wants. Again, the objective is to make the link between any such self-injurious behaviour or intention with sexually offensive behaviour.

PA7. Relationship Problems

- Like the HCR-20, the SVR-20 confines this item to romantic and intimate relationships and explicitly excludes relationships with friends and family. In a study of a community forensic ID service, Lindsay, Smith, Law, Quinn, Anderson, Smith and Allan (2004) reported that only around 2 per cent of male ID offenders had been in a stable intimate relationship.
- If the item is based on the importance of stable social support, the ability of an individual to take advantage of such support and the protective effect of stable social support against further violence, then this item needs to be expanded for ID application. For individuals with ID, it is appropriate to consider their general attachment ability and style with individuals in their life irrespective of whether or not these relationships are romantic. As such, prior relationships with peers, siblings and caseworkers are all likely to be important in considering this item.
- For ID clients who have not had the opportunity (or do not have the skill or functioning level) to develop any sort of intimate relationship, we should look at their ability to initiate/maintain any sort of appropriate close relationship (friends, family, carers, support workers, housemates). We should contrast appropriate relationship-seeking with attempts to develop inappropriate relationships. If an ID individual seeks an appropriate friendship with a staff member or peer, that is to be welcomed, but if the object of his desire is a child or if he attempts to transgress clearly defined boundaries, particularly when the issue is explained, there is reason for concern. Further, if the person engages in stable, but inappropriate relationships (e.g., is sexually violent in the context of friendships or intimate relationships) then clearly stable social relationships may be indicative of increased risk.
- A basic point here is that stable, supportive social relationships mitigate the risk of violence by showing that the person can maintain a stable relationship (thereby suggesting the importance of reasonable interpersonal skills and the converse – that violent interactions reduce the likelihood of support people remaining supportive).

- When scoring this item, a person who is able to maintain stable and positive relationships but has had limited opportunity to develop intimate relationships should score 0. A score of 1 would be appropriate where the client shows some difficulty maintaining their relationships (e.g., reports from contacts indicate that the client is difficult to get along with) but have not lost supports as a result of their behaviour or personality or that they have had some opportunity but failed to engage in intimate relationships. A 2 is appropriate in cases in which the person has a history of difficulty in maintaining supports or where the person has not had their autonomy limited and by definition should have been able to develop intimate relationships but appears not to have been able to do so.

PA8. Employment Problems

- Lindsay (2008) has argued that for sex offenders with ID, engagement with society is not only desirable in itself but also a crucial aspect of treatment. These theoretical positions are based on empirical work demonstrating that sex offenders seem satisfied with more impoverished relationships and a lower level of engagement with society than do other individuals (Steptoe, Lindsay, Forrest & Power, 2006). Therefore, the person's record of ability to engage with occupation and education services throughout their adult life is relevant to this item and should be considered in the scoring.
- ID considerations may include any regular daytime occupation, whether paid employment, education training, or ID day programmes; associated challenging behaviours that compromise attendance to programmes or place of work.
- Lindsay and Taylor (2008) opined that most individuals with ID have the opportunity to engage in supported activities through ID services, such as attendance at voluntary or paid employment placements, attendance at special needs college courses, attendance at social work resource centres, day programmes and so on. The ID individual's ability to engage with these occupation centres should be reviewed in a similar light to open employment for mainstream offenders. Therefore, the person's record of ability to engage with occupation, education and recreation services throughout their adult life is relevant to this item and should be considered in the scoring.
- Employment problems should be extended to meet the broadened definition of employment. Regular lateness or failure to attend (differentiated, of course, from problems in attending or arriving on time arising from difficulties with transport or staffing issues) should score 1, and refusing to attend or being dismissed from programmes because of behaviour or attitude would count as 2 for this item.

PA9. Past Non-sexual Violent Offences

- The SVR-20 manual cites evidence showing that non-sexual violence (actual, attempted or threatened harm) is a risk factor for criminality and violence for criminals (including sexual offenders) and forensic patients.
- The SVR-20 manual indicates that self-report and reports from credible collateral sources should be considered, along with all violence which occurred in any psychiatric or correctional facility. This assumes non-litigated but credible reports of violent behaviour. Therefore, for ID clients, we would include not just offences but staff-recorded incidents of violence.

- Other ID considerations could include collateral damage from temper tantrums (sometimes staff or other residents get in the way of the upset ID person and are hurt) or an individual with ID 'striking out' at objects instead of people.

PA10. Past Non-violent Offences

- A history of general (non-sexual, non-violent) offending is a risk factor for violence and sexual violence among offenders and forensic patients. The SVR-20 manual indicates that self-report and reports from credible collateral sources should be considered, along with all violence that has occurred in any psychiatric or correctional facility.
- In terms of ID considerations, once again 'recorded incidents' are clearly relevant; it is necessary to differentiate between annoying behaviours such as stealing other ID individual's belongings to tease or annoy someone and 'real' stealing. Similarly, lighting a fire (e.g., a chair or paper) in one's room should be considered differently to trying to burn down the group home.

PA11. Past Supervision Failures

- The SVR-20 manual says to score '0' if the person has never had a period of institutional or community supervision – legally imposed restrictions. Many ID clients with violent behaviour do not end up having contact with the criminal justice system because of the tolerance of violence of staff in support services (Lyall, Holland & Collins, 1995). This means that many people with an ID would not have had legally-imposed restrictions if their violent behaviour was classified as challenging as opposed to being an offence. Furthermore, many courts might redirect a client to treatment services rather than impose a court order. However, if restrictions were placed on a person to restrict his opportunity to commit problematic sexual behaviour and he disregarded the restriction (regardless of understanding) we would suggest scoring a 1, and for more serious failures (e.g., a new sexual offence or other illegal activity) we would suggest scoring a 2.
- With ID clients, this item should include any sort of imposed supervision, not necessarily just those imposed for criminal activity. This would then include supervision or imposed restrictions resulting from challenging or offensive behaviour.
- The scoring of this item should vary with the client's level of understanding of his restrictions, including not just what the restrictions are, but also why the restrictions were imposed. With non-ID clients, supervision failure may be for nefarious reasons more often than is the case with ID clients, for whom the supervision failure may be because the person did not understand or know what or why there was a restriction (so the supervision failure may not be the result of any sort of antisocial motive but purely because of ignorance of the rules). On the other hand, a client may actually refuse to follow residential rules in a care setting or actively decide to not abide by a treatment or care plan.
- In almost all jurisdictions, community service orders and treatment plans are meted out to ID clients. Most of the items in such orders have to do with such things as community access privileges (e.g., going for walks), housekeeping issues and time structuring for the client. There may be explicit issues related to mitigating risk for violence in such orders and this may have an in-house consequence of loss of restrictions. If related to risk, these sorts of

issues should be recognised as a supervision failure (scoring 1 point), though some assessors might forget or ignore these types of supervision.

- We emphasise that the supervision issues of most concern in this item have to do with issues related to sexually violent behaviour. We would not include such non-compliance with direction as absconding from a house to buy cigarettes, or simply not following the direction of staff to turn off a TV, for instance, as worthy of scoring as a supervision failure. A qualifier to this would be if the person going unsupervised to obtain their cigarettes has a history of committing sexually violent or sexually offensive challenging acts when unsupervised.

- Finally, 'recorded incidents' are clearly relevant; the assessor needs to differentiate between annoying behaviours such as stealing other ID individual's belongings to tease someone and 'real' stealing. Similarly, lighting a fire (e.g., setting light to a chair or paper) in one's room should be differentiated from setting fire to the group home (intent is an issue – depending on outcome!).

Sexual Offending Items[4]

SO12. High Density Sex Offences

- The number of past sexual offences is very reliably associated with sexual recidivism among offenders and forensic patients. This is a risk factor that is likely to reflect the presence of sexual deviation and attitudes that support or condone sexual violence.

- It is commonly held that ID offenders commit more sexual offences than non-ID offenders (e.g., Murphy, Coleman & Haynes, 1983), but another possible reason that the proportion of ID offenders in jail is higher than their relative numbers in the general community is simply over-incarceration for any number of reasons (including inadequate legal representation, as suggested by a number of authors, including Hayes, 1997). At the present time, it appears that we do not know the base rates of sexual or other types of violent offending for the different types of ID sex offenders (or the different types of ID clients for that matter).

- Perhaps the simplest way to solve this lack of empirical knowledge is for large treatment enterprises to report some up-to-date epidemiological data in this regard to provide some guidance as to what constitutes low, moderate and high rates of offending. It would also be helpful to know the frequency of challenging sexual behaviour for a range of ID clients. Thus, for this item, and all following items, we also would code 'recorded incidents' – those instances of sexually inappropriate or challenging or offensive behaviour that did not result in charges, but were clearly inappropriate enough to warrant a file entry.

SO13. Multiple Sex Offence Types

- We recommend that this item be scored as suggested in the manual with several caveats. Firstly, it is possible that ID clients may have a broader spectrum of sexually inappropriate

---

[4] For all of these items, we would also code 'recorded incidents' – those instances of behaviour that warranted a file entry of sexually violent behaviour, whether considered 'challenging' or 'offensive', or which warranted an external charge by the police. There is a dearth of baseline information on the frequency of sexually challenging behaviour which complicates the relative scoring for ID clients. Hopefully, research efforts will help to alleviate this and other risk-related issues.

behaviour, but there is no agreement in this regard in the literature (to our knowledge). Perhaps the sexual behaviour of the ID client is simply more observable because of the constraints of their living situations. Finally, we would suggest recording all sexual misbehaviour, including behaviours such as inappropriate masturbation (e.g., in public view as opposed to in his room or the toilet), *if* it is clear that the client knows that it is inappropriate and does it anyway.

SO14. Physical Harm to Victim(s) in Sex Offences

- We recommend that this item be scored as suggested in the manual with one general caveat. That is, the notes from the SVR-20 item indicate that intent is irrelevant to this item and therefore the issue of premeditation is merely hypothetical. However, if the harm is accidental (e.g., the result of weight or size difference or lack of coordination) or occurs as collateral damage during a temper tantrum or as a result of a scuffle with another resident or staff member, we feel this should be noted.

SO15. Uses Weapons or Threats of Death in Sex Offences

- We recommend that this item be scored as suggested in the manual with a general caveat. That is, we have doubts about the ability of some ID persons to understand or form the intent to use weapons or make serious threats of death. Some ID clients say things like 'I hate you' or 'I wish you were dead' during a temper tantrum, in a childish fashion. Others may grab a knife during anger and run around with it – often putting themselves in harm's way as opposed to being an actual threat to anyone else. However, if it is clear that the threats are not posturing or temper-related, or the weapon use is manipulative for sexual purposes, then this is certainly scoreable. And, again, if the behaviour is not intentional but is risk-related, it should be scored accordingly as a risk issue.

SO16. Escalation in Frequency or Severity of Sex Offences

- This item may not need to be adapted for ID application, but one should be certain that any observed escalation is in fact a real change in frequency or severity of the offending behaviour and not simply the result of increased identification or reporting of the behaviour. The basic problem of lack of accurate baseline data to differentiate one ID sexual offender from another remains a problem for this and other items that require knowledge of relative frequency, severity or the sexual behavioural spectrum of the ID persons being considered.

SO17. Extreme Minimisation or Denial of Sex Offences

- The meta-analyses by Hanson and Morton-Bourgon (2004, 2005) suggest that minimisation and denial are poor predictors of sexual offending. However, according to many professional reviews (e.g., Polizzi, MacKenzie & Hickman, 1999) and most current treatment texts (e.g., Marshall, Anderson & Fernandez, 1999), denial of responsibility is still considered an important issue. In our view, extreme minimisation or denial serves in a number of possible roles, including (and these are not necessarily mutually exclusive) an explicit risk factor; a factor limiting the development of insight – hence a more distal risk factor, or a factor acting as a barrier to treatment – thus, an even more distal risk factor (assuming treatment is effective).

- While we recommend that this item be scored as suggested in the manual, there are some ID offender considerations. These would include possible refusal to acknowledge offending because of memory deficits (competency versus motivation) or inaccurate reporting owing to confabulation (not being able to remember the full picture and making up some of the details to 'help out' or please the interviewer). This might be assessed by looking at the client's memory capacity for other events that occurred at the same time but are unrelated to the offensive behaviour and are of a benign nature. It is possible that if a client does not understand or cannot remember the offending he is of higher risk as he may also be unable to identify and manage risk factors (although the former does not necessarily result in the latter). Certainly, the *why* and *how* of denial and minimisation need to be ferreted out for the individual client to accurately portray their risk – and manage it.

SO18. Attitudes That Support or Condone Sex Offences

- We recommend that this item be scored as suggested in the manual with two general caveats. Firstly, the issue of opportunity for sexual expression – little opportunity may result in inappropriate expressions of sexuality (e.g., public masturbation may occur where opportunities for private masturbation is limited), and the understanding that this is acceptable may result depending on the consequences. Secondly, while attitudes about sexually offensive behaviour are often quite peer-driven they are either supported or opposed by staff. The importance of the staff setting appropriate norms cannot be neglected in this regard.

Future Plans

FP19. Lacks Realistic Plans

- As noted in the previous chapter, this item is similar to that of the PCL-R Item 13 or PCL-SV Item 9. As Morrissey (2006) suggested in her guidelines, this item should take into account what is appropriate for persons according to their 'level of ability and adaptive skills, and in terms of the person's comprehension of what is . . . (reasonably) attainable for them' (p. 8).
- Like the HCR-20 and PCL-R, this item on the SVR-20 is mainly related to post-release plans and this ignores the fact that many ID clients are not in custody and that many of those in the community are actually in long-term placement. Further, it may also be more difficult for people to judge what is realistic for an ID client, in that people often underestimate their abilities or ability to learn. As a result, we encourage assessors to focus not only on feasibility but ability and willingness. If a client is willing and able to discuss and engage in planning goals, and if they are able to formulate good plans or adjust plans to make them realistic with a little support, then a 0 is warranted.
- Higher scores should be given when the goals are unrealistic, unattainable and this lack of realism and ability to either achieve the goal or realise the inherent infeasibility of the goal actually contributes to the risk the client presents to the community.

FP20. Negative Attitude toward Intervention

- This item is quite similar to the HCR-20 item R4, namely, 'Noncompliance with Remediation Attempts' and therefore many of the same concerns apply here. For example, interventions (or 'remediation attempts') in disability services refer to behaviour intervention plans implemented by support services and the administration of medication. In the assessment of the attitude of the client toward intervention, it is most likely that attitude is being inferred from compliance with proposed intervention plans, and it is compliance with those aspects related to reducing sexually offensive behaviour that are of greatest concern.
- Although this item is concerned with the individuals predicted level of future noncompliance with intervention, the item assumes that there are plans for or have been previous attempts at intervention by which to assess the client's future risk. Services supporting those with ID will often not have any intervention plans in place or plans for such for the future. Reasons for this include lack of recognition that this is something the client actually requires or the fact the ID services often operate in crisis mode and future planning is not always a high priority or reality.
- Intent is an issue for this item. Not all ID clients have a negative attitude towards intervention because of a hidden agenda to keep offending; sometimes it is simply because being in treatment is uncomfortable psychologically (that is, they find it embarrassing to talk about things).
- Obviously, where non-compliance with treatment is clearly intentional it should be scored in the same way as for mainstream offenders. The level of ID will also impact on the on the level of intentional non-compliance. The outcome of the non-compliance, whether or not it appears to have been intentional, and how it affects risk should be the focus here. The type of remediation or intervention and its relationship to offending should be taken into consideration in terms of intent when scoring this item. It is suggested that the probability of noncompliance to planned future interventions not directly related to offending behaviour be scored as a 1 (e.g., managing daily routines, skill-building, management of other challenging behaviours – all of which may have more distal impact on risk) and those directly related to offending (e.g., direct or 'line of sight' supervision) a 2.
- This item specifically mentions medical intervention. Individuals with an ID are more likely to be on medication than are members of the mainstream population. In scoring this item it is suggested that if the medication is not related to offending and predicted non-compliance may be for a valid reason, (e.g., not wanting to take the medication because of side effects), then a 0 is given. If the medication is not related to offending & the reason for noncompliance relates to attitudes or personality factors that are consistent with re-offending (e.g., being disagreeable) a 1 is scored. If the medication is being refused is directly related to offending then a score of 2 is given regardless of the reason for refusal.

'Item 21' – Other Considerations

- The SVR-20 manual has an 'unofficial' item 21 for 'rare but important risk factors not included as separate items'. The manual provides some examples, such as acute mental disorder, recent loss of social support (e.g., family, employment) and frequent contact with potential victims. These risk factors are considered 'case-specific', that is, unique to the individual client.

- The possible ID client special considerations include (among probably endless possibilities): encouragement of denial/minimisation by family or support system of sexual incidents; placement with vulnerable people; access to supervision; mobility and access to services; anti-libidinal medication access or misuse; ongoing activities that provide access to potential victims (e.g., delivering catalogues); different spectra of offensive behaviours across different diagnoses (e.g., autism – exposure common, less commonly physically violent; foetal alcohol spectrum disorder – the opposite).
- Also, it is outside the scope of this chapter to make any conclusions as to whether certain developmental disorders have greater or lesser risk valences than others as a result of the disorders themselves because of a lack of information in the literature (apart from some published case studies). For example, with some autistic clients we have noticed more offensive exposure incidents, but these clients seem less likely to be physically or sexually violent.

CONCLUSIONS

There is limited data supporting the use of the SVR-20 with sexually violent ID offenders in terms of predictive accuracy as opposed to theoretical congruence (e.g., Lambrick, 2003). However, for the assessment of risk for ID individuals with actual charges or convictions for sexual offences we suggest that the literature provides tentative and theoretical support for the use of the SVR-20 in combination with an actuarial instrument for a convergent risk assessment (Boer, 2006).

Unfortunately, neither the SVR-20 manual nor any of the relevant actuarial risk assessment instruments provide much in terms of ID-specific risk assessment or management information, whether for individuals charged with offences or those who simply present challenging behaviours. And, given that the *raison d' être* of risk assessment is presumably to inform risk management, clearly this is a shortcoming of current risk assessment methodologies, particularly when applied to ID individuals.

In order to use the SVR-20 more appropriately with ID clients who either offend sexually or show sexually challenging behaviour, we have offered some suggestions to conceptualise or expand the current SPJ items within an ID context. We suggest that the convergence of the risk posed by the original and parallel sets of variables will help to provide an overall picture of the level of risk posed by the individual in the context of the environmental variables that comprise the individual's current circumstances. It is our opinion that only by contextualising the individual's risk within an ecological framework can an accurate portrayal of current dynamic risk (and hence the management of that risk) be construed.

REFERENCES

Blanchard, R., Watson, M.S., Choy, A., Dickey, R., Klassen, P., Kuban, M. & Ferren, D.J. (1999). Pedophiles: Mental retardation, maternal age, and sexual orientation. *Archives of Sexual Behavior*, *28* (2), 111–27.

Boer, D.P. (2006). Sexual offender risk assessment strategies: is there a convergence of opinion yet? *Sexual Offender Treatment, 1,* 1–4.

Boer, D.P., Hart, S.D., Kropp, P.R. & Webster, C.D. (1997). *Manual for the sexual violence risk – 20: Professional guidelines for assessing risk of sexual violence.* Vancouver, BC: The Mental Health, Law, and Policy Institute.

Collacott, R.A., Cooper, S.A., Branford, D. & McGrother, C. (1998). Epidemiology of self-injurious behaviour in adults with learning disabilities. *British Journal of Psychiatry, 173,* 428–32.

Day, K. (1994). Male mentally handicapped sex offenders. *British Journal of Psychiatry, 165,* 630–9.

de Vogel, V., de Ruiter, C., van Beek, D. & Mead, G. (2004). Predictive validity of the SVR-20 and Static-99 in a Dutch sample of treated sex offenders. *Law and Human Behavior, 28,* 235–51.

Dempster, R.J. (1998). Prediction of sexually violent recidivism: A comparison of risk assessment instruments. Master's thesis, Simon Fraser University, Burnaby, British Columbia, Canada.

Doyle, D.M. (2004). The differences between sex offending and challenging behaviour in people with an intellectual disability. *Journal of Intellectual and Developmental Disability, 29* (2), 107–18.

Emerson, E. (2001). *Challenging behaviour: Analysis and intervention in people with severe intellectual disabilities,* 2nd edn. Cambridge, UK: Cambridge University Press.

Gray, N.S., Hill, C., McGleish, A., Timmons, D., MacCulloch, M.J. & Snowden, R.J. (2003). Prediction of violence and self-harm in mentally disordered offenders: A prospective study of the efficacy of HCR-20, PCL-R, and psychiatric Symptomatology. *Journal of Consulting and Clinical Psychology, 71* (3), 443–51.

Gray, N.S., Fitzgerald, J., Taylor, J.L. & Snowden, R.J. (2007). *Predicting future reconviction in offenders with intellectual disabilities: The predictive efficacy of VRAG, PCL-SV and the HCR-20.* Paper presented at the Third International Congress of Law and Mental Health.

Hanson, R.K. & Bussière, M.T. (1996). *Predictors of sexual offender recidivism: A meta-analysis.* (User Report No. 1996-04). Ottawa: Department of the Solicitor General of Canada. Also available electronically from www.sgc.gc.ca/epub/corr/e199604/e199604.htm.

Hanson, R.K. & Morton-Bourgon, K. (2004). *Predictors of sexual recidivism: An updated meta-analysis.* Public Works and Government Services Canada. Cat. No.: PS3-1/2004-2E-PDF. ISBN: 0-662-36397-3.

Hanson, R.K. & Morton-Bourgon, K.E. (2004). *Predictors of sexual recidivism: An updated meta-analysis.* Corrections User Report No. 2004-02: Public Safety and Emergency Preparedness, Ottawa, Canada. Available from www.psepc-sppcc.gc.ca/publications/corrections/pdf/200402_e.pdf.

Hanson, R.K. & Morton-Bourgon, K.E. (2005). The characteristics of persistent sexual offenders: A meta-analysis of recidivism studies. *Journal of Consulting and Clinical Psychology, 73,* 1154–63.

Hanson, R.K. & Thornton, D. (1999). *Static 99: Improving actuarial risk assessments for sex offenders* (User report 1999-02). Ottawa: Department of the Solicitor General of Canada.

Hare, R.D. (2003). *The Hare Psychopathy Checklist – Revised* 2nd edn. Toronto, Ontario: Multi-Health Systems.

Hart, S.D., Cox, D.N. & Hare, R.D. (1995). *The Hare PCL:SV.* Toronto, Ontario: Multi-Health Systems.

Harris, G.T., Rice, M.E. & Quinsey, V.L. (1993). Violent recidivism of mentally disordered offenders: The development of a statistical prediction instrument. *Criminal Justice and Behavior, 20,* 315–35.

Hayes, S. (1997). Prevalence of intellectual disability and local courts. *Journal of Intellectual and Developmental Disability, 22,* 71–85.

Kerker, B.D., Owens, P.L., Zigler, E. & Horwitz, S.M. (2004). Mental health disorders among individuals with mental retardation: Challenges to accurate prevalence estimates. *Public Health Reports, 119,* 409–17.

Lambrick, F. (2003). Issues surrounding the risk assessment of sexual offenders with an intellectual disability. *Psychiatry, Psychology & Law, 10*, 353–8.

Langevin, R. & Pope, S. (1993). Working with learning disabled sex offenders. *Annals of Sex Research, 6*, 149–60.

Lindsay, W.R. (2008). *A treatment programme for sex offenders with intellectual disability*. Chichester: John Wiley.

Lindsay, W.R., Elliott & Astell (2004). Predictors of sexual offence recidivism in offenders with intellectual disabilities. *Journal of Applied Research in Intellectual Disabilities, 17*, 299–305.

Lindsay, W.R., Law, J., Quinn, K., Smart, N. & Smith, A.H.W. (2001). A comparison of physical and sexual abuse: histories of sexual and non-sexual offenders with intellectual disability. *Child Abuse & Neglect, 25*, 989–95.

Lindsay, W.R., Smith, A.H.W., Law, J., Quinn, K., Anderson, A., Smith, A. & Allan, R. (2004). Sexual and nonsexual offenders with intellectual and learning disabilities: A comparison of characteristics, referral patterns, and outcome. *Journal of Interpersonal Violence, 19* (8), 875–90.

Lindsay, W.R. & Taylor, J.L. (2008). Assessment and treatment of offenders with intellectual and developmental disabilities. In K. Soothill, P. Rogers, and M. Dolan (Eds), *Handbook of Forensic Mental Health*, UK: Willan Press.

Lyall, I., Holland, A.J. & Collins, S. (1995). Offending by adults with learning disabilities and the attitudes of staff to offending behaviour: Implications for service development. *Journal of Intellectual Disability Research, 39* (6), 501–8.

Martin, P. & Guth, C. (2005). Unusual devastating self-injurious behaviour in a patient with a severe learning disability: treatment with citalopram. *Psychiatric Bulletin, 29*, 108–10.

Marshall, W.L., Anderson, D. & Fernandez, Y. (1999). *Cognitive behavioural treatment of sexual offenders*. Chichester: John Wiley & Son.

Morrissey, C. (2006). Guidelines for assessing psychopathy in offenders with intellectual disabilities using the PCL-R and PCL:SV. Available from the author at catrin.morrissey@nottshc.nhs.uk.

Morrissey, C., Hogue, T., Mooney, P., Allen, C., Johnston, S., Hollin, C., Lindsay, W.R. & Taylor, J.L. (2007). Predictive validity of the PCL-R in offenders with intellectual disability in a high secure hospital setting: Institutional aggression. *Journal of Forensic Psychiatry and Psychology, 18*, 1–15.

Murphy, W.D., Coleman, E.M. & Haynes, M.R. (1983). Treatment and evaluation issues with the mentally retarded sex offender. In J.G. Greer and I.R. Stuart (Eds), *The Sexual Aggressor: Current Perspectives on Treatment*. New York: Van Nostrand.

Polizzi, D.M., MacKenzie, D.L. & Hickman, L.J. (1999). What works in adult sex offender treatment? A review of prison and non-prison-based treatment programs. *International Journal of Offender Therapy and Comparative Criminology, 43*, 357–74.

Royal College of Psychiatrists (2001). *Diagnostic Criteria for Learning Disability (DC-LD)*. London: Gaskell.

Steptoe, L., Lindsay, W.R., Forrest, D. & Power, M. (2006). Quality of life and relationships in sex offenders with intellectual disability. *Journal of Intellectual and Developmental Disabilities, 31* (1), 13–19.

Swanson, J.W. (1994). Mental disorder, substance abuse, and community violence: An epidemiological approach. In J. Monahan & H.J. Steadman (Eds), *Violence and mental disorder: Developments in risk assessment* (pp. 101–36). Chicago: University of Chicago Press.

Thompson, D. (1997). Profiling the sexually abusive behaviour of men with intellectual disabilities. *Journal of Applied Research in Intellectual Disabilities, 10*, 125–39.

Thompson, D. & Brown, H. (1997). Men with intellectual disabilities who sexually abuse: A review of the literature. *Journal of Applied Research in Intellectual Disabilities, 10*, 140–58.

Webster, C.D., Douglas, K.S., Eaves, D. & Hart, S.D. (1997). *HCR-20: Assessing Risk for Violence (version 2)*. Burnaby, British Columbia, Canada: The Mental Health, Law, and Policy Institute of Simon Fraser University.

White, P., Chant, D., Edwards, N., Townsend, C. & Waghorn, G. (2005). Prevalence of intellectual disability and comorbid mental illness in an Australian community sample. *Australian and New Zealand Journal of Psychiatry, 39* (5), 395–400.

PART FOUR

Assessing Treatment Need and Deviancy

12

Psychometric Assessment of Sexual Deviancy in Sexual Offenders with Intellectual Disabilities

LEAM A. CRAIG AND WILLIAM R. LINDSAY

INTRODUCTION

The assessment of deviant sexual interest in sexual offenders has repeatedly been shown to be a strong discriminating factor between those sexual offenders who go on to commit further sexual offences (Hanson & Bussière, 1998; Hanson & Morton-Bourgon, 2005). Perhaps not surprisingly a wide range of assessments have been developed to assess for deviant sexual interests, including phallometric technology (Marshall & Fernandez, 2003), attention-based measures (Gress & Laws, 2009), self-report sexual interests (Laws, Hanson, Osborn & Greenbaum, 2000) and psychometric measures (Craig & Beech, 2009). Their cost-effectiveness and easy-to-use design has resulted in the greatest proliferation of assessment protocols being in the field of psychometric testing.

Indeed, assessment resources for non-intellectually disabled (ID) sexual offenders are plentiful with a wide range of psychometric measures available to assess any number of psychological constructs (see Beech, Fisher, Thornton, 2003; Craig & Beech, 2009). Such measures include assessing sexual interests and appetites, cognitive distortions, affectivity and impulsivity and self-management. In contrast to those for non-ID sexual offenders, empirically tested psychometric resources for sexual offenders with ID have been scarce, which has often hampered accurate assessment of treatment need and cognitive shift (Lindsay, 2002). However,

Assessment and Treatment of Sexual Offenders with Intellectual Disabilities: A Handbook
Edited by Leam A. Craig, William R. Lindsay and Kevin D. Browne
© 2010 John Wiley & Sons, Ltd.

it is only since the 1990s that clinicians and researchers have begun to develop, and empirically validated, a range of psychometric measures specifically designed for sexual offenders with ID. The purpose of this chapter is to review the available psychometric measures commonly used when assessing psychological constructs in sexual offenders with ID and to organise these measures into an assessment framework which can later be empirically validated. However, before describing the measures currently available it is important to first consider some psychometric properties.

PSYCHOMETRIC PRINCIPLES

A major objective of psychometric testing is to, as far as is possible, objectively measure some psychological construct accurately and reliably. Not only must the psychometric test assess the construct (construct validity) but, for a psychological test to be useful, it must have been standardised on the population it is to be used with and provide normative data by which an individual can be compared. This allows comparison between the subject and the study population so that judgements can be made as to how closely the subject's score relates to the mean within a normal distribution. The process of standardisation has two elements: first the need to obtain information on the test scores of the general population by taking appropriate samples, and second the need to obtain a set of principles by which raw data from the test can be transformed to give a set of data which has a normal distribution. The latter becomes particularly important if the scores are to be subject to statistical analysis (Rust & Golombok, 1989). One of the difficulties in using many tests with sexual offenders with ID is that they frequently lack standardisation with appropriate norms. This makes any comparisons between subjects questionable as there is no way to know whether the test has construct validity and can discriminate between groups (i.e., sex offenders and non-sex offenders). Crucial to the process of standardising psychometric tests is the sample from which the norms are to be taken. However, many tests used to measure constructs in sexual offenders have been standardised on samples of college samples (for example, the Nowicki-Strickland Internal-External Locus of Control Scale; Nowicki, 1976). Fisher, Beech and Browne (1999) point out that part of the problem of standardisation is the question of how valid a sample is. For example, to what extent can a sample of college students, or male factory workers in the case of the Burt Rape Myth Acceptance Scale (Burt, 1980), as a normed sample, compare with a sample of sexual offenders, as the two samples may differ in terms of social class etc. A further consideration when using psychometric measures relates to the characteristics of the sample from which the test was standardised. Where specific groups are being sampled, a sample size of many hundreds is usually considered the norm (Kline, 1986). This is often a difficulty in standardisation studies of sexual offenders with ID as most assessment and treatment studies are limited to small groups or case studies (Courtney, Rose & Mason, 2006; Craig, Stringer & Moss, 2006).

Having normative data on measures used to assess attitudes, values and beliefs of sexual offenders with ID is crucial to the assessment of treatment need and risk and they must include a wide range of psychological constructs. Before describing psychometric assessment of sexual deviancy in sexual offenders with ID, we will first consider current alternative methods.

ALTERNATIVE APPROACHES TO ASSESSING SEXUAL DEVIANCY IN SEXUAL OFFENDERS WITH INTELLECTUAL DISABILITIES

Penile Plethysmograph

Although sexual preference should be considered as a motivating factor in sexual offenders with ID (Tudway & Darmoody, 2005), in comparison to non-ID sexual offenders, there are few measures designed to assess sexual deviancy in adult sexual offenders with ID. The assessment of sexual preference in this client group is primarily limited to the clinical assessment of sexual interests and appetites (Craig, Stringer & Hutchinson, 2009; Swaffer, Hollin, Beech, Beckett & Fisher, 2000). Within the literature a common method used for assessing sexual arousal is the penile plethysmograph (PPG) (Serin, Mailloux & Malcolm, 2001). Some studies report that the arousal to deviant stimuli is considered to be one of the best predictors of sexual re-offence (Hanson & Morton-Bourgon, 2005) while others report the predictive validity of phallometric assessments to be limited (see Marshall & Fernandez, 2003) and question the validity of phallometric assessment (Laws, 2003).

The assessment of sexual interest in sexual offenders with ID is considered to pose a greater challenge than the like assessment of mainstream sexual offenders, (Gardner, Graeber & Machkovitz, 1998). Tudway and Darmoody (2005) suggest that a lack of consistency in stimulus sets, poor discrimination abilities and problems with regard to the nature and constitution of the populations in the studies using PPG mean that such measures may be problematic with ID groups. Indeed, phallometric assessment with sexual offenders with ID is rarely with only a few studies being published (e.g., Rea, DeBriere, Butler & Saunders, 1998; Reyes *et al.*, 2006). Reyes *et al.* (2006) administered the PPG to 10 sexual offenders with ID held in a state treatment facility (*M* IQ = 61.6). They recorded changes in penile circumference to various categories of stimuli both appropriate and inappropriate. They found some participants showed differentiated deviant arousal or higher levels of arousal to specific inappropriate stimuli ('deviant' is a term used in the existing sex-offender literature to describe this type of arousal) while others showed undifferentiated deviant arousal, in which case they showed non-specific arousal to inappropriate stimuli. They argue that using such assessments can yield clear outcomes with sex offenders with ID. However, notwithstanding the caution when using PPG technology (see Laws, 2003; Marshall & Fernandez, 2003), such equipment is not always readily available in probation or community health settings.

Blanchard *et al.* (1999) completed an important study on phallometric assessment that has had significant research consequences over the following decade. In a study of 950 sexual offenders they reported that those who had offended against prepubescent children had lower IQ scores than those without prepubescent victims. Of those sexual offenders with prepubescent victims, those with male victims had lower IQ scores than those with only female victims. These authors then reported on a small subgroup of 32 offenders with a measured intellectual disability. All 32 had offended against prepubescent children and phallometrically assessed age and gender preferences correlated significantly with sex offence history. Therefore, sex offenders with ID were more likely to offend against younger children, male children and across victim categories than were non-disabled sex offenders. In a subsequent study, this research group, Cantor, Blanchard, Robichaud and Christensen (2005), conducted a detailed meta-analytic study of previous reports which had included reliable data on IQ and sexual offending. Their reanalysis of 25,146 sex offenders and controls found a robust relationship between lower IQ and sexual offending, but specifically, lower IQ and paedophilia. They hypothesised that 'a third variable – a perturbation of prenatal or childhood brain development – produces both paedophilia and low IQ' (p. 565). These authors accepted that psychological influences are likely to be important but incomplete in explaining paedophilia, emphasising the value of investigating the range of hypotheses presented for the perpetration of sexual offences. Addressing the criticism of referral bias, Blanchard *et al.* (2007) demonstrated with 832 participants from a range of sources that this finding holds irrespective of referral source.

Developing this work further, Rice, Harris, Lang and Chaplin (2008) have used phallometry to investigate the relative sexual interests of 69 sex offenders with ID (average IQ 59.4) and 69 controlled sex offenders (average IQ 102). They also included a further control group of 69 community volunteers (non-offenders). They found that sex offenders with ID exhibited their largest phallometric response to prepubescent girls in contrast to community volunteers whose highest response was to adult women and the mainstream sex offenders whose highest response was to pubescent females. A similar pattern was seen to male stimuli with the sex offenders with ID exhibiting the largest response to prepubescent boys while community volunteers and mainstream sex offenders had their highest average response to adults and pubescent males respectively. These authors (as with others conducting this vein of research) concluded that, like mainstream sex offenders, sex offenders with ID commit offences largely because of the deviant sexual interests.

One interesting development in the field of deviant sexual interest as measured by phallometry is the screening assessment developed by Seto and Lalumiere (2001). This is a brief screening scale to identify paedophilic interest in the absence of phallometric assessment. They developed a screening scale for paedophilic interests (SSPI), which consists of four items: male victim, more than one victim, victim aged 11 or younger, unrelated victim. They found that the SSPI had a significant correlation with paedophile interest as measured by phallometry ($r = 0.34$) and, in a further analysis of results, showed that individuals with the highest SSPI scores were more than five times as likely to show paedophilic interest as individuals receiving the lowest scores. They recommended that the SSPI might be used as a screening for deviant sexual interests. In a pilot correlational study on 32 sex offenders with ID, Lindsay, Michie and Scott (2003) found that the SSPI had a significant positive correlation with the offences against children scale on the questionnaire on attitudes consistent with sexual offending (see later). It did not, however, correlate significantly with measures of risk for future sexual offending.

Social and Emotional Continuum

An alternative approach to assessing deviancy in sexual offenders with ID was suggested by Craig and Moss (2006) (for a more detailed description see, Craig, in press). Where an ID is apparent there is usually a degree of interplay between the person's social and emotional development. This may result in a marked distinction between the individual's chronological age and developmental level. A person with an ID, therefore, may be functioning at a significantly lower level in terms of their emotional and social development than their chronological age would suggest. Craig and Moss (2006) assessed sexually inappropriate behaviour in the context of the developmental level in sexual offenders with ID and compared their results to a four-group continuum of 'normal-to-deviant' sexual behaviour in children. The term 'normal' is used to describe behaviours that occur naturally throughout sexual development, as a result of biological and physiological changes. 'Abnormal' or 'pathological' are terms used to describe sexual behaviours that one would not expect to occur within the natural development. These kinds of behaviours are indicative of a disturbance of the natural development (Araji, 1997). They used a dimensional framework ranging from normal to deviant sexual behaviour in children developed by Johnson and Feldmeth (1993). These four groups do not comment on the aetiology of the behaviours, merely the characteristics of the behaviours.

- Group 1 Normal Sexual Exploration or 'Sex Play'
- Group 2 Sexually Reactive Behaviours
- Group 3 Extensive Mutual Sexual Behaviours
- Group 4 Children Who Molest

Craig and Moss (2006) compared the inappropriate sexual behaviours in 20 male sex offenders with ID in terms of developmental and chronological levels on a four group 'normal-to-deviant' continuum. They assessed developmental age using the Vineland's Adaptive Behaviour Scales (VABS) (Sparrow, Balla & Cicchetti, 1984). The VABS assesses the developmental level of ID populations and provides an estimate of the person's developmental level in each of the three areas of communication, daily living skills and socialization along with a general estimate of developmental functioning based on the aggregate of these three scores. The VABS provides a maximum developmental age of 18, at which point the person is assessed as adult and therefore in possession of the necessary skills in order to function independently within a community setting. The majority of the sample had an assessed mean developmental age that was lower than their chronological age. There was a significant difference between the mean chronological age (31.5 years) and the mean developmental age, which was 9 years. When the sexually inappropriate behaviour was examined in the context of chronological and developmental levels, there was a significant difference between the categorization of behaviours within the two contexts. In this study 55 per cent of the sample's sexualised behaviour was re-categorized when assessed in terms of their mean developmental age, 40 per cent had a shift of 2 categories, 15 per cent shifted by one category. Nevertheless, in 60 per cent of the sample the sexual behaviour was considered deviant when it was re-assessed in the context of the developmental age.

In terms of deviant behaviour, two groups of sexual offenders emerged. In one group behaviour was assessed as being significantly less deviant when considered in the context of the individual's developmental level, indicating age appropriate behaviour in terms of a model of normal sexual development in children. In the second group, behaviour was identified as being deviant irrespective of the developmental level of the individual when compared to normal sexual behaviour exhibited by children of a similar developmental level. Under these circumstances, the clients in the first group would require social and personal education that facilitated developmental maturation and relationships training whereas the second group would require additional therapeutic input to address 'deviant appetites'. This is broadly consistent with the observations made by Coleman and Haaven (2001) who emphasise the importance of understanding the function and motivation of the behaviour in sexual offenders with ID.

The results are also consistent with the Counterfeit Deviance Hypothesis (Hingsburger, Griffiths & Quinsey 1991), which suggests that some sexually deviant behaviour by men with

ID has its root in a lack of social and sexual knowledge rather than aberrant sexual preferences. In addition, Lunsky, Frijters, Griffiths, Watson and Williston (2007) assessed the sexual knowledge of two groups of sex offenders with ID. They compared offenders who showed persistent deviant sexual preferences (violent offenders and offenders against children) to those who had committed naive and inappropriate sexual acts (indecent exposure, public masturbation). They found that the latter group had poorer sexual knowledge than non-sexual offenders with ID and concluded that inappropriate offenders were more in need of social and personal education that would promote a better understanding of relationships and developmental maturation. As with the Craig and Moss (2006) study, two groups emerge, one for which the data suggest lower (or the absence of) sexual deviancy and who may have problems with developmental maturation and poor socio-sexual knowledge and another who show greater levels of sexual deviancy.

While the results from Craig and Moss (2006) raise important questions regarding the assessment of deviant behaviour, it is important not to misinterpret this study. Although the behaviours, when re-assessed, were found to be less deviant, they are still deviant and do not conform directly to a model of normal sexual development in children. As the behaviour is seen to be deviant, which therefore justifies the referral for a risk assessment, it cannot be assumed that there were any willing participants to engage in sexual behaviour with the referred individual. Two assumptions have been made during the course of the study, the first being that all targets of the sexual behaviour were unwilling participants and, the second, that the individual had to employ a degree of coercion or manipulation to engage in the behaviour with their 'targeted' person. Although the motivation to engage in sexual experimentation may be similar for some adults with ID to that with children (i.e., curiosity driven) (Gil, 1993) this cannot be assumed, and neither can it be assumed that the intensity, arousal and affect regarding sexuality between adults with ID and children are the same. Nevertheless, although Craig and Moss (2006) recognise the methodological limitations in the research, this study raises important questions on understanding the motivation of sexually inappropriate behaviour in people with ID.

ASSESSMENT OF THE CONSTRUCT OF 'SEXUAL DEVIANCY'

An alternative approach to measuring sexual deviancy is the use of psychometric measures as part of a structured approach to risk assessment. Two systems have been developed in the UK that look at stable-dynamic 'need' factors. The Sex Offender Treatment Evaluation Project (STEP) test battery (Beech, Fisher & Beckett, 1999) used by the probation services in England and Wales to measure 'deviancy' in child abusers and the Initial Deviance Assessment (IDA) from Thornton's (2002) Structured Risk Assessment model for use with sex offenders in the English and Welsh prison service. The deviancy construct in the STEP test battery was originally developed by Beech (1998), who classified child abusers according to their levels of problems on a battery of psychometric measures. The two main types of abusers identified using this system were termed *High Deviancy* and *Low Deviancy* in terms of the differences between groups on psychometric measures.

- *High Deviancy* child abusers are defined as having a high level of treatment need as measured by high levels of pro-offending attitudes and social adequacy problems.

- *Low Deviancy* child abusers appear to have lower level treatment need than High Deviancy men and did not show globalised cognitive distortions about children, nor did they show the high levels of emotional identification with children seen in High Deviancy offenders.

Thornton's (2002) Structured Risk Assessment (SRA) model is a research guided multi-step framework for assessing the risk presented by a sex offender and provides a systematic way of going beyond static risk classification. The full scheme covers static and a deviancy assessment (IDA), an evaluation of progress based on treatment response and risk management based on offence specialisation and acute risk factors. Thornton argues that combining the psychological factors identified in the IDA with static assessment allows better predictive accuracy than using static assessment alone. The IDA itself considers empirically derived dynamic psychological and behavioural factors. Deviance is defined in terms of the extent to which the offender's functioning is dominated by the psychological factors that contribute to his offending. It is postulated that the main dynamic risk factors fall into four domains: Sexual Interests, Distorted Attitudes, Social and Emotional Functioning and Self-Management – here high deviancy means that the dynamic risk factors underlying offending are relatively intense and pervasive (Thornton, 2002).

Domain 1 – Sexual Interests

This domain refers to both the direction and the strength of sexual interests and considers offence-related sexual preferences and sexual preoccupation both factors identified as predictive of sexual recidivism (Hanson & Bussière, 1998; Hanson & Morton-Bourgon, 2005; Pithers, Kashima, Cunningham & Beal, 1988; Proulx, Pellerin, McKibben, Aubut & Ouimet, 1999).

Domain 2 – Distorted Attitudes

This domain refers to sets of beliefs about offences, sexuality or victims that can be used to justify sexual offending behaviour. Denial or minimisation of a particular offence is not considered relevant unless it can be linked to more general attitudes. Distorted beliefs in sexual offenders are well supported within the literature (Beech, Fisher & Beckett, 1999; Hanson & Harris, 2000; Hanson & Scott; 1995; Pithers, Kashima, Cumming & Beal, 1988; Ward, Louden, Hudson & Marshall, 1995) as offence precursors consistent in both child abusers (Beech, Fisher & Beckett, 1999; Hanson & Scott, 1995) and rapists (Malamuth & Brown, 1994; Hanson & Scott, 1995). Consistent with this, Hanson and Morton-Bourgon's (2005) meta-analysis found denial and minimisation unrelated to sexual recidivism, while more general attitudes tolerant of sexual crime were associated with sexual recidivism.

Domain 3 – Social and Emotional Functioning

This domain refers to the ways of relating to other people and to motivating emotions felt in the context of these interactions. Negative emotional states such as anxiety, depression and low self-esteem (Pithers, Kashima, Cumming & Beal, 1988; Proulx, Pellerin, McKibben, Aubut & Ouimet 1999), and especially anger (Hanson & Harris, 2000), have been found to be offence precursors. Factors such as low self-esteem, loneliness and external locus of control seem to distinguish child abusers from comparison groups (Beech, Fisher & Beckett, 1999). Meta-analytical results support the recidivism relevance of emotional congruence/emotional over-identification with children and to a lesser extent hostility as being important factors related to recidivism (Hanson & Morton-Bourgon, 2005).

Domain 4 – Self-Management

This domain refers to an individual's ability to plan, problem-solve and regulate dysfunctional impulses that might otherwise lead to relapse (Pithers, Kashima, Cumming & Beal, 1988; Ward, Hudson & Keenan, 1998). Antisocial behaviour and lifestyle impulsivity have been identified as precursors of sexual re-offending (Prentky & Knight, 1991). Thornton likens this construct to that of Factor 2 in the PCL-R (Hare, 1991), which has been found to predict sexual recidivism (Firestone, Bradford, McCoy, Greenberg, Larose & Curry, 1999; Rice & Harris, 1997).

In testing the IDA assessment, Thornton (2002) compared offenders with previous convictions for child molestation (Repeat) against offenders who had been convicted for child sexual offences for the first time (Current Only) on a range of psychometric measures. Repeat offenders tended to score more highly on indicators of distorted attitudes, and obtained poorer scores on the socio-affective functioning and poorer self-management than the Current Only group. In terms of risk of sexual offence recidivism, Thornton combined the psychometric indicators into levels of deviancy: high, moderate and low. None of the 40 low deviance offenders, 5 per cent (2 of 43) of the moderate deviance offenders, and 15 per cent (5 of 34) of the high deviance offenders were reconvicted for sexual offences. Therefore, the repeat offenders showed greater risk and treatment need.

In extending this work, Craig, Thornton, Beech and Browne (2007) recently considered the effectiveness of psychometric markers of risk in approximating the deviancy domains described in the SRA model and how these measures of dynamic risk could be used to predict sexual reconviction compared with actuarial risk scales. They used psychometric markers from the Special Hospitals Assessment of Personality and Socialisation (SHAPS) (Blackburn, 1982), and the Multiphasic Sex Inventory (MSI) (Nichols & Molinder, 1984) to approximate the four deviancy domains from which they were able to calculate a psychological deviance index (PDI). The PDI reflects the number of dysfunctional domains an individual has ranging from zero to four. When the PDI was organised into deviancy levels (viz., Low (0), Moderate (1–2 domains) and High (3+ domains)), it was found the degree of PDI and rates of sexual reconviction were linear at 3 per cent, 18 per cent and 40 per cent respectively. That is to say, there was a linear relationship between the number of deviant domains an individual had and the rate of sexual reconviction.

The approach of using psychometric data to assess stable dynamic treatment need, sexual deviancy and risk in sexual offenders has proved useful and is now widely used throughout prison and probation settings in the UK. We will now explore to what extent this methodology of assessing treatment need and deviancy can be used with sexual offenders with ID.

ASSESSING SEXUAL DEVIANCY AS A CONSTRUCT IN SEXUAL OFFENDERS WITH INTELLECTUAL DISABILITIES

It is only since the 1990s that a number of psychometric measures have been developed and validated specifically for sexual offenders with ID. Table 12.1 lists the psychometric measures for sexual offenders with ID organised into the four deviancy domains. The development of

Table 12.1 Psychometric measures used to assess sexual deviancy as a construct
in sexual offenders with ID

Domains	Psychometric Measures
Sexual Interests	*Multiphasic Sex Inventory* (MSI) (Nichols & Molinder, 1984) – Sexual Obsession and Paraphilia scales *Sexual Attitudes and Knowledge Assessment* (SAK) (author unknown)
Distorted Attitudes	*MSI Cognitive Distortions and Immaturity, and Justifications scales* *Adapted Victim Empathy* (Beckett & Fisher, 1994) *The Adapted Victim Consequences Task* - adapted from the Victim Empathy Questionnaire (Bowers, Mann & Thornton, 1995) *Abel and Becker Cognition Scale* (Abel, Becker & Cunninghan-Rathner, 1984) *Questionnaire on Attitudes Consistent with Sexual Offenders* (QACSO: Lindsay, Neilson, Morrison & Smith, 1998; Broxholme & Lindsay, 2003) *Sex Offenders Opinion Test* (SOOT: Bray, 1997) *Sex Offences Self-Appraisal Scale* (SOSAS: Bray & Forshaw, 1996)
Social and Emotional Functioning	*Adapted Self Esteem Questionnaire* – adapted version of Thornton's Brief Self Esteem Scale (Thornton, Beech & Marshall, 2004) *Adapted Emotional Loneliness Scale* – adapted from the Russell, Peplan and Cutrona's (1980) UCLA Emotional Loneliness scale *The Nowicki-Strickland Internal-external Locus of Control Scale* (Nowicki, 1976)
Self-Management	*Adapted Relapse Prevention Interview* (Beckett, Fisher, Mann & Thornton, 1997) *The Psychopathic Checklist-Revised* (PCL-R: Hare, 1991) – Factor 2 (adapted by Morrissey, 2003)

these questionnaires raises the possibility of applying the SRA model to sexual offenders with ID using the method described above. We will now describe the psychometric measures organised into deviancy domains.

Sexual Interests Domain

MSI (Nichols & Molinder, 1984) – Sexual Obsession and Paraphilia Scales

The MSI is a 300-item psychometric measure specially designed to assess psychosexual characteristics of sexual offenders (rapists, child molesters, exhibitionists). The MSI provides information that is independent of personality and psychopathology tests and has been found to provide data that corroborates with physiological indices of arousal (Bernard, Fuller, Robbins & Shaw, 1989). It has good psychometric properties and risk assessment properties (see Craig,

Browne, Beech & Stringer, 2006, Craig, Thornton, Beech & Browne, 2007). Craig, Browne, Beech and Stringer (2006) found that the sexual obsessions scale (auc)[1] = 0.85), child molest scale (auc = 0.74), Rape scale (auc = 0.74) and the paraphilia scale (auc = 0.74) obtained good results in predicting sexual reconviction two-year follow-up. Although this measure was primarily designed for non-ID sexual offenders, it has been used to measure cognitive shift in low-functioning sexual offenders (mean IQ = 70) who have completed treatment (Craig, Stringer & Moss, 2006). In particular, Craig, Stringer and Moss were able to show that treatment of low-functioning sexual offenders generated significant changes on important variables, such as sexual knowledge and honesty about their sexual interests, using the MSI scales. However, they note measures such as the MSI were standardized on non-ID populations and it is not clear to what extent these can translate to ID groups. It is possible such measures are not sensitive to subtle changes in cognitive shift in clients with ID.

Sexual Attitudes and Knowledge Assessment (SAK, author unknown)

This protocol is designed to assess knowledge of sexual matters, sexual anatomy and relationships across four domains: sexual awareness, assertiveness, understanding relationships and social interaction. Participants are asked to respond to a series of questions, each accompanied by a picture. The SAK can be used in several ways: to identify learning needs in individuals to determine the specific goals and strategies for group treatment; to complete pre- and post-treatment evaluations of a participant and assess programme effectiveness; and to design a one-to-one training programme for an individual.

Distorted Attitudes Domain

Adapted Victim Empathy (Beckett & Fisher, 1994)

This protocol is designed to assess a sexual offender's expression of empathy toward their victim. Scores are expressed as percentages, where the higher the percentile score, the lower the level of empathy expressed toward the victim. Keeling, Rose and Beech (2007) adapted and evaluated a number of assessments for offenders with special needs including the Victim Empathy Scale. They reported that the adapted scale had psychometric equivalence when compared to the original with good internal consistency and a significant correlation with a very large effect size between the adapted and original scale. There was also good retest reliability and high correlations with other adapted empathy scales suggesting good convergent validity.

A recent treatment evaluation study demonstrated the effectiveness of this measure in assessing a change in attitudes towards the victim following cognitive-behavioural intervention for sexual offenders with ID (Murphy, Sinclair, Hays, Heaton & SOTSEC-ID members, 2006; Murphy, Powell, Guzman & Hays, 2007).

---

[1] The area under the curve (auc) of the Receiver Operating Characteristic (ROC) analysis is the preferred analysis used to measure the predictive accuracy of a scale. This analysis plots the data points and compares the *sensitivity* or 'hit rate' (the percentage of re-offenders correctly identified as high-risk on assessment) with *specificity* (the percentage of non-re-offenders correctly identified as low-risk). A perfectly accurate test would yield a ROC hit rate of 1.0 (no overlap between recidivists and non-recidivists) and 0.50 indicating prediction no better than chance. Graphically represented, the 'curve' for a perfect test would travel up the vertical axis then along the top of the box until it reaches the top right-hand corner, whereas a diagonal line (i.e., useless test) is 0.50.

The Adapted Victim Consequences Task

The Adapted Victim Consequences Task is a nine-item interview requiring participants to list the good and bad things that happened to their victim as a result of the offence. It is an adaptation from the Victim Empathy Questionnaire (Bowers, Mann & Thornton, 1995).

Abel and Becker Cognition Scale (Abel, Becker & Cunninghan-Rathner, 1984)

The Abel and Becker Cognition Scale consists of 29 items chosen from statements offenders have actually made in treatment. Agreement with any of the items represents an example of distorted cognitions to be addressed in therapy. This scale is used clinically and is not formally scored. Kolton, Boer and Boer (2001) used the scale with sex offenders with ID and found the response options of the test needed to be changed from a 4-choice system (1 = agree, 4 = strongly disagree) to a dichotomous system (agree/disagree) to reduce extremity bias of the sample. The revised assessment provided 'adequate' total score to item correlations and test–retest reliability, and internal consistency was 'acceptable'.

Questionnaire on Attitudes Consistent with Sexual Offenders (QACSO) (Lindsay, Neilson, Morrison & Smith, 1998; Lindsay, Michie, Whitefield, Martin, Grieve & Carson 2006; Broxholme & Lindsay, 2003; Lindsay, Whitefield & Carson 2007)

The QACSO is a 63-item questionnaire specifically designed for use with sex offenders who have ID. This protocol is designed to measure cognitive distortions commonly expressed by sexual offenders across eight domains: Rape and Attitudes to Women, Voyeurism, Exhibitionism, Dating Abuse, Homosexual Assault, Offences against Children, Stalking and Sexual Harassment and Social Desirability. The QACSO has been standardised on sexual offenders with ID, non-sexual offenders with ID, non-offenders with ID and mainstream males. The measure has been shown to discriminate sexual offenders with ID from non-offenders indicating particular cognitive distortions which facilitate offending behaviour in sexual offenders. The QACSO has adequate test–retest reliability for all groups with the exception of 'rape' and 'attitudes towards women' for non-sexual offenders without learning disabilities. The measure has good internal reliability and construct validity. The QACSO can be used to assess individuals who have been identified as at risk of offending sexually and to reassess individuals who attend treatment to identify risk of re-offending. The measure can also be used for research purposes examining core themes and attitudes held by offenders (Broxholme & Lindsay, 2003; Lindsay, Whitefield & Carson 2007). Internal consistency of each scale revealed alphas of around 0.8.

In addition to discriminating between groups, the protocol has been used to monitor treatment progress (Lindsay & Smith, 1998; Rose, Jenkins, O'Connor, Jones & Felce, 2002; Murphy & Sinclair, 2009). There is also some preliminary evidence that the QACSO may differentiate between offenders against children and offenders against adults, with the latter scoring significantly lower on the offences against children scale (Lindsay, Michie, Whitefield, Martin, Grieve and Carson, 2006). The psychometric properties of the QACSO were recently cross validated in two studies (ibid.). In both studies, the offenders against adults reported higher levels of attitudes consistent with sexual offending in the area of rape and attitudes to women. In both studies, offenders against children reported significantly higher levels of cognitive distortions in the area of offences against children.

In a study that compared treated and untreated sex offenders with ID, Langdon and Talbot (2006) found that the treatment group had significantly fewer cognitive distortions as measured by the QACSO when compared to a no treatment group. They felt that the results suggested that psychological treatment was effective in reducing levels of cognitive distortions. The scale has also demonstrated its ability to assess change in pro-sexual assault attitudes towards sexual behaviour following cognitive-behavioural intervention for men with ID (Murphy, Sinclair, Hays, Heaton & SOTSEC-ID, 2006; Murphy, Powell, Guzman & Hays 2007). As has been mentioned, Lindsay, Michie and Scott (2003) reported a significant correlation between the SSPI (Seto & Lalumiere, 2001) and the QACSO.

Sex Offenders Opinion Test (SOOT) (Bray, 1997)

The original Sex Offenders Opinion Test (SOOT) is a 28-item instrument measuring attitudes about victims of sexual offences in general. Of the 28 items, 7 items measure lying with the remaining 21 items being scored using a five-point Likert scale. Total scores relate to levels of distortions: the higher the score, the greater the distortions about victims of sexual offences. The scale has been shown to have good measures of internal consistency and is sensitive to treatment effects (Williams, Wakeling & Webster, 2007). A factor analysis revealed two factors: Factor 1 contained 15 items, which seemed to represent 'Deceitful Women and Children', and Factor 2 contained 5 items, defined by 'Children, Sex and the Law'.

Sex Offences Self-Appraisal Scale (SOSAS) (Bray & Forshaw, 1996)

This 20-item protocol is designed to assess attitudes known to be prevalent among sexual offenders using statements which form attractive excuses and are therefore likely to illicit agreement. As well as a total score, the scale also provides information on six domains: social desirability, victim blaming, denial, blame, minimisation and realism. The measures assess openness and objectivity, identifying levels of denial, blame or minimisation in relation to offending. Using a five-point Likert scale, from 1 = strongly disagree through to 5 = strongly agree, item responses are summed to give a total SOSAS score, with higher scores relating to greater denial/distortions (range: 0–95). The scale has been shown to have good measures of internal consistency and a factor analysis revealed two distinct factors, denial of responsibility and denial of future risk (Williams, Wakeling & Webster, 2007). It has also been shown to measure cognitive shift following intervention and distinguish between high- and low-risk groups and has been used with sexual offenders with ID (Murphy, Sinclair, Hays, Heaton & SOTSEC-ID, 2006; Murphy, Powell, Guzman & Hays 2007).

Conclusion

Of the various assessments reviewed here, the QACSO has the most relevant research base targeted on offenders with ID. It has also been used in a number of studies by different research groups. The Adaptive Victim Empathy Scale, the SOOT and the SOSAS have also been shown to have reasonably psychometric properties with good internal consistency when employed with sex offenders with ID. Therefore, these various assessments are likely to have utility in assessment and treatment in this client group.

Social and Emotional Functioning Domain

Adapted Self-Esteem Questionnaire

The Adapted Self-Esteem Questionnaire is an adapted version of Thornton's Brief Self-Esteem Scale (Thornton, Beech & Marshall, 2004). The measure consists of eight items used to evaluate levels of self-esteem. The items have been re-worded using simpler phrasing and respondent's rate items on a dichotomous yes/no scale. High scores relate to high self-esteem (range: 0–8). The measure is used by Her Majesty's Prison Service, it has been shown to have good internal consistency and is sensitive to treatment effect with participants scoring higher post treatment, indicative of increased self-esteem.

Adapted Emotional Loneliness Scale

This scale is used in Her Majesty's Prison Service assessment battery and consists of 18 items measuring the participants' feelings of emotional loneliness. Adapted from the Russell, Peplan, and Cutrona's (1980) UCLA Emotional Loneliness scale, items measure an awareness of the participants' own feelings. Respondents rate each item on a three-point scale: 'yes', 'no' and 'don't know'. High scores equate to greater emotional loneliness (range 0–18). This measure is currently used in the adapted assessment battery in Her Majesty's Prison Service as a retrospective tool where participants are asked to think about 'how their life was six months prior to offending'. Although this scale showed good internal consistency it was not shown to be sensitive to treatment effects (see Williams, Wakeling & Webster, 2007). It is suggested that the scale could be used as part of a pre-treatment measure of emotional loneliness only to help inform clinical practice rather than a measure of cognitive shift or sexual deviancy.

The Nowicki-Strickland Internal-external Locus of Control Scale (Nowicki, 1976)

The Nowicki-Strickland Internal-External Scale was designed to quantify the extent to which a person believes that events occur either as a result of their own behaviour (internal locus of control) or as a consequence of events outside of their control, such as luck or fate (external locus of control). The scale has 40 items requiring a 'yes' or 'no' response, and test–retest reliability has been reported to be $r = 0.83$ (Nowicki & Duke, 1974). The Nowicki-Strickland measure of locus of control is one of the most widely used measures of locus of control and has been previously used with adults with ID (Wehmeyer, 1994; Wehmeyer & Palmer, 1997), including adults with ID who have a history of sexual offending (Langdon & Talbot, 2006; Rose, Jenkins, O'Conner, Jones & Felce, 2002) along with sex offenders without an ID (Fisher, Beech & Browne, 1998). Fisher, Beech and Browne (1998) have derived cut-off scores for this measure where scores of 11 or less represent the endorsement of an internal locus of control whereas scores of 12 or more represent an external locus of control. Interestingly, Rose, Jenkins, O'Connor, Jones and Felce (2002) reported an increase in perceived external locus of control for sex offenders with ID who had undergone a comprehensive treatment programme.

Lindsay (2008), in the development of a theoretical model for sexual offending in men with ID, suggested that this might represent a more realistic appraisal of legal and societal censure for sexual offending.

Self-Management Domain

Adapted Relapse Prevention Interview (Beckett, Fisher, Mann & Thornton, 1997)

This measure is an interview schedule designed for people with ID and can be used either at the point of assessment for group inclusion or within the first week of group attendance. It should be administered and scored by the person who has clinical responsibility for the treatment programme. The measure was originally developed for use in the Sex Offender Treatment Evaluation Project (STEP) (Beckett, Beech, Fisher & Fordham, 1994) as a research tool to measure to what extent individuals participating in treatment programmes were aware of their risk factors and risk situations. It is divided into questions that focus on awareness of risk factors and questions that focus on the use of appropriate strategies to avoid risky scenarios, escape them or, if necessary, cope safely with them. The tool is able to distinguish between different areas of relapse knowledge and can inform on the effectiveness of a relapse prevention intervention. The scale used in Her Majesty's Prison Service treatment programme for sexual offenders with ID has been adapted and has been shown to have a good measure of internal consistency and is very sensitive to treatment intervention (Williams, Wakeling & Webster, 2007).

The Psychopathic Checklist-Revised (Hare, 1991)

Factor 2 measures lifestyle impulsivity. This administration and scoring of this measure has been adapted for offenders with ID (see Morrissey, 2003; Morrissey *et al.*, 2005; see Chapter 9).

CONCLUSIONS

The assessment of sexual preferences and deviancy, attitudes, values and beliefs in people with ID who display sexually aggressive behaviour is complex and at present no particular measurement methodology is accepted universally within applied forensic practice. Such an assessment is likely to rely on a combination of clinical information and psychometric data. As discussed here, with the recent development and standardisation of a number of psychometric measures designed for sexual offenders with ID, one approach may be to assess sexual deviancy in sexual offenders with ID as part of an IDA advocated by Thornton (2002). Such an approach to assessment may help structure limited and valued resources based on the '*risk*, *need* and *responsivity*' principle in determining the course of treatment or management for a particular individual (Andrews & Bonta, 2003). That is to say that the most intensive treatment or management resources should be offered to the highest risk offenders with the greatest psychological need.

REFERENCES

Abel, G.G., Becker, J.V. & Cunninghan-Rathner, J. (1984). Complications, consent and cognitions in sex between children and adults. *International Journal of Law and Psychiatry*, 7, 89–103.

Andrews, D.A. & Bonta, J. (2003). *The psychology of criminal conduct*, 3rd edn. Cincinnati, OH: Anderson.

Araji, S.K. (1997). *Sexually aggressive children: Coming to understand them*. London: Sage Publications.

Beckett, R., Beech, A.R., Fisher, D. & Fordham, A.S. (1994). *Community-based treatment for sex offenders: An evaluation of seven treatment programmes.* A report for the Home Office. Available from Home Office Publications Unit, 50, Queen Anne's Gate, London, SW1 9AT, England.

Beckett, R. & Fisher, D. (1994) Victim empathy measure. In R. Beckett, A. R. Beech., D. Fisher. & A. S. Fordham, *Community-based treatment for sex offenders: An evaluation of seven treatment programmes*. A report for the Home Office. Available from Home Office Publications Unit, 50, Queen Anne's Gate, London, SW1 9AT, England.

Beckett, R., Fisher, D., Mann, R. & Thornton, D. (1997). The relapse prevention interview. In H. Eldridge (Ed.), *Therapists guide for maintaining change: Relapse prevention manual for adult male perpetrators of child sexual abuse*. Thousand Oaks, CA: Sage Publications.

Beech, A.R. (1998). A psychometric typology of child abusers. *International Journal of Offender Therapy and Comparative Criminology*, 42, 319–39.

Beech, A.R., Fisher, D. & Beckett, R.C. (1999). *An evaluation of the prison sex offender treatment programme*. U.K. Home Office Occasional Report. Home Office Publications Unit, 50, Queen Anne's Gate, London, SW1 9AT, England. Available electronically from homeoffice.gov.uk/rds/pdfs/occ-step3.pdf.

Beech, A.R., Fisher, D.D. & Thornton, D. (2003). Risk assessment of sex offenders. *Professional Psychology: Research and Practice*, 34, 339–52.

Bernard, G., Fuller, A., Robbins, L. & Shaw, T. (1989). *The child molester*. New York: Brunner/Mazel.

Blackburn, R. (1982). The special hospital assessment of personality and socialization (SHAPS). Park Lane Hospital. Unpublished manuscript. Available from School of Psychology, University of Liverpool, Liverpool, UK.

Blanchard, R., Kolla, N.J., Cantor, J.M., Klaasen, P.E., Dickey, R., Kuban, M.E. & Blak. T. (2007). I.Q., handedness, pedophelia in adult male patients stratified by referral source. *Sexual Abuse: A Journal of Research and Treatment*, 19, 285–309.

Blanchard, R., Watson, M.S., Choy, A., Dickey, R., Klaasen, P., Kuban, M. & Christensen, B.A. (1999). Paedophiles: Mental retardation, maternal age and sexual orientation. *Archives of Sexual Behaviour*, 28, 111–27.

Bowers, Mann, R.E. & Thornton, D. (1995) Victim empathy/consequences task. Unpublished manuscript. Available from Offending Behaviour Programmes Unit, Home Office, London.

Bray, D.G. (1997). The sex offenders opinion test (SOOT). North Warwickshire NHS Trust. Unpublished.

Bray, D. & Forshaw, N. (1996). Sex offender's self appraisal scale. version 1.1. Lancashire Care NHS Trust/North Warwickshire NHS Trust. Unpublished.

Broxholme, S. & Lindsay, W.R. (2003). Development and preliminary evaluation of a questionnaire on cognitions related to sex offending for use with individuals who have mild intellectual disability. *Journal of Intellectual Disability Research*, 47, 472–82.

Burt, M.R. (1980). Cultural myths and supports for rape. *Journal of Personality and Social Psychology*, 38 (2), 217–30.

Cantor, J.M., Blanchard, R., Robichaud, L.K. & Christensen, B.K. (2005). Quantitative reanalysis of aggregate data on IQ in sexual offenders. *Psychological Bulletin*, 131, 555–68.

Coleman, E.M. & Haaven, J. (2001). Assessment and treatment of intellectual disabled sexual abusers. In M.S. Carich & S.E. Mussack (Eds), *Handbook for sexual abuser assessment and treatment*. Vermont: Safer Society Foundation, Inc.

Courtney, J., Rose, J. & Mason, O. (2006). The offence process of sex offenders with intellectual disabilities: A qualitative study. *Sexual Abuse: A Journal of Research and Treatment, 18* (2), 169–92.

Craig, L.A.(in press). Controversies in assessing risk and deviancy in sex offenders with intellectual disabilities. *Psychology, Crime & Law*.

Craig, L.A. & Beech, A.R. (2009). Psychometric assessment of sexual offenders. In A.R. Beech, L.A. Craig & K.D. Browne (Eds), *Assessment and treatment of sex offenders: A handbook*. John Wiley & Son.

Craig, L.A., Browne, K.D., Beech, A. & Stringer, I. (2006). Psychosexual characteristics of sexual offenders and the relationship to reconviction. *Psychology, Crime & Law, 12* (3), 231–44.

Craig, L.A. & Moss, T.E. (2006). Categorising sexually inappropriate behaviour in men with learning disabilities. Paper presented at the 15th Annual Conference, Division of Forensic Psychology, Preston, UK, June 20th – 22nd.

Craig, L.A., Stringer, I. & Hutchinson, R. (2009). Core assessments of adult sex offenders with learning disabilities. In M. Calder (Ed.), *The complete guide to sexual abuse assessments* (2nd edn.). Russell House Publishing.

Craig, L.A., Stringer, I. & Moss, T. (2006). Treating sexual offenders with learning disabilities in the community: A critical review. *International Journal of Offender Therapy and Comparative Criminology, 50*, 369–90.

Craig, L.A., Thornton, D., Beech, A. & Browne, K.D. (2007). The relationship of statistical and psychological risk markers to sexual reconviction in child molesters. *Criminal Justice & Behavior., 34* (3), 314–29.

Firestone, P., Bradford, J.M., McCoy, M., Greenberg, D.M., Larose, M.R. & Curry, S. (1999). Prediction of recidivism in incest offenders. *Journal of Interpersonal Violence, 14*, 511–31.

Fisher, D., Beech, A.R. & Browne, K.D. (1998). Locus of control and its relationship to treatment change in child molesters. *Legal and Criminological Psychology, 3*, 1–12.

Fisher, D., Beech, A.R. & Browne, K.D. (1999). Comparison of sex offenders to non-sex offenders on selected psychological measures. *International Journal of Offender Therapy and Comparative Criminology, 43*, 473–91.

Gardner, W.I., Graeber, J.L. & Machkovitz, S.J. (1998). Treatment of offenders with mental retardation. In R.M. Wettstein (Ed), *Treatment of offenders with mental disorders*. (pp. 329–64). New York: Guilford.

Gil, E. (1993). Age-appropriate sex play versus problematic sexual behaviours. In E. Gil & T.C. Johnson (Eds), *Sexualized children: Assessment and treatment of sexualized children and children who molest* (pp. 21–40). Rockville, MD: Launch Press.

Gress, C. L. Z. & Laws, D.R. (2009). Measuring sexual deviance: Attention-based measures. In A.R. Beech, L.A. Craig & K.D. Browne (Eds), *Assessment and Treatment of Sex Offenders: A Handbook*. John Wiley & Son.

Hanson, R.K. & Bussière, M.T. (1998). Predicting relapse: A meta-analysis of sexual offender recidivism studies. *Journal of Consulting and Clinical Psychology, 66* (2), 348–62.

Hanson, R.K. & Harris, A. J. R. (2000). Where should we intervene? Dynamic predictors of sexual offense recidivism. *Criminal Justice and Behavior, 27*, 6–35.

Hanson, R.K. & Morton-Bourgon, K. (2005). The characteristics of persistent sexual offenders: A meta-analysis of recidivism studies. *Journal of Consulting and Clinical Psychology, 73*, 1154–63.

Hanson, R.K. & Scott, H. (1995). Assessing perspective-taking among sexual offenders, non-sexual criminal and non-offenders. *Sexual Abuse: A Journal of Research and Treatment, 7*, 259–77.

Hare, R.D. (1991). *Manual for the Revised Psychopathy Checklist*. Toronto, Ontario: Multi-Health Systems Inc.

Hingsburger, D., Griffiths, D. & Quinsey, V. (1991). Detecting counterfeit deviance: Differentiating sexual deviance from sexual inappropriateness. *Habilitation Mental Health Care Newsletter, 10,* 51–4.

Johnson, T.C. & Feldmeth, J.R. (1993). Sexual behaviours: A continuum. In E. Gil & T.C. Johnson (Eds), *Sexualized children: Assessment and treatment of sexualized children and children who molest* (pp. 21–40). Rockville, MD: Launch Press.

Keeling, J.A., Rose, J.L. & Beech, A.R. (2007). A preliminary evaluation of the adaptation of four assessments for offenders with special needs. *Journal of Intellectual and Developmental Disability, 32,* 62–73.

Kline, P. (1986). *A handbook of test construction.* New York: Methuen.

Kolton, D. J. C., Boer, A. & Boer, D.P. (2001). A revision of the Abel and Becker cognition scale for intellectually disabled sexual offenders. *Sexual Abuse: A Journal of Research and Treatment, 13* (3), 217–19.

Langdon, P.E. & Talbot, T.J. (2006). Locus of control and sex offenders with an intellectual disability. *International Journal of Offender Therapy and Comparative Criminology, 50* (4), 391–401.

Laws, D.R. (2003). Penile plethysmography: Will we ever get it right? In T. Ward, D.R. Laws & S.M. Hudson (Eds), *Sexual deviance: Issues and controversies* (pp. 82–102). CA: Sage Publications Inc.

Laws, D.R., Hanson, R.K., Osborn, C.A. & Greenbaum, P.E. (2000). Classification of child molesters by plethysmographic assessment of sexual arousal and a self-report measure of sexual preference. *Journal of Interpersonal Violence, 15,* 1297–312.

Lindsay, W.R. (2002). Research and literature on sex offenders with intellectual disabilities. *Journal of Intellectual Disability Research, 46,* 74–85.

Lindsay, W.R. (2008). *The treatment of sex offenders with developmental disabilities: A practice workbook.* Chichester: Wiley-Blackwell.

Lindsay, W.R., Michie, A.M. & Scott, M. (2006). Cognitive distortions, deviant sexual interest and assessed risk in sexual offenders with intellectual disability. Paper presented to the Third Annual Seattle Conference, Edinburgh.

Lindsay, W.R., Michie, A.M., Whitefield, E., Martin, V., Grieve, A. & Carson, D. (2006). Response patterns on the questionnaire on attitudes consistent with sexual offending in groups of sex offenders with intellectual disabilities. *Journal of Applied Research in Intellectual Disabilities, 19,* 47–53.

Lindsay, W.R., Neilson, C. & Smith, A. H. W. (1988). The treatment of six men with a learning disability convicted of sex offences with children. *British Journal of Clinical Psychology, 37,* 83–98.

Lindsay, W.R. & Smith, A. H. W. (1998). Responses to treatment for sex offenders with learning disability: A comparison of men with 1 and 2 year probation sentences. *Journal of Learning Disability Research, 42,* 346–53.

Lindsay, W.R., Whitefield, E. & Carson, D. (2007). An assessment for attitudes consistent with sexual offending for use with offenders with intellectual disability. *Legal and Criminological Psychology, 12,* 55–68.

Lunsky, Y., Frijters, J., Griffiths, D.M., Watson, S.L. & Williston, S. (2007). Sexual knowledge and attitudes of men with intellectual disabilities who sexually offend. *Journal of Intellectual and Developmental Disability, 32,* 74–81.

Malamuth, N.M. & Brown, L.M. (1994). Sexually aggressive men's perception of women's communication: Testing three explanations. *Journal of Personality and Social Psychology, 67,* 699–712.

Marshall, W.L. & Fernandez, Y.M. (2003). *Phallometric testing with sexual offenders: Theory, research, and practice* Brandon, VT: The Safer Society Press.

Morrissey, C. (2003). The use of the PCL-R in forensic populations with learning disability. *British Journal of Forensic Practice, 5,* 20–4.

Morrissey, C., Hogue, T., Mooney, P., Lindsay, W.R., Steptoe, L., Taylor, J. & Johnston, S. (2005). Applicability, reliability, and validity of the psychopathy checklist-revised in offenders with intellectual disabilities: Some initial findings. *International Journal of Forensic Mental Health, 4,* 207–20.

Murphy, G.H., Powell, S., Guzman, A.-M. & Hays, S.J. (2007). Cognitive-behavioural treatment for men with intellectual disabilities and sexually abusive behaviour: A pilot study. *Journal of Intellectual Disabilities Research, 51*, 902–12.

Murphy, G.H. & Sinclair, N. (2009). Treatment of sex offenders with intellectual disabilities: The SOTSEC ID programme. In A.T. Beech, C. Craig & K. Brown (Eds), *Assessment and treatment of sex offenders: A handbook*. Chichester: John Wiley.

Murphy, G.H., Sinclair, N., Hays, S-J, Heaton, K. & SOTSEC-ID members. (2006). Effectiveness of group cognitive-behavioural treatment for men with learning disabilities at risk of sexual offending. Final report to the Department of Health. Available from Tizard Centre, University of Kent, Canterbury, Kent, CT2 9JA.

Nichols, H.R. & Molinder, I. (1984). *Manual for the multiphasic sex inventory*. Available from, Nichols & Molinder, 437 Bowes Drive, Tacoma, WA 98466-70747 USA).

Nowicki, S. (1976). Adult Nowicki-Strickland internal-external locus of control scale. Test Manual available from S. Nowicki, Jr., Department of Psychology, Emory University, Atlanta, GA 30322, USA. Also available in Salter, A. C. (1988). *Treating child sex offenders and victims: A practical guide*. CA: Sage Publications.

Nowicki, S. & Duke, M.P. (1974). A locus of control scale for noncollege as well as college adults. *Journal of Personality Assessment, 38*, 136–7.

Pithers, W.D., Kashima, K.M., Cumming, G.F. & Beal, L.S. (1988). Relapse prevention: A method of enhancing maintenance of change in sex offenders. In A.C. Salter (Ed), *Treating child sex offenders and victims: A practical guide* (pp. 131–70). Newbury Park, CA: Sage.

Prentky, R.A. & Knight, R.A. (1991). Identifying critical dimensions for discriminating among rapists. *Journal of Consulting and Clinical Psychology, 59*, 643–61.

Proulx, J., Pellerin, B., McKibben, A., Aubut, J. & Ouimet, M. (1999). Recidivism in sexual aggressors: Static and dynamic predictors of recidivism in sexual aggressors. *Sexual Abuse: A Journal of Research and Treatment, 11*, 117–29.

Rea, J.A., DeBriere, T., Butler, K. & Saunders, K.J. (1998). An analysis of four sexual offenders' arousal in the natural environment through the use of a portable penile plethysmograph. *Sexual Abuse: A Journal of Research and Treatment, 10*, 239–55.

Reyes, J.R., Vollmer, T.R., Sloman, K.N., Hall, A., Reed, R., Jansen, G., Carr, S., Jackso, K. & Stoutimore, M. (2006). Assessment of deviant arousal in adult male sex offenders with developmental disabilities. *Journal of Applied Behavior Analysis, 39*, 173–88.

Rice, M.E. & Harris, G.T. (1997). Cross-validation and extension of the violence risk appraisal guide for child molesters and rapists. *Law and Human Behavior, 21*, 231–41.

Rice, M.E., Harris, G.T., Lang, C. & Chaplin, T.C. (2008). Sexual preference and recidivism of sex offenders with mental retardation. *Sexual Abuse: A Journal of Research Treatment, 20*, 409–25.

Rose, J., Jenkins, R., O'Conner, C., Jones, C. & Felce, D. (2002). A group treatment for men with learning disabilities who sexually offend or abuse. *Journal of Applied Research in Learning Disabilities, 15*, 138–50.

Russell, D., Peplan, C.A. & Cutrona, C.A. (1980). The revised UCLA Loneliness Scale: Concurrent and discriminant validity evidence. *Journal of Personality and Social Psychology, 39*, 472–80.

Rust, J. & Golombok, S. (1989). *Modern psychometrics: The science of psychological assessment*. London: Routledge.

Serin, R.C., Mailloux, D.L. & Malcolm, P.B. (2001). Psychopathy, deviant sexual arousal, and recidivism among sexual offenders. *Journal of Interpersonal Violence, 16* (3), 234–46.

Seto, M.C. & Lalumiere, M.L. (2001). A brief screening scale to identify paedophilic interests among child molesters. *Sexual Abuse: A Journal of Research and Treatment, 13*, 15–25.

Sparrow, S.S., Balla, D.A. & Cicchetti, D.V. (1984). *Vineland's Adaptive Behaviour Scales; Interview Edition, Expanded Form*. American Guidance Service Inc., Circle Pines, MN.

Swaffer, T., Hollin, C., Beech, A., Beckett, R. & Fisher, D. (2000). An exploration of child sexual abusers' sexual fantasies before and after treatment. *Sexual Abuse: A Journal of Research and Treatment, 12,* 61–8.

Thornton, D. (2002). Constructing and testing a framework for dynamic risk assessment. *Sexual Abuse: A Journal of Research and Treatment, 14,* 137–51.

Thornton, D., Beech, A. & Marshall, W.L. (2004). Pretreatment self-esteem and posttreatment sexual recidivism. *International Journal of Offender Therapy and Comparative Criminology, 48,* 567–99.

Tudway, J.A. & Darmoody, M. (2005). Clinical assessment of adult sexual offenders with ID. *Journal of Sexual Aggression, 3,* 277–87.

Ward, T., Hudson, S.M. & Keenan, T. (1998). A self-regulation model of the sexual offence process. *Sexual Abuse: A Journal of Research and Treatment, 10,* 141–57.

Ward, T., Louden, K., Hudson, S.M. & Marshall, W.L. (1995). A descriptive model of the offence chain for child molesters. *Journal of Interpersonal Violence, 10,* 452–72.

Wehmeyer, M.L. (1994). Perceptions of self-determination and psychological empowerment of adolescents with mental retardation. *Education and Training in Mental Retardation and Developmental Disabilities, 29,* 9–21.

Wehmeyer, M.L. & Palmer, S.B. (1997). Perceptions of control of students with and without cognitive disabilities. *Psychological Reports, 81,* 195–206.

Williams, F., Wakeling, H. & Webster, S. (2007). Psychometric study of six self-report measures for use with sexual offenders with cognitive and social functioning deficits. *Psychology, Crime & Law, 13* (5), 505–22.

13

Assessing Treatment Need in Sexual Offenders with Intellectual Disabilities

PETER E. LANGDON AND GLYNIS H. MURPHY

INTRODUCTION

The accurate and theoretically driven formulation of any problem rests upon accurate and well conducted assessment, nested within the scientific method. Together, assessment and formulation effectively drive intervention, and the success or failure of any intervention can often be attributed to poorly conducted assessment leading to poor hypothesis generation and formulation. The purpose of this chapter is to outline a process of effective assessment that should be employed with a sex offender with an intellectual disability (ID) in order to ensure that formulation is properly informed, helping to maximise treatment success.[1]

ASSESSMENT

The assessment of sexual offending has to be multifaceted covering a variety of areas of bio-psycho-social functioning. Beech, Fisher and Thornton (2003) argue that when assessing risk of sexual offending, dispositional, historical, contextual and clinical factors, incorporating dynamic and actuarial risk assessment, should be considered. They suggest that functional analysis of behaviour should help to inform this process. Bearing this in mind, the overriding

---

[1] When referring to sexual offenders with ID, we mean men with ID who engage in sexually inappropriate behaviour, regardless of whether or not they have been convicted of a sexual offence. This is because in some areas criminal justice agencies are reluctant to initiate proceedings against sexual offenders with ID.

Assessment and Treatment of Sexual Offenders with Intellectual Disabilities: A Handbook
Edited by Leam A. Craig, William R. Lindsay and Kevin D. Browne
© 2010 John Wiley & Sons, Ltd.

goal of assessment is to develop an effective formulation of a presenting problem which should naturally inform psychological treatment, and the information contained within the formulation should come from a variety of sources.

The assessment of sexual offending by people with ID is no different from that used when assessing non-disabled sexual offenders, as suggested by Beech, Fisher and Thornton (2003). However, some additional factors should be considered, and this assessment procedure should involve: (i) a clinical interview and mental state examination (ii) functional analysis of the presenting problem as appropriate (iii) an assessment of dynamic risk factors and (iv) consideration of actuarial risk assessment tools, bearing in mind the potential problems this technology has when employed with sex offenders with ID. We would also consider that teams working with people with ID need to recognise that this population has a high rate of mortality (Harris & Barraclough, 1998) and are 2.5 times more likely to have health problems than people without ID (van Schrojenstein Lantman-de Valk, Metsemakers, Haveman & Crebolder, 2000). People with ID are more likely to be suffering from neurological and psychological problems as well as eye and ear problems, obesity problems and sexually transmitted diseases (ibid.). As a consequence, any clinician working with people with ID needs to be acutely aware of the health risks faced by people with ID.

CLINICAL INTERVIEW AND MENTAL STATE EXAMINATION

The assessment of any individual with a presenting problem, whether it be sexual offending or otherwise, should start with a careful clinical interview, which ensures that the clinician is able to collect valuable information that will aid formulation of the presenting problem. Traditionally, such interviews involve extracting a clinical history and conducting a mental state examination in order to gain a better understanding of the presenting problem. This initial clinical interview offers the clinician an opportunity to observe the client and collect evidence which can be used to support or refute aspects of a formulation.

Clinical history-taking involves skill and an ability to form a relationship with a client quickly. Considering people with ID, who may have significant difficulties with expressive and receptive speech, as well as memory and understanding, clinical interviews may often be challenging for a clinician, and a third party (e.g., carer, parent or sibling) and records (e.g., witness statements), may prove vital for forming an accurate clinical history. The specific areas of interest when taking a clinical history may vary depending on the client, but generally speaking, they should cover several broad areas as presented in Table 13.1.

The prevalence of medical and psychiatric disorders is thought to be elevated among people with ID and borderline ID (Deb, Thomas & Bright, 2001a, 2001b; Hassiotis et al., 2008; van Schrojenstein Lantman-de Valk, 2005), and clinical psychologists and psychiatrists are well trained to conduct a mental state examination and assess mental health problems. An effective mental state examination is conducted during a clinical interview and involves observing a person's behaviour, speech and mood as well as their general presentation, including their appearance. Non-verbal communication, including gesture and facial expression, are also of interest as it may as it help a clinician to determine mood. The quantity and quality of speech may provide further clues about a person's mental state, and thought content and thought

Table 13.1 Areas to address when taking a clinical history

Broad Area	Specific Aspects
The Presenting Problem	A clear and concise description of the inappropriate sexual behaviour should be gained detailing the frequency, severity and intensity of the problem. Information regarding the history of the problem should also be gained, as well as information regarding the contextual factors affecting the occurrence of the problem.
Personal History	This includes a description of the person's early development where possible. This information may have to come from third-party sources but can be helpful when considering the presence of some developmental disorders. Information about childhood, education, occupation and relationships, including friendships, should also be collected. A clinician should pay particular attention to the development of sexual behaviour, romantic relationships and their sexual history and interests. Past medical, psychiatric and forensic history should be gathered.
Family History	This includes gaining information about parents and siblings as well as other members of the family (e.g., grandparents) who may be relevant. A family history should also provide information on psychiatric and medical disorders within the family, as well as their social functioning within the community.
Current Circumstances	A person's current social circumstances are of marked importance. This includes information regarding housing, social care, financial concerns and occupation. Information regarding their use of community facilities and peer groups is also important.
Other Variables	Other specific variables of interest include general intellectual functioning and adaptive behaviour which can provide a wealth of information pertaining to a person's abilities, language ability, neuropsychological functioning, personality and any information pertaining to the aetiology of an ID (e.g., specific genetic disorders, teratogenic agents or trauma). A careful assessment of a person's mental state is also required.

processes are relevant, and concern should be given to specific symptomatology such as delusions, hallucinations, obsessions and nightmares. A careful and considerate clinician would, of course, recognise that speech and language difficulties may make a number of questions aimed at assessing mental state difficult for many people with ID. Therefore, questions should be simple and jargon-free. People with ID may also tend to acquiesce more and to say yes to closed questions (Heal & Sigelman, 1995), which may further complicate the assessment process. It may also be relevant to rely upon a third party who knows the individual well in order to gain access to additional information.

One of the crucial parts of any mental state examination is assessing the level of insight into the presenting problem. Some individuals with severe and profound ID may not have the mental capacity to recognise that some sexual behaviour is inappropriate (e.g., public masturbation), and as a consequence it becomes difficult to describe their inappropriate sexual behaviour as 'sexual offending', although the behaviour may have a negative impact upon society. Some of these individuals may never develop insight into the inappropriateness of their behaviour, and any resulting formulation and intervention should consider this. Others with mild to moderate ID may have the ability to understand that their sexual behaviour is in fact inappropriate but may resist or deny that such behaviour has a negative impact upon victims or society, and consequentially this should appropriately inform the assessment and formulation process.

FUNCTIONAL ANALYSIS

One technique that should be familiar to any psychologist working with people who have ID is functional analysis. This is a process by which a clinician rigorously applies the scientific method to our understanding and treatment of behavioural problems, and it is generally underpinned by behavioural theory, including models of operant conditioning. The process is vital to applied behavioural analysis and has to be driven by theory. The broad aim of functional analysis is to understand the 'purpose or function' of a behaviour. Many clinicians consider functional analysis to be a process of determining the (A)ntecedents that precede a behaviour, followed by information about the (B)ehaviour, coupled with a description of the (C)onsequences of a behaviour (O'Leary & Wilson, 1975), and many clinical psychologists will be familiar with the use of ABC charts (Murphy, 1987). ABC charts are likely to be a useful aide memoire to clinicians and forensic practitioners when trying to formulate a person's offending behaviour. However, it is important to note that, as some have pointed out, 'functional analysis isn't as easy as ABC' (Owens & Mackinnon, 1993, p. 225), and many would argue that the process is complex, given the chaotic nature of behaviour and the secretive nature of sexual behaviour, and that it is therefore limited in terms of its predictive validity. As such, formal training in applied behaviour analysis is required before undertaking such work.

Considering this, psychologists need to be well trained in the process of functional analysis and the limitations before using such methodologies. Beech, Fisher and Thornton (2003) suggest that this process may be difficult with sexual offenders who are denying their offence, but nevertheless, rigorous functional analysis should be informed by a process of clinical interview and history-taking, coupled with a review of relevant sources of information, and psychometric assessment in order to derive the 'purpose' or function that sexual offending serves for a person with ID (see Craig, Stringer & Hutchinson, 2009).

ACTUARIAL AND DYNAMIC RISK ASSESSMENT

Following on from clinical interviews and functional analysis, actuarial and dynamic risk assessment should also be considered. Actuarial risk assessment is a standardised assessment of static risk factors drawn from research and aims to consider the probability of someone being reconvicted of a sexual offence. Static risk factors are generally those which are historical and do not change (e.g., number of previous convictions, age or victim choice). Examples of such tools, some of which also incorporate dynamic risk assessment, include the Structured Anchored Clinical Judgement (SACJ) (Grubin, 1998; Hanson & Thornton, 2000), Rapid Risk Assessment for Sexual Offense Recidivism (RRASOR) (Hanson, 1997), Risk Matrix 2000 (RM2000) Thornton *et al.*, 2003), the Static 99 (Hanson & Thornton, 2000), and the Sexual

Violence Risk-20 (SVR-20) (Boer, Hart, Kropp & Webster, 1997). None of these tools, nor many others, have explicitly included populations of people with ID within their standardisation samples. This is a potential weakness of these instruments when using them with sex offenders with ID, but some authors have suggested that these tools could be used bearing such problems in mind (Harris & Tough, 2004). There is some emerging evidence that the RRASOR and the Static-99 may adequately categorise the level of risk presented by sex offenders with ID (Tough, 2001 cited in Harris & Tough, 2004), and Boer, Tough and Haaven (2004) have recommended the use of the RRASOR with sex offenders with ID. Lambrick and Glaser (2004) report on how they have used the SVR-20 with sex offenders with ID, commenting on the inappropriateness of some of the items, which are in the process of being revised by the original authors to reflect people with ID more accurately. Lindsay *et al.* (2008) reported that the Static-99 significantly predicted inappropriate sexual incidents among people with ID, while the RM2000 did not.

Other studies have suggested that actuarial and other risk assessment tools aimed at predicting violence such as the Violence Risk Appraisal Guide (VRAG) (Quinsey, Harris, Rice & Cormier, 1998), Psychopathy Checklist – Screening Version (PCL-SV) (Hart, Cox & Hare, 1995) and History, Clinical, Risk Management-20 (HCR-20) (Webster, Douglas, Eaves & Hart, 1997) work reasonably well at predicting future violence within a sample of people with ID who have been discharged from hospital (Gray, Fitzgerald, Taylor, MacCulloch & Snowden, 2007). Lindsay *et al.* (2008) also demonstrated that the VRAG and the HCR-20 have predicative validity with regards to violent incidents exhibited by people with ID, as did Quinsey, Book and Skilling (2004).

Others have suggested that the Psychopathy Checklist- Revised (PCL-R) (Hare, 1991) may predict future violence exhibited by people with ID (Morrissey *et al.*, 2005). However, Morrissey, Hogue, Mooney, Allen, Johnston, Hollin *et al.* (2007) further reported that the PCL-R did not relate to institutional violence exhibited by people with ID, while the HCR-20 and the Emotional Problem Scales: Behaviour Rating Scale (Prout & Strohmer, 1991) predicted violence effectively. However, in a related study Morrissey, Mooney, Hogue, Lindsay and Taylor (2007) found that the PCL-R successfully predicted patient transfers from lower security to higher security settings and *vice versa*. Gray, Fitzgerald, Taylor, MacCulloch and Snowden (2007) noted that people with ID tended to re-offend at a much slower rate, indicating that the prevailing base rate of re-offending among people with ID was rather different from that among people without ID, which has implications for the calculation of risk probability using actuarial risk assessment tools.

Dynamic risk assessment refers to the assessment of factors (e.g., distorted cognitions) that are associated with a risk of sexual offending but may be amenable to treatment and as a consequence may change, in which case risk may subsequently reduce. Beech, Fisher and Thornton (2003) further classify dynamic risk factors into two categories: (i) stable factors, or those factors that may only change slowly following treatment, such as victim empathy or distorted cognitions and (ii) acute factors, or those factors that can change rapidly and suggest a person is at significant risk of committing a sexual offence in the near future – for example, recent substance misuse or a lack of supervision.

In the United Kingdom, the assessment of stable dynamic risk employed within the probation and prison service revolves around the assessment of sexual interests, offence supportive attitudes, relationships and self-management. This assessment of stable dynamic risk has its foundations within psychometric assessment research, and studies have demonstrated that factors such as pro-offending attitudes, sexual deviancy, poor empathy and socio-affective problems are associated with risk (Beech, 1998; Fisher, Beech & Browne, 1999; Thornton, 2002).

Some researchers have attempted to employ a structured rating methodology with regards to the assessment of stable and acute dynamic risk. Hanson and Harris (2000, 2001) have developed the Sex Offender Need Assessment Rating (SONAR), which examines five stable factors (intimacy deficits, negative social influences, attitudes toward sexual offending, sexual and general self-regulation) and four acute factors (substance misuse, negative mood, anger and victim access). Harris and Tough (2004) suggest that SONAR could be used as an aide with respect to decision-making involving sexual offenders who have ID, considering that most of the structured risk assessment tools within this area have not been standardised using populations of people with ID.

Boer, McVilly and Lambrick (2007) and Boer, Tough and Haaven (2004) proposed a structure of dynamic risk factors that can be used as a guide when assessing sexual offenders with ID. They included five stable dynamic items and four acute dynamic items that relate to staff and environmental factors, as well as twelve stable dynamic factors and nine acute dynamic factors that relate to sexual offenders with ID. These items have subsequently been combined by Douglas Boer to form the Assessment of Risk and Manageability for Individuals with Developmental, Intellectual, or Learning Limitations who Offend (ARMIDILLO). Examples of items include staff attitudes toward sex offenders with ID, victim access, offender attitude toward supervision, and coping skills. Although there is no validation or reliability data available, this assessment methodology appears promising.

A similar dynamic risk assessment tool aimed at predicting violence, rather than sexual offending, among people with ID is the Dynamic Risk Assessment and Management System (DRAMS) (Lindsay, Murphy et al., 2004; Steptoe, Lindsay, Murphy & Young, 2008). The items within the DRAMS cover areas such as mood, antisocial behaviour, self-regulation, victim access and compliance among others. Lindsay et al. (2004, 2008) reported that the DRAMS scores were elevated prior to the day of an aggressive incident, and they demonstrated that it has good internal consistency, reliability and validity. Although not a specific assessment meant to assess sexual offending, this assessment tool has use with regards to predicting aggressive and challenging behaviour incidents among offenders with ID and should be considered when such issues are of concern.

Research examining the use of structured dynamic risk assessment and actuarial risk assessment for sexual offending and aggressive behaviour exhibited by people with ID is in its infancy in comparison to studies using these tools with sexual offenders without ID. There are some emerging attempts to develop specific tools which can be used with sexual offenders with ID (Boer, McVilly & Lambrick, 2007; Boer, Tough & Haaven 2004) and evidence to suggest that some existing actuarial tools may predict future recidivism reasonably well (Lindsay et al., 2008). However, the use of these tools with individuals should occur with a full knowledge of the potential weaknesses. Hart, Michie and Cooke (2007) demonstrated that the confidence intervals associated with the assessment of group risk for different categories of sexual offenders using the VRAG (Quinsey, Harris, Rice & Cormier, 1998) and the Static-99 (Hanson & Thornton, 2000) may overlap, while confidence intervals associated with an individual assessment of risk were of such a magnitude that the risk estimate was of no value. The findings of this study are potentially damning for actuarial risk assessment tools, and the researchers recommend that clinicians should use these tools with caution when attempting to estimate an individual's level of risk. They suggest that these measures are ethically problematic and may not be appropriate for use within legal proceedings, and they conclude that they lack precision. This has led to some healthy debate on theoretical principles, and Doren (2007), Mossman and Sellke (2007) and Harris, Rice and Quinsey (2007) have all expressed concern over the methodology of the Hart *et al.* (2007) study. Nevertheless, these problems must be considered when employing actuarial risk assessment tools, and any clinician must be aware of them. Evaluations need to be made regarding the representativeness of the standardisation sample, the validity of the instrument, and the potential drawbacks and positives to labelling an individual using such instruments. This is specifically problematic when using these instruments with individuals who have ID given that very few of the standardisation samples have included people from this population, and this population is well-versed in being labelled.

PSYCHOMETRIC ASSESSMENT

Although there are many problems associated with the use of actuarial risk assessment tools, dynamic risk assessment tools originally have their grounding in research in comparative studies examining psychological factors that differ between populations of offenders and non-offenders. Such descriptive comparative methodologies may appear simplistic, but they are very valuable in that they provide a source of sound information for formulating more complex and valid psychological theories. For example, Lindsay, Elliot and Astell (2004) correlated static and dynamic variables with sexual re-offending or suspected re-offending, reporting that antisocial attitude, poor relationship with mother and allowances being made by staff were associated with actual sexual re-offending, while denial of crime, sexual abuse in childhood, erratic attendance and allowances made by staff predicted suspected re-offending.

However, other studies have also examined factors which are thought to relate to sexual offending risk, including variables such as sociosexual knowledge, sexual interest, distorted cognitions, impulsivity, self-esteem and empathy. Many of these variables have been found to differ between populations of sex offenders and non-offenders without ID (e.g., Fisher, Beech & Browne, 1999). Keeling, Beech and Rose (2007) have reviewed some of the assessment tools that may be used with sex offenders who have ID. However, we would add to this list, and therefore aim to review below, further instruments and the associated rationale for using them with sex offenders with ID.

Socio-Sexual Knowledge

The notion of counterfeit deviance (Hingsburger, Griffiths & Quinsey, 1991) implies that inappropriate sexual behaviour is caused by a lack of sufficient knowledge of the social rules governing the expression of sexuality (see Chapter 2). This assumption has potential relevance to formulating sexual offending among people with ID, as it is not beyond the realm of possibility that some sexual offenders with ID may engage in inappropriate sexual behaviour because they have not effectively internalised the social rules governing sexual behaviour. However, Talbot and Langdon (2006), Michie, Lindsay, Martin and Grieve (2006) and

Lockhart, Guerin and Coyle (2010) all demonstrated that sexual offenders with ID have higher levels of sexual knowledge than non-offenders with ID, refuting, to a certain degree, the assumption underlying counterfeit deviance. Lunsky, Frijters, Griffiths, Watson and Williston (2007) also examined this possibility by comparing sexual offenders with ID who they thought had a deviant sexual interest to two groups: people with ID who they thought had engaged in inappropriate sexual behaviour through naivety and people with ID who were non-offenders. The findings indicated that sexual offenders have higher sexual knowledge than non-offenders, and as previously suggested by Talbot and Langdon (2006) this may be attributable to sex education training. Lunsky, Frijters, Griffiths, Watson and Williston (2007) also argued that there may be a subgroup of sexual offenders with ID who engaged in inappropriate sexual behaviour as a consequence of a lack of sociosexual knowledge. This may be the case, but it may be limited to people with ID who have severe or profound ID, and as a consequence their inappropriate sexual behaviour would not be construed as a sexual offence but would nevertheless be considered inappropriate.

There are many instruments that can be used to assess sociosexual knowledge of sex offenders with ID. Talbot and Langdon (2006) revised the Bender Sexual Knowledge Questionnaire, creating the General Sexual Knowledge Questionnaire (GSKQ), which was used with sex offenders with ID and non-offenders with and without ID. They reported the internal consistency for the entire measure to by high at 0.94, and the split-half reliability to be good at 0.80. Both Michie, Lindsay, Martin and Grieve (2006) and Lunsky, Frijters, Griffiths, Watson and Williston (2007) used the Socio-Sexual Knowledge and Attitudes Assessment Tool (SSKAAT), which was originally developed by Wish, McCombs and Edmondson (1980). The SSKAAT was revised by Griffiths and Lunsky (2003) and has been shown to have good psychometric properties. Other measures are available, including the Sex Knowledge, Experience, Feelings and Needs Scale (SexKen-ID) (McCabe, 1994), which has also been shown to have good psychometric properties (McCabe, Cummins & Deeks, 1999). There is also the Assessment of Sexual Knowledge (ASK) (Galea, Butler, Iacono & Leighton, 2004), which has been developed for use with people who have ID, and the Sexual Attitudes and Knowledge Scale (SAK) (Heighway & Webster, 2007), which has been shown to have excellent internal consistency (Langdon, Maxted, Murphy & SOTSEC-ID, 2007) and has been used with sexual offenders with ID (ibid.; Murphy, Powell, Guzman & Hays, 2007; SOTSEC-ID, in press), although may be subject to ceiling effects with some individuals.

Sexual Deviance and Sexual Interest

There is very little in the way of standardised, valid and reliable measures of sexual deviance and sexual interest that can be used with sex offenders who have ID (for a review see Craig, in press). Keeling, Beech and Rose (2007) mention that Boer, Gauthier, Watson, Dorward and Kolton (2005) recommend the use of the Multiphasic Sex Inventory (MSI) (Nichols & Molinder, 1984, 2000) with sex offenders with ID, and further comment that O'Connor (1996) used the Wilson Sex Fantasy Questionnaire (WSFQ) (Wilson, 1988) with sex offenders with ID, but some of the participants found completion of the test difficult. There are also likely to be difficulties employing the MSI with sex offenders with ID given the large number of items, the complexity of the language and the length of time needed to administer the test (Craig, Stringer & Moss, 2006). Keeling, Beech and Rose (2007) noted that the items can be administered aurally using a tape, but this does not reduce the time associated with administration, nor may it improve comprehension of some of the complex items.

Keeling, Beech and Rose commented that the use of phallometry may be equally problematic in use with sex offenders with ID as it is with sex offenders without ID, and, sensibly, they raise additional concerns regarding consent in use with people who have ID, who in some circumstances may have difficulties with mental capacity. Excluding the use of phallometry, there are ipsative viewing time methodologies to assess sexual interest which can be employed with sexual offenders with ID. Affinity (Glasgow, 2007) is a computer-based assessment tool in which respondents are asked to rate their sexual interest in images of people of varying ages while, during this time, covert viewing-time data is collected. The premise to the assessment is that people spend longer looking at images that they find sexually appealing. However, the measure is considered to be idiographic and this makes it difficult to develop reliability and validity data from group-based studies. Moreover, there are important ethical issues raised when collecting covert viewing-time data.

Cognitive Distortions and Empathy

There are several instruments available that serve to assess distorted cognitions among sex offenders with ID. Keeling, Beech and Rose (2007) reviewed the use of the Abel-Becker Cognition Scale (ABCS) (Abel, Becker & Cunningham-Rathner, 1984) and associated literature with sex offenders with ID, concluding that it does not reliably distinguish between sex offenders and non-offenders with ID and is too transparent.

Alternatively, the Questionnaire on Attitudes Consistent with Sexual Offending (QACSO) (Broxholme & Lindsay, 2003; Lindsay, Michie, Whitefield, Martin, Grieve & Carson, 2006; Lindsay, Whitefield & Carson, 2007) was specifically developed to examine the cognitive distortions among sexual offenders with ID. The questionnaire requires respondents to answer 'yes' or 'no' in response to a question (e.g., 'Do you think that women who go around without a bra on or in tight clothes want to have sex?'), and that scale has been shown to have good test–retest reliability and discriminant validity between sexual offence types (Broxholme & Lindsay, 2003). However, some of the items may not adequately consider the reported sexuality of respondents. For example, the item 'If a man approached you for sex would you hit him or tell him you are not gay?' makes the assumption that respondents are heterosexual.

There are other measures of cognitive distortions that have been employed with sexual offenders who have ID. Langdon, Maxted, Murphy and SOTSEC-ID (2007) used the Sexual Offenders Self-Appraisal Scale (SOSAS) (Bray & Forshaw, 1996) within a study investigating the offence pathways of sexual offenders with ID. They reported that the internal consistency of the SOSAS was 0.68, which is substantial. This measure requires participants to respond using a five-point Likert scale indicating agreement with various statements about their offending. Williams, Wakeling and Webster (2007) also used the SOSAS and reported that the internal consistency of the SOSAS was 0.76, which is also substantial, and the increase may reflect the inclusion of men without ID within their participant sample. They also subjected the SOSAS to factor analysis, extracting two factors which accounted for only 39.9 per cent of the variance. This study made use of sexual offenders within UK prisons and included participants without an actual ID; however, it is unclear from the study how many participants included actually did and did not have a formal ID. One of the main problems with the SOSAS is that it has items that have double negatives, which are likely to be confusing for some people with ID.

There is also the Sex Offenders Opinion Test (SOOT) (Bray, 1997), which aims to examine the attitudes of sexual offenders toward victims of sexual offences. Williams, Wakeling and Webster (2007) reported that the SOOT had very good internal consistency at 0.82, and they also subjected this instrument to factor analysis, extracting two factors accounting for 36.5 per cent of the variance. Again, their sample of participants included men without an ID.

Considering victim empathy, Keeling, Beech and Rose (2007) suggest the use of the Victim Empathy Scale (Beckett & Fisher, 1994) with sex offenders with ID, but this measure has been revised with the permission of the original authors for use specifically with sex offenders with ID and was used within the studies of Langdon, Maxted, Murphy and SOTSEC-ID (2007), Murphy, Powell, Guzman and Hays (2007) and SOTSEC-ID (in press). The revised measure has been called the Victim Empathy Scale – Adapted (VESA), and some of the items have been modified by removing double negatives and simplifying the wording. Responses are rated on a four-point Likert scale represented by four columns of varying heights to indicate the degree of agreement or disagreement. Langdon and colleagues (2007) reported that the internal consistency of this scale was excellent at 0.91. Keeling, Rose and Beech (2007) have also adapted this measure and it is unclear whether or not their version is similar to the version used by Langdon, Maxted, Murphy and SOTSEC-ID (2007) and Murphy, Powell, Guzman and Hays (2007). However, they examined the psychometric properties of the measure they used, reporting internal consistency at $k = 0.77$, and test–retest reliability at $r = 0.88$.

Williams, Wakeling and Webster (2007) made use of the Adapted Victim Empathy Consequences task with sex offenders with and without ID. This is a nine-item interview in which respondents are asked to report their perception of the benefits and drawbacks of their sexual offending with regard to their victim. Reponses are scored according to a judgement regarding how much empathy is thought to be evidenced. The internal consistency of this questionnaire was reported to be 0.75 and a principal components analysis found one factor explaining 36.9 per cent of the variance (ibid.).

Some other authors (Proctor & Beail, 2007) have adapted the Interpersonal Reactivity Index (IRI) (Davis, 1983) by simplifying the measure and removing some wording. Proctor and Beail (2007) did not explicitly include sexual offenders with ID, but they found no differences between a group of offenders and non-offenders with ID who were matched for full scale IQ, on the IRI. They also examined differences between a group of offenders and non-offenders using the Test of Emotional Perception (Moffatt, Hanley-Maxwell & Donnellan, 1995) and several theory of mind tests. They found no difference between offenders and non-offenders with ID on a first order theory of mind test, suggesting a ceiling effect on this measure, while offenders tended to perform better on a second order theory of mind test. Offenders with ID also performed significantly better than non-offenders with ID on the Test of Emotional Perception. These results are counterintuitive in that it was expected that offenders with ID would have more difficulty with these tasks than non-offenders with ID.

Socio-Affective Functioning

There are several measures that aim to assess aspects of socio-affective functioning, including constructs such as self-esteem, emotional loneliness, locus of control and impulsivity. For example, Williams, Wakeling and Webster (2007) reported on the use of the Adapted Self-Esteem Questionnaire with sexual offenders with and without ID and found the internal consistency to be 0.77, with a principal components analysis revealing one factor explaining 38.4 per cent of the variance. They also reported (ibid.) on the use of an Adapted Emotional Loneliness measure which was found to have good internal consistency and one factor accounting for 29.9 per cent of the variance.

Keeling, Rose and Beech (2007), in a study of sexual offenders with and without 'special needs' reported on the adaptation of several measures that could potentially be used with sexual offenders with ID. However, their sample included only 16 participants with 'special needs' and not all of them had an ID. They revised the Social Intimacy Scale (Miller & Lefcourt, 1982), which measures a person's experiences of intimacy, and the Relationship Scales Questionnaire (Griffin & Bartholomew, 1994), which aims to assess attachment. The Social Intimacy Scale was reported to have good internal consistency and reliability and to be correlated with the UCLA Loneliness Scale (Russell, 1996). However, there were some difficulties with the Relationship Scales Questionnaire in terms of internal consistency and validity, and none of these measures of socio-affective functioning have yet been shown to be associated with sexual offending.

Treatment Amenability

Locus of control (Rotter, 1966) is a construct that is measured along the external *vs* internal dimension. An internal locus of control has been defined as the 'perception of events, whether positive or negative, as being a consequence of one's own actions and thereby potentially under personal control' (Lefcourt, 1976, p. 29), while an external locus of control has been defined as 'the perception of positive or negative events as being unrelated to one's own behaviour and thereby beyond personal control' (ibid., p. 29). Locus of control is considered to be an important construct as it is considered to be linked to treatment outcome for sexual offenders without ID (Fisher, Beech & Browne, 1998), while Page and Scalora (2004) suggest that the construct may be used as a indicator of treatment amenability with young offenders. However, Langdon and Talbot (2006) demonstrated that locus of control among sex offenders with ID who had received treatment, sex offenders with ID who had not received treatment and non-offenders with ID did not differ; all groups endorsed an external locus of control. Rose, Jenkins, O'Connor, Jones and Felce (2002) demonstrated that locus of control may have actually become more external among a group of sexual offenders with ID as a result of treatment. Langdon and Talbot (2006) suggested that locus of control may not relate to treatment outcome with sex offenders who have ID because the measures being used may not be sensitive enough to detect change with this population. They also suggested that people with ID may have difficulties with perceived competence, self-esteem, choice and locus of control as nested within theoretical approaches to self-determination (Wehmeyer, 1997, 1998, 2001), and as a consequence, many people with ID may endorse an external locus of control.

Goodman, Leggett and Garrett (2007) developed a new measure of locus of control for use with people who have ID which was based upon the Nowicki-Strickland Locus of Control Scale (Nowicki & Duke, 1974). The internal consistency of the new measure was poor at 0.53 and the factor structure problematic. However, they reported that there was no difference between people with ID who had contact with criminal justice and those who had no contact with criminal justice. However, they further demonstrated that those with convictions reported higher external locus of control than non-offenders. This could be explained by considering that those who are subject to convictions have a reduced sense of control over their own lives and consequently report a greater external locus of control. Overall, it would appear that using measures of locus of control as an index of treatment amenability is problematic for people with ID and should be used with caution.

When considering whether or not people with ID are likely to be amenable to psychological interventions it is important to note that there has been a general assumption in the past that many people with ID are unlikely to derive benefit from therapy because of difficulties with cognitive ability and communication (Hurley, Pfadt, Tomasulo & Gardner, 1996). However, there have been successful case reports of cognitive-behavioural therapy for depression (Lindsay, Howells & Pitcaithly, 1993) and group-based cognitive-behavioural therapy for depression (McGillivray, McCabe & Kershaw, 2008) and anger (Taylor, Novaco, Gillmer & Thorne, 2002). There have also been reports that group-based cognitive-behavioural treatment of sexual offending by people with ID may reduce levels of cognitive distortions and improve victim empathy and sexual knowledge and may reduce recidivism (Lindsay & Smith, 1998; Murphy, Powell, Guzman & Hays, 2007; SOTSEC-ID, in press).

However, Hatton (2002) suggested there were three prior types of ability that were needed for cognitive-behavioural therapy, (i) cognitive ability, (ii) emotional recognition and (iii) comprehension of the cognitive model. Some authors have attempted to explore whether or not people with ID have the capacity to take part in some of the proposed components of cognitive behavioural therapy. However, several studies have emerged which have demonstrated that people with ID may be able to recognise basic emotions but may have difficulty with more complex tasks, such as cognitive mediation, which tends to be associated with language ability and general intellectual functioning (Dagnan & Chadwick, 1997; Dagnan, Chadwick & Proudlove, 2000; Joyce, Globe & Moody, 2006; Sams, Collins & Reynolds, 2006). However, in a recent study Bruce, Collins, Langdon, Powlitch and Reynolds (in press) have demonstrated that a single one-hour session of training regarding skills needed for cognitive-behavioural therapy significantly improved the ability of people with ID to engage in cognitive-mediation but did not improve their ability to recognise thoughts, feelings and behaviour. The findings suggest that training in these skills may be helpful for people with ID who are engaging in cognitive behavioural therapy.

Issues associated with general intellectual functioning and verbal abilities may be pivotal in determining whether or not a sexual offender with an ID may be able to participate in group-based treatment. However, the work of Bruce and colleagues (in press) suggests that work around the necessary skills needed to complete some of the tasks required for cognitive-behavioural therapy would be useful and should be incorporated into treatment programmes. Clinicians and forensic practitioners should cover such aspects in their assessment and should incorporate them into their formulations to ensure that interventions are effectively designed to address the treatment needs of their clients.

Relapse Prevention

The probation service and the prison service in the United Kingdom make use of a relapse prevention questionnaire (Beckett, Fisher, Mann & Thornton, 1997) which is completed by a respondent and asks a series of questions about their thoughts, feelings and behaviours regarding their actual sexual offending and about the strategies and plans they have in order reduce their risk of re-offending. The questionnaire can also take the form of an interview, and this has been adapted for people with a full scale IQ of less than 80 by the Offending Behaviour Programmes Unit, HM Prison Service. According to Williams, Wakeling and Webster (2007), the interview consists of 17 items that aim to assess a person's ability to recognise risk and develop coping strategies. One item asks a person to indicate their perceived probability of committing another sexual offence. Responses are subsequently coded and converted into a score; higher scores are meant to suggest greater knowledge of relapse prevention strategies. Williams and colleagues (ibid.) reported that the internal consistency of this interview was excellent and factor analysis led to the extraction of a single factor accounting for 31.4 per cent of the variance. However, follow-up data is yet to be made available.

CONCLUSIONS

The process of assessing sexual offenders with ID is multifaceted, covering several areas of bio-psycho-social functioning. Inclusive within this are aspects of medical health, which should be dealt with by appropriately qualified professionals. Aspects of psychological and social functioning should also be assessed by appropriately qualified professionals, and should make use of a full clinical interview and mental state examination, which may draw on some aspects of functional analysis. Sexual offending behaviour should be covered through this process and further examined by making use of existing psychometric assessment tools and dynamic and actuarial risk assessment tools. However, there are significant problems with the use of actuarial risk assessment tools that clinicians and forensic practitioners need to be aware of before they can be applied to people with ID. A variety of psychometric assessment tools are available that assess sociosexual knowledge, distorted cognitions, victim empathy, socio-affective functioning and relapse prevention. There are currently few reliable and valid assessment tools for deviant sexual interests among people with ID, although there are some computer-based idiographic tools available. Examining treatment amenability among sexual offenders with ID is problematic given the difficulties this population have with concepts such as self-determination. However, there is some emerging evidence to suggest that people with ID can complete some of the necessary tasks of cognitive-behavioural therapy with additional training, and a number of studies have shown that cognitive-behavioural treatment is effective at improving sexual knowledge and victim empathy, as well as reducing the distorted cognitions among, sexual offenders with ID (Murphy, Powell, Guzman & Hays, 2007; SOTSEC-ID, in press).

REFERENCES

Abel, G.G., Becker, J.V. & Cunningham-Rathner, J. (1984). Complications, consent, and cognitions in sex between children and adults. *International Journal of Law and Psychiatry*, 7, 89–103.

Beckett, R. & Fisher, D. (1994). Victim empathy measure. In R. Beckett, A. Beech, D. Fisher & A.S. Fordham (Eds), *Community-based Treatment for sex offenders: An evaluation of seven treatment programmes* (pp. 136–40). London: Home Office.

Beckett, R., Fisher, D., Mann, R. & Thornton, D. (1997). The relapse prevention questionaire and interview. In H. Eldridge (Ed.), *Therapists guide for maintaining change: Relapse prevention manual for adult male perpetrators of child sexual abuse.* Thousand, Oaks, CA: Sage Publications.

Beech, A.R. (1998). A psychometric typology of child abusers. *International Journal of Offender Therapy and Comparative Criminology, 42,* 319–39.

Beech, A.R., Fisher, D.D. & Thornton, D. (2003). Risk assessment of sex offenders. *Professional Psychology Research and Practice, 34* (4), 339–52.

Boer, D.P., Gauthier, C.M., Watson, D.R., Dorward, J. & Kolton, D.J.C. (2005). The assessment and treatment of intellectual disabled sex offenders: The regional psychiatric centre (Pacific) 'Northstar' treatment and relapse prevention program. Paper presented at the Towards a National Strategy: A Conference on Intervention with Sex Offenders, Toronto.

Boer, D.P., Hart, S.D., Kropp, P.R. & Webster, C.D. (1997). *Manual for the sexual violence risk-20: Professional guidelines for assessing risk of sexual violence.* Vancouver: The British Columbia Institute Against Family Violence.

Boer, D.P., McVilly, K.R. & Lambrick, F. (2007). Contextualizing risk in the assessment of intellectually disabled individuals. *Sexual Offender Treatment, 2,* 1–5.

Boer, D.P., Tough, S. & Haaven, J. (2004). Assessment of risk manageability of intellectually disabled sex offenders. *Journal of Applied Research in Intellectual Disabilities, 17,* 275–83.

Bray, D. (1997). *The sex offenders opinion test (SOOT).* Preston, UK: Lancashire Care NHS Trust.

Bray, D. & Forshaw, N. (1996). *Sex Offenders Self Appraisal Scale (Version 1.1.).* Preston, UK: Lancashire Care NHS Trust.

Broxholme, S.L. & Lindsay, W.R. (2003). Development and preliminary evaluation of a questionnaire on cognitions related to sex offending for use with individuals who have mild intellectual disabilities. *Journal of Intellectual Disability Research, 47,* 472–82.

Bruce, M., Collins, S., Langdon, P.E., Powlitch, S. & Reynolds, S. (in press). Does training improve understanding of core concepts in cognitive behaviour therapy by people with intellectual disabilities? A randomised experiment. *British Journal of Clinical Psychology.*

Craig, L.A. (in press). Controversies in assessing risk and deviancy in sex offenders with intellectual disabilities. *Psychology, Crime & Law.*

Craig, L.A., Stringer, I. & Hutchinson, R. (2009). Core assessment of adult sex offenders with a learning disability. In M. Calder (Ed.), *The complete guide to sexual abuse assessments – second edition* (pp. 228–49). Russell House Publishing Ltd.

Craig, L.A., Stringer, I., Moss, T. (2006). Treating sexual offenders with learning disabilities in the community: A critical review. *International Journal of Offender Therapy and Comparative Criminology, 50,* 369–90.

Dagnan, D. & Chadwick, D. (1997). Cognitive-behaviour therapy for people with learning disabilities: Assessment and intervention. In B. Stenfert-Kroese, D. Dagnan & K. Loumidis (Eds), *Cognitive-behaviour therapy for people with learning disabilities* (pp. 110–23). London: Routledge.

Dagnan, D., Chadwick, D. & Proudlove, J. (2000). Toward an assessment of suitability of people with mental retardation for cognitive therapy. *Cognitive Therapy and Research, 24,* 627–36.

Davis, M. (1983). Measuring individual differences in empathy: Evidence for a multidimensional approach. *Journal of Personality and Social Psychology, 44,* 113–26.

Deb, S., Thomas, M. & Bright, C. (2001a). Mental disorder in adults with intellectual disability 1: Prevalence of functional psychiatric illness among a community-based population aged between 16 and 64 years. *Journal of Intellectual Disability Research, 45,* 495–505.

Deb, S., Thomas, M. & Bright, C. (2001b). Mental disorder in adults with intellectual disability. 2: The rate of behaviour disorders among a community-based population aged between 16 and 64 years. *Journal of Intellectual Disability Research, 45*, 506–14.

Doren, D. (2007). A critique of Hart, Michie & Cooke (2007). The precision of actuarial risk instruments. *British Journal of Psychiatry* (July).

Fisher, D., Beech, A. & Browne, K. (1998). Locus control and its relationship to treatment change and abuse history in child sexual abusers. *Legal & Criminological Psychology, 3* (Part 1), 1–12.

Fisher, D., Beech, A.R. & Browne, K. (1999). Comparison of sex offenders to nonoffenders on selected psychological measures. *International Journal of Offender Therapy and Comparative Criminology, 43* (4), 473–91.

Galea, J., Butler, J., Iacono, T. & Leighton, D. (2004). The assessment of sexual knowledge in people with intellectual disability. *Journal of Intellectual & Developmental Disability, 29* (4), 350–65.

Glasgow, D.V. (2007). *The Affinity Measure of Sexual Interest – Version 2.5*. Victoria, BC: Pacific Psychological Assessment Corporation.

Goodman, W., Leggett, J. & Garrett, T. (2007). Locus of control in offenders and alleged offenders with learning disabilites. *Journal of Learning Disabilities, 35*, 192–7.

Gray, N.S., Fitzgerald, S., Taylor, J., MacCulloch, M.J. & Snowden, R.J. (2007). Predicting future reconviction rates in offenders with intellectual disabilities: The predictive efficacy of VRAG, PCL-SV, and the HCR-20. *Psychological Assessment, 19* (4), 474–9.

Griffin, D. & Bartholomew, K. (1994). Models of the self and other: Fundemental dimensions underlying measure of adult attachment. *Journal of Personality and Social Psychology, 67*, 430–45.

Griffiths, D. & Lunsky, Y. (2003). *Socio-sexual knowledge and attitudes assessment tool – revised (SSKAAT-R)*. Wooddale, IL: Stoelting Company.

Grubin, D. (1998). *Sex offending against children: Understanding the risk*. London: Research Development Statistics.

Hanson, R.K. (1997). *The development of a brief actuarial risk scale for sexual offence recidivism*. (User Report 97-04), Ottawa: Department of the Solicitor General of Canada.

Hanson, R.K. & Harris, A.J.R. (2000). Where should we intervene? Dynamic predictors of sexual offense recidivism. *Criminal Justice and Behavior, 27*, 6–35.

Hanson, R.K. & Harris, A.J.R. (2001). A structured approach to evaluating change among sexual offenders. *Sex Abuse: A Journal of Research and Treatment, 13*, 105–22.

Hanson, R.K. & Thornton, D. (2000). Improving risk assessments for sex offenders: A comparison of three actuarial scales. *Law and Human Behavior, 24* (1), 119–36.

Hare, R.D. (1991). *The Psychopathy Checklist-Revised*. Toronto, Multi-Health Systems.

Harris, A.J.R. & Tough, S. (2004). Should actuarial risk assessments be used to sex offenders who are intellectually disabled? *Journal of Applied Research in Intellectual Disabilities, 17*, 235–41.

Harris, E.C. & Barraclough, B. (1998). Excess mortality of mental disorder. *British Journal of Psychiatry, 173*, 11–53.

Harris, G.T., Rice, M.E. & Quinsey, V.L. (2007). Abandoning evidence-based risk appraisal in forensic practice: Comments on Hart *et al. British Journal of Psychiatry* (August).

Hart, S.D., Cox, D.N. & Hare, R.D. (1995). *The Psychopathy Checklist – Screening Version (PCL-SV)*. Toronto: Multi-Health Systems.

Hart, S.D., Michie, C. & Cooke, D.J. (2007). Precision of actuarial risk assessment instruments. *British Journal of Psychiatry, 190* (suppl. 49), s60–s65.

Hassiotis, A., Strydom, A., Hall, I., Ali, A., Lawrence-Smith, G., Meltzer, H., *et al.* (2008). Psychiatric morbidity and social functioning among adults with borderline intelligence living in private households. *Journal of Intellectual Disability Research, 52*, 95–106.

Hatton, C. (2002). Psychosocial interventions for adults with intellectual disabilities and mental health problems: A review. *Journal of Mental Health, 11* (4), 357–73.

Heal, L.W. & Sigelman, C.K. (1995). Response biases in interviews of individuals with limited mental ability. *Journal of Intellectual Disability Research, 39,* 331–40.

Heighway, S.M. & Webster, S.K. (2007). *STARS: Skills training for assertiveness, relationship-building and sexual awareness.* Arlington, TX: Future Horizons, Inc.

Hingsburger, D., Griffiths, D. & Quinsey, V. (1991). Detecting counterfeit deviance: Differentiating sexual deviance from sexual inappropriateness. *Habilitative Mental Healthcare Newsletter, 10,* 51–4.

Hurley, A.D., Pfadt, A., Tomasulo, D. & Gardner, W.I. (1996). Counseling and psychotherapy. In J. Jacobson & J. Mulick (Eds), *Manual of diagnosis and professional practice in mental retardation* (pp. 371–80). Washington, DC: American Psychological Association.

Joyce, T., Globe, A. & Moody, C. (2006). Assessment of component skills for cognitive therapy in adults with intellectual disability. *Journal of Applied Research in Intellectual Disabilities, 19,* 17–23.

Keeling, J.A., Beech, A.R. & Rose, J.L. (2007). Assessment of intellectual disabled sexual offenders: The current position. *Aggression and Violent Behavior, 12,* 229–41.

Keeling, J.A., Rose, J.L. & Beech, A.R. (2007). A preliminary evaluation of the adaptation of four assessments for offenders with special needs. *Journal of Intellectual and Developmental Disability, 32* (2), 62–73.

Lambrick, F. & Glaser, W. (2004). Sex offenders with an Intellectual Disability. *Sexual Abuse: A Journal of Research and Treatment, 16,* 381–92.

Langdon, P.E., Maxted, H., Murphy, G.H. & SOTSEC-ID (2007). An exploratory evaluation of the Ward and Hudson offending pathways model with sex offenders who have intellectual disability. *Journal of Intellectual and Developmental Disability, 32* (2), 94–105.

Langdon, P.E. & Talbot, T.J. (2006). Locus of control and sex offenders with an intellectual disability. *International Journal of Offender Therapy and Comparative Criminology, 50,* 391–401.

Lefcourt, H.M. (1976). *Locus of control: Current trends in theory and research.* Hillsdale, NJ: Lawrence Erlbaum.

Lindsay, W.R., Elliot, S.F. & Astell, A. (2004). Predictors of sexual offence recidivism in offenders with intellectual disabilities. *Journal of Applied Research in Intellectual Disabilities, 17* (4), 299–305.

Lindsay, W.R., Hogue, T.E., Taylor, J.L., Steptoe, L., Mooney, P., O'Brien, G., *et al.* (2008). Risk assessment in offenders with intellectual disability: A comparison across three levels of security. *International Journal of Offender Therapy and Comparative Criminology, 52,* 90–111.

Lindsay, W.R., Howells, L. & Pitcaithly, D. (1993). Cognitive therapy for depression with individuals with intellectual disabilities. *British Journal of Medical Psychology, 66,* 135–41.

Lindsay, W.R., Michie, A.M., Whitefield, E., Martin, V., Grieve, A. & Carson, D. (2006). Response patterns on the questionnaire on attitudes consistent with sexual offending in groups of sex offenders with intellectual disabilities. *Journal of Applied Research in Intellectual Disabilities, 19* (1), 47–53.

Lindsay, W.R., Murphy, L., Smith, G., Murphy, D.G.M., Edwards, Z., Chittock, C., *et al.* (2004). The dynamic risk assessment and management system: An assessment of immediate risk of violence for individuals with offending and challenging behaviour. *Journal of Applied Research in Intellectual Disabilities, 17,* 267–74.

Lindsay, W.R. & Smith, A.H.W. (1998). Responses to treatment for sex offenders with intellectual disability: a comparison of men with 1- and 2-year probation sentences. *Journal of Intellectual Disability Research, 42,* 346–53.

Lindsay, W.R., Whitefield, E. & Carson, D. (2007). An assessment for attitudes consistent with sexual offending for use with offenders with intellectual disabilities. *Legal and Criminological Psychology, 12* (1), 55–68.

Lockhart, K., Guerin, S. and Coyle, K. (2010). Expanding the test of counterfeit deviance: Are sexual knowledge, experience and needs a factor in the sexualised challenging behaviour of adults with intellectual disability? *Research in Developmental Disabilities, 31,* 117–30.

Lunsky, Y., Frijters, J., Griffiths, D.M., Watson, S.L. & Williston, S. (2007). Sexual knowledge and attitudes of men with intellectual disability who sexually offend. *Journal of Intellectual and Developmental Disability, 32* (2), 74–81.

McCabe, M.P. (1994). *Sexual knowledge, experience, feelings and needs scale for people with intellectual disability (SexKen-ID)*. Burwood, Australia: Deakin University.

McCabe, M.P., Cummins, R.A. & Deeks, A.A. (1999). Construction and psychometric properties of sexuality scales: Sex knowledge, experience and needs scales for people with intellectual disabilities (SexKen-ID), people with physical disabilities (SexKen-PD), and the general population (SexKen-GP). *Research in Developmental Disabilities, 20*, 241–54.

McGillivray, J.A., McCabe, M.P. & Kershaw, M.M. (2008). Depression in people with intellectual disability: An evaluation of a staff-administered treatment program. *Research in Developmental Disabilities, 29*, 524–36.

Michie, A.M., Lindsay, W.R., Martin, V. & Grieve, A. (2006). A test of counterfeit deviance: A comparison of sexual knowledge in groups of sex offenders with intellectual disability and controls. *Sex Abuse: A Journal of Research and Treatment, 18*, 271–8.

Miller, R.S. & Lefcourt, H.M. (1982). The assessment of social intimacy. *Journal of Personality Assessment, 46*, 514–18.

Moffatt, C.W., Hanley-Maxwell, C. & Donnellan, A.M. (1995). Discrimination of emotion, affective perspective-taking and empathy in individuals with intellectual disability. *Education and Training in Mental Retardation and Developmental Disabilities, 30*, 76–85.

Morrissey, C., Hogue, T., Mooney, P., Allen, C., Johnston, S., Hollin, C., *et al.* (2007). Predictive validity of the PCL-R in offenders with intellectual disability in a high secure hospital setting: Institutional aggression. *Journal of Forensic Psychiatry and Psychology, 18*, 1–15.

Morrissey, C., Hogue, T.E., Mooney, P., Lindsay, W.R., Steptoe, L., Taylor, J., *et al.* (2005). Applicability, reliabilty, and validity of the Psychopathy Checklist – Revised in offenders with intellectual disabilities: Some initial findings. *International Journal of Forensic Mental Health, 4*, 207–20.

Morrissey, C., Mooney, P., Hogue, T.E., Lindsay, W.R. & Taylor, J.L. (2007). Predictive validity of the PCL-R for offenders with intellectual disability in a high security hospital: Treatment progress. *Journal of Intellectual and Developmental Disability, 32* (2), 125–33.

Mossman, D. & Sellke, T.M. (2007). Avoiding errors about 'margins of error'. *British Journal of Psychiatry* (July).

Murphy, G. (1987). Direct observation as an assessment tool in functional analysis and treatment. In J. Hogg & N.V. Raynes (Eds), *Assessment in Mental Handicap: A Guide to Assessment Practices, Tests, and Checklists* (pp. 190–238). London: Croom Helm.

Murphy, G., Powell, S., Guzman, A.M. & Hays, S.J. (2007). Cognitive-behavioural treatment for men with intellectual disabilities and sexually abusive behaviour: A pilot study. *Journal of Intellectual Disability Research, 51* (11), 902–12.

Nichols, H.R. & Molinder, I. (1984). *Multiphasic sex inventory manual*. Tacoma, WA: Nichols & Molinder.

Nichols, H.R. & Molinder, I. (2000). *Multiphasic sex inventory-II manual*. Tacoma, WA: Nichols & Molinder.

Nowicki, S. & Duke, M.P. (1974). A locus of control scale for noncollege as well as college adults. *Journal of Personality Assesment, 38*, 136–7.

O'Connor, W. (1996). A problem-solving intervention for sex offenders with an intellectual disability. *Journal of Intellectual & Developmental Disability, 21*, 219–35.

O'Leary, K.D. & Wilson, G.T. (1975). *Behavior therapy: Application and outcome*. Englewood Cliffs, NJ: Prentice Hall.

Owens, R.G. & Mackinnon, A. (1993). The functional analysis of challenging behaviours: Some conceptual and theoretical problems. In R.S.P. Jones & C. Eayrs (Eds), *Challenging behaviour and intellectual disability: A psychological perspective* (pp. 224–39). Clevedon, Avon: British Institute of Learning Disabilities.

Page, G.L. & Scalora, M.J. (2004). The utility of locus of control for assessing juvenile amenability to treatment. *Aggression and Violent Behavior, 9* (5), 523–34.

Proctor, T. & Beail, N. (2007). Empathy and theory of mind in offenders with intellectual disability. *Journal of Intellectual and Developmental Disability*, *32* (2), 82–93.

Prout, H.T. & Strohmer, D.C. (1991). *The emotional problem scales*. Odessa, FL: Psychological Assessment Resources.

Quinsey, V.L., Book, A. & Skilling, T.A. (2004). A follow-up of deinstitutionalised developmentally handicapped men with histories of antisocial behaviour. *Journal of Applied Research in Intellectual Disabilities*, *17*, 243–54.

Quinsey, V.L., Harris, G.T., Rice, M.E. & Cormier, C. (1998). *Violent offenders: Appraising and managing risk*. Washington, DC: American Psychological Association.

Rose, J., Jenkins, R., O'Connor, C., Jones, C. & Felce, D. (2002). A group treatment for men with intellectual disabilities who sexually offend or abuse. *Journal of Applied Research in Intellectual Disabilities*, *15* (2), 138–50.

Rotter, J.B. (1966). Generalised expectancies for internal versus external control of reinforcement. *Psychological Monographs*, *80*, 1–28.

Russell, D.W. (1996). The UCLA loneliness scale (version 3): Reliability, validity and factor structure. *Journal of Personality Assessment*, *66*, 20–40.

Sams, K., Collins, S. & Reynolds, S. (2006). Cognitive therapy abilities in people with learning disabilities. *Journal of Applied Research in Intellectual Disabilities*, *19*, 25–33.

SOTSEC-ID (in press). Effectiveness of group cognitive-behavioural treatment for men with intellectual disabilities at risk of sexual offending. *Journal of Applied Research in Intellectual Disabilities*.

Steptoe, L., Lindsay, W.R., Murphy, L. & Young, S.J. (2008). Construct validity, reliability and predictive validity of the dynamic risk assessment and management system (DRAMS) in offenders with intellectual disability. *Legal and Criminological Psychology*, *13*, 309–21.

Talbot, T.J. & Langdon, P.E. (2006). A revised sexual knowledge assessment tool for people with intellectual disabilities: Is sexual knowledge related to sexual offending behaviour? *Journal of Intellectual Disability Research*, *50* (7), 523–31.

Taylor, J.L., Novaco, R.W., Gillmer, B. & Thorne, I. (2002). Cognitive-behavioural treatment of anger intensity among offenders with intellectual disabilities. *Journal of Applied Research in Intellectual Disabilities*, *15* (2), 151–65.

Thornton, D. (2002). Constructing and testing a framework for dynamic risk assessment. *Sexual Abuse: A Journal of Research and Treatment*, *14*, 139–54.

Thornton, D., Mann, R.E., Webster, S.D., Blud, L., Travers, R., Friendship, C., *et al.* (2003). Distinguishing and combining risks for sexual and violent recidivism. *Annals of the New York Academy of Sciences*. *989*, 225–35.

Tough, S. (2001). Validation of two standard assessments (RRASOR, 1997; STATIC-99, 1999) on a sample of adult males who are intellectually disabled with significant cognitive deficits. Master's Thesis. University of Toronto, Toronto, ON, Canada.

van Schrojenstein Lantman-de Valk, H.M.J. (2005). Health in people with intellectual disabilities: Current knowledge and gaps in knowledge. *Journal of Applied Research in Intellectual Disabilities*, *18*, 325–33.

van Schrojenstein Lantman-de Valk, H.M.J., Metsemakers, J.F.M., Haveman, M.J. & Crebolder, H.F.J.M. (2000). Health problems in people with intellectual disability in general practice: a comparative study. *Family Practice*, *17*, 405–7.

Webster, C.D., Douglas, K.S., Eaves, D. & Hart, S.D. (1997). HCR-20: Assessing risk for violence (version 2). Vancouver: Simon Fraser University.

Wehmeyer, M.L. (1997). Self-determination and educational outcome: A definitional framework and implications for intervention. *Journal of Developmental and Physical Disabilities*, *9*, 175–209.

Wehmeyer, M.L. (1998). Self-determination and individuals with significant disabilities: Examining meanings and misinterpretations. *Journal of the Association for Persons with Severe Handicaps, 23,* 5–16.

Wehmeyer, M.L. (2001). Self-determination and mental retardation. *International Review of Research in Mental Retardation, 24,* 1–48.

Williams, F., Wakeling, H. & Webster, S. (2007). A psychometric study of six self-report measure for use with sexual offenders with cognitive and social functioning deficits. *Psychology, Crime and Law, 13,* 505–22.

Wilson, G.D. (1988). Measure of sex fantasy. *Sexual and Marital Therapy, 3,* 45–55.

Wish, J.R., McCombs, K.F. & Edmonson, B. (1980). *The socio-sexual knowledge and attitudes test.* Wooddale, IL: Stoelting Company.

PART FIVE

Provisions and Treatment

14

Staff Support and Development when Working with Sexual Offenders with Intellectual Disabilities

SHAWN MOSHER

INTRODUCTION

Staff support and development is one of the most important components of working with persons with an Intellectual Disability (ID). This arguably becomes even more important when staff members are asked to work with people with an ID who are also labelled as sex offenders. Such work, as suggested by Perini (2004), stands at the interface of mental health, with its therapeutic and remediative aspirations, and the criminal justice system, with its emphasis on deterring offenders and public protection, and as such can be fraught with difficult professional and treatment issues.

Many of the front-line staff who deal with ID persons will have had little experience of, or training in, working with this population and even less in working with ID sex offenders. Indeed, services have traditionally tended to 'desexualise' persons with an ID (Craft, 1987), even those who have engaged in sexually offensive behaviour. While this may serve the short-term functions of lessening potential staff stress and reducing the felt necessity for specialist support or training, there is the potential danger of longer term negative effects such as increased staff burnout or a lack of skills necessary to reduce risk or lead to effective therapeutic change. This is especially important when one considers the close scrutiny carers of such people often come under from external agencies.

Although it may seem intuitively sensible to offer support and development to those staff working with ID sex offenders, the literature has surprisingly little to say on this issue. This seems rather surprising given the research findings, which suggest that burnout is a significant problem for staff working in the ID field generally (Dyer & Quine, 1998; Skirrow &

Assessment and Treatment of Sexual Offenders with Intellectual Disabilities: A Handbook
Edited by Leam A. Craig, William R. Lindsay and Kevin D. Browne
© 2010 John Wiley & Sons, Ltd.

Hatton, 2007) and that it can be ameliorated at least partially by, for instance, social support (Gill-Monte & Peiro, 1998) and training (Tierney, Quinlan & Hastings, 2007).

ISSUES REQUIRING TRAINING AND SUPPORT

It is acknowledged that working with persons with ID can be challenging. The nature of the client group, especially in non-community settings, is such that staff members are often asked to deal with a wide variety of challenging behaviour, including, but not restricted to, sexually inappropriate acts. Severe challenging behaviour, such as found in ID services, can be particularly stressful (Hastings, 2002). This stress can lead to a number of detrimental feelings in care staff, including negative emotional reactions (Langdon, Yaguez & Kuipers, 2007; Mossman, Hastings & Brown, 2002) and fear (Rose & Cleary, 2007), which can result in high staff turnover (Hatton & Emerson, 1998). These negative reactions can in their turn have an effect on the organisations in which the staff work and, crucially, on the service users themselves. Indeed, up to one-third of people working with ID clients have stress levels high enough to indicate a potential mental health problem (Hatton *et al.*, 1999a). Such a high level of stress in so many workers will have an inevitable knock-on effect on the people who these workers support.

Many of these difficulties could potentially be dealt with using staff training and support (Dyer & Quine, 1998), but there are few examples in the literature demonstrating the efficacy of these interventions. However, training has been shown to reduce negative emotions among care staff (Dowey, Toogood, Hastings & Nash, 2007; Mosher, Auge & Hebb, n.d.), which is in turn linked to lower stress and burnout levels (Snow, Langdon & Reynolds, 2007). Cognitive behavioural models of intervention with staff have shown some evidence of success (Rose, Jones & Fletcher, 1998), theoretically doing so by identifying and then seeking to correct maladaptive decision making and negative cognitions about the service users. Gardener, Rose, Mason, Tyler & Cushaway (2005) sought to reduce the stress of persons working with challenging behaviour by offering instruction on how to identify and then modify negative automatic thoughts, using positive self-talk and teaching relaxation imagery. The same authors also note that interventions that were primarily behavioural in nature – using training in assertion and problem solving skills along with progressive muscle relaxation – was also effective in reducing stress. There is also emergent evidence that using a more emotion-focused approach, in contrast to cognitive or behavioural methods, can also reduce stress (Bond & Bunce, 2000), although this is yet to be comprehensively assessed when applied to the field of ID.

Skirrown and Hatton (2007) have considered the problem of burnout for those working with ID clients. Burnout is conceptualised as being a potential result of stress and as being a state of mental, physical or emotional exhaustion brought on by experiences in emotionally demanding situations (Aitken & Schloss, 1994). As with stress, this difficulty arises not just because of its prevalence among staff but also because of the implications it can have on service users. In addition, Hastings (2002) has pointed out that employing organisations have a legal and moral duty to provide for the welfare, including mental health, of their employees. This may be of interest because burnout rates, in addition to being linked to challenging behaviour, have also been linked to a feeling among staff that they put more into an organisation than the organisation gives back (Chung, Corgett & Cumella, 1996; Skirrow & Hatton, 2007). This implies that staff training for stress can be positive but is also unlikely to ameliorate stress and burnout on its own. Rather, direct care workers will also need to feel valued and supported by their employing organisation. There are several ways that employers can foster a feeling of being valued and supported in their employees.

STAFF SELECTION

Specialist resources that offer intervention for persons with ID who sexually offend are by the very nature of the client group few and far between. This intervention often takes place in secure or semi-secure settings, where attrition rates for direct-care staff can approach or even exceed 50 per cent per year. These settings are often highly specialised, which could restrict the potential pool of staff recruits. It is therefore important for organisations to be able to select, train and retain motivated staff if they are to have employees who have acquired and developed the specialist skills needed in order to offer appropriate and effective therapeutic support (Perini, 2004).

A skilled and motivated workforce is obviously important to any organisation but, given the challenges and costs of replacing high numbers of staff and of training new staff in specialist skills, initial selection and induction is crucial to working with ID persons. There are a number of factors to be taken into account in attracting appropriate staff to work with such potentially challenging clients. These include

- Opportunities for career advancement: employees may feel more loyalty to and appreciation of employers if they feel that their careers are supported by those who employ them'
- Flexible working and attractive shift patterns: large organisations such as the National Health Service have realised that such flexibility on their part can be more important to some employees than rate of pay.
- Competitive wage and benefit structures: workers in such a challenging field need to know that their effort will be rewarded in a financially competitive manner.
- 'Family friendly' policies: employment strategies that encompass flexible working hours and a healthy work and personal-life balance acknowledge individuality and are valued by employees.
- A good reputation both locally and nationally for clinical excellence: a sense of acknowledge worth and justified pride in the workplace fosters employee satisfaction.
- High-quality working environments: staff may feel more motivated and likely to achieve if the areas in which they work are safe and pleasant for themselves and those with whom they work.
- Opportunities to take part in ongoing development and further specialist and general training: both direct and professional staff will benefit from knowing that their employing organisation supports the development of new skills.
- Research and teaching opportunities: chances for personal and career extension may be of value for qualified staff.
- A sense of collaboration and sharing of therapeutic values so that all members of staff feel appreciated: research shows that employees who are disenfranchised are less productive and less motivated.
- Formal and informal systems of confidential support: both peer and line management supervision can be included as support mechanisms; both are linked to job satisfaction and reduced stress.

- A coherent system of debrief following traumatic or particularly difficult incidents: assaults on staff and client restraint are not uncommon in ID services and confidence in oneself and one's employers can be enhanced if workers know that specific mechanisms of support are available following challenging episodes.
- The opportunity to participate in decision making: a worker who feels disempowered and unimportant may be more stressed and less satisfied in his or her job.

Any selection process should include service user involvement. This gives service users a necessary voice in who is going to support them. It will also allow other members of the selection panel to consider the quality of the interactions between prospective employer and service user, thereby perhaps assisting the process of selecting only those people comfortable in working with persons with an ID.

Research has shown (Blumenthal, Lavender & Hewson, 1998; Chung, Corgett & Cumella, 1996; Hatton *et al.*, 1999a; Hertzburg, 1966; Holmstrom & Elf, 2004) that attending to such factors can improve job satisfaction, may lead organisations to attract quality staff in the first instance and can improve retention and burnout rates. Organisations can support staff by enabling them to feel valued, by clearly promoting the shared goals and values of those in the organisation and by offering a variety of relevant employment benefits, many of which do not have to be monetary. Many of the issues discussed here could be held in common with any organisation regardless of the type of work it does. However, there are also specific types of support that need to be tailored to the specific requirements of work in the field of ID and they will be discussed below.

GENERAL INTELLECTUAL DISABILITY TRAINING

Attracting staff in both suitable quantity and quality is not sufficient to retain and motivate workers, many of whom, despite previous training, will be new to the specialist field of ID and sex offending. Indeed, it must be assumed that many staff, even those with professional qualifications or previous experience in the social care field, may be new to working with ID generally.

There are few organisations in the UK that do not speak of the importance of training and which do not offer some form of further training once staff are in post. Training and development must be part of the organisational culture in order for it to be considered important to staff of all grades and occupations. However, it can be difficult to foster such a culture, especially if direct-care staff feel they are overworked or unappreciated by other members of the team and by management.

Some organisations that work in the field of ID and sex offending offer structured periods of induction of one or two weeks duration; during this time company policy, procedure, philosophy and work practices are discussed. Other organisations, by reasons of scale or geography, may have a less formalised and structured approach to inducting new staff. Regardless of the structure of the induction period, there are several elements that would benefit new employees.

Any induction should include an exposition of the nature of ID, including its aetiology, course and the impact this difficulty can have on people's cognitions, behaviours and life experiences. This information could, in turn, have a positive impact on the way in which staff members interact with the persons in their care and how they attribute challenging behaviours (Rose & Cleary, 2007; Snow, Langdon & Reynolds, 2007). Such training could, for example, lead staff to attribute certain negative behaviours to the nature of the ID rather than to maliciousness on the part of the service user. There is an increased trend towards disseminating this type of basic yet crucial information via electronic means (so called e-learning), thereby allowing staff working at small or geographically isolated units to engage in less structured forms of induction.

It is widely acknowledged that specialist ID units, by their nature, must deal with a high degree of challenging behaviour. Instruction in the management of these problems is crucial to both ongoing quality care of residents and to staff morale (Perini, 2004). Effective training can help staff understand behaviour, grasp its communicative function and devise practical means of assisting clients to change their behaviours. Such training can normalise behaviours previously considered deliberate and aggressive, with one result being better relationships with clients. This training must include elements not only of understanding challenging behaviour but also gaining some understanding of the complex series of emotional responses these behaviours can engender within staff and of guarding against negative reactions to the clients in question (Brown & Brown, 1997). Part of this might include training on the issues of transference and counter-transference.

Appropriate training on challenging behaviour will also enable staff to be open-minded about their biases and about what they think can be done about the presenting problem. Functional assessment and functional analyses (see Sturmey, 1996) are specialist forms of intervention, but all direct workers would benefit from tuition in the basics of these core approaches as they can explain reasons for challenging behaviour and reduce staff frustrations. Staff would also benefit from being exposed to various easy-to-apply techniques to change the service user's immediate environment and thereby possibly interrupt a difficult behaviour.

At times, however, these behaviours may not be manageable by de-escalation techniques or environmental manipulation alone. There are times when, despite the best efforts of all involved, issues escalate. This could necessitate the use of hands-on restraint techniques. It will therefore be important for incoming direct-care staff of all grades to be taught a government approved method, such as Maybo, of dealing physically with challenging behaviour. This could increase staff confidence in dealing with such behaviour, which is linked in turn to reduced burnout and attrition rates (Skirrow & Hatton, 2007).

It is important that staff do not come to feel that violence towards them is expected or tolerated by their organisation. This is obviously more important for those members of staff who are most exposed to service users and therefore most at risk of being assaulted. Any incidents of violent behaviour towards staff must be carefully recorded and the worker in question be given the option to pursue the matter through the police. This option will enable the worker to feel that the incident is being taken seriously and will also allow them to exercise some control over their unfortunate situation. Any consideration of prosecution must be supported by management and direct supervisory personnel. Of course, it is also crucial that any form of physical violence on the part of workers to service users be dealt with by immediate suspension followed by investigation and, where necessary, by police involvement.

It has long been recognised by government in the UK that a competenc-based system of learning and certification would be a valuable way of not only developing but also recognising the evolving skills of direct-care staff who would not have obtained previous qualifications (Perini, 2004). There are two such systems available to people working in the field of ID. One is known as Learning Disability Qualification (LDQ, formerly known as Learning Disability Awards Framework – LDAF). This is a competency-based process consisting of four phases, successful completion of which can lead to a Higher Professional Diploma in Learning

Disability Services. The LDQ is broken down further into small units of instruction that can be completed at the learner's own pace. This learner-friendly approach is considered important in maximising training uptake (Jewell, Corry, Snyder, Kulju, Stewart & Silverstein, 2001).

The other competency-based system is that of the wider National Vocational Qualification (NVQ). This is based on nationally recognised vocational standards and consists of a combination of specific training and on-the-job assessment. The five levels in the NVQ provide recognised qualifications up to degree level. A similar system, known as Scottish Vocational Qualifications, operates in Scotland.

Both of these competency-based structures are intended for persons who do not hold previous qualifications in the specialist filed of ID. Specialist training is, however, also expected in clinical fields. For example, the Royal College of Psychiatrists administers a training scheme involving three to four years of post-qualification training in the psychiatry of ID (Day, 2001). Similarly, the nursing profession coordinates a post-qualification training programme in ID nursing and psychologists also complete a period of postgraduate clinical training that involves an ID component.

It may be very useful for organisations to implement a mentoring system for new staff. While formal training in ID is considered crucial in specialist settings (Department of Health, 2001), the support offered by experienced staff may play an important role in reducing feelings of frustration and burnout as well as increasing feelings of efficacy and improving morale. Little research has been done in this area, however, and the mechanism of this support remains to be determined as well as its level of efficacy, if any.

Many persons with an ID have communication difficulties (Money, 1997). The great majority of people new to this field, even highly qualified professionals, will have little experience of specialist communication training in systems such as Makaton or in visual communication systems such as Boardmaker. Support and training in this area, particularly for the frontline staff who will do most of the interacting with ID service users, can have a positive impact on levels of reciprocal understanding between client and worker and could have a significant positive impact on quality of care. Indeed, research (Chatterton, 1999; Purcell, McConkey & Morris, 2000) suggests that communication workshops can increase staff responsiveness to service users as well as improve the quality of staff–client communication. Government publications in this area support the efficacy of improved communication and indeed now consider this to be good practice (Department of Health, 2001).

Training is a valuable tool to assist staff to feel important to, and valued by, the organisation. However, it is a truism that considerable theoretical knowledge cannot take the place of experience and experiential learning. To this end, general staff training would ideally provide for a period of time during which new staff members can be supernumerary on the 'shop floor'. This will allow workers the opportunity to observe how more experienced members of staff handle a variety of situations as well as to come to know the people they will be supporting without the pressure of having to make decisions or intervene when they may be lacking in confidence and practical awareness.

SPECIALIST TRAINING

As important as general training in preparing staff to work with ID sex offenders is, it is highly specialist work that requires specialist levels of support and training. However, staff training has not always been accorded the emphasis that is required despite high numbers of staff in even non-specialist ID facilities reporting having encountered sexually inappropriate behaviour. McConkey and Ryan (2001) note that the percentage of staff trained in areas of sexuality tends to be far lower than the percentage who have received training in the area of ID generally. Christian, Stinson and Dotson (2002) record a familiar refrain when they report that many units that cater for persons with ID who have a sexual offence history feel that there are more important things to focus on than training in areas of sex, sexuality and offending. Given that many units also deal with significant levels of challenging behaviour as well as high absentee rates this attitude may not be a surprise. Other issues may appear to take priority. Several authors point out that some members of staff, and indeed, some management teams, have expressed concerns that such training could have undesirable consequences (Carr, 1995) or happens in an incidental and almost accidental fashion (Ager & Littler, 1998).

However, there is literature that describes and, to a limited extent, evaluates the impact on specialist training in the area of ID. This research shows that even brief workshop interventions with frontline staff can alter their opinions and knowledge about ID challenging behaviour and sexuality generally and sexual offending more specifically (Dagnan & Cairns, 2005; Hames, 1996; Jones & Hastings, 2003). Dowey, Toogood, Hastings and Nash (2007) report that a one-day workshop on challenging behaviour significantly altered staff member's causal explanations for a variety of challenging behaviours. Participants were better able to offer correct behavioural interpretations for client behaviours than they were before the training. The authors comment that this means that causal thinking about challenging behaviours can be altered with training. Similarly, Kalsy and colleagues (Kalsy, Heath, Adams & Oliver 2007) report that brief training interventions with frontline staff can positively shift staff attributions for the challenging behaviour of service users. Other work suggests that brief training about sexuality in people with an ID can also have a positive effect (Hogg, Campbell, Cullen & Hudson, 2001). There is evidence to suggest that longer training courses can effect more complex changes in staff and improve confidence (Allen & Tynan, 2000; Tierney, Quinlan & Hastings, 2007).

There is less evidence of the effects training has on those staff working with sexually offending persons with an ID, although there is awareness that there has not been enough emphasis on gathering this evidence (Epps, 2003). While it has been noted that attitudes towards sexuality and ID have become increasingly liberal since the mid 1980s (Murray & Minnes, 1994; Yool, Langdon & Garner, 2003), attitudes towards ID men who have sex offending histories are considerably more hardened (Yool, Langdon & Garner, ibid.). This less flexible and understanding attitude could have negative implications for the care and treatment of this vulnerable population.

Attitudes towards the client group are important in ID generally, but particularly so when working with ID sex offenders. The nature of their offences is considered abhorrent by society. Many workers, by virtue of their participation in wider society, will be exposed to and possibly share aspects of this dislike. Professional detachment is important but personal attitudes and resulting emotional involvement perhaps inevitably cloud professional judgement. Strong emotions, either positive or negative, do not help the service user and excessive detachment can also be detrimental to the working relationship (Roundy & Horton, 1990).

In a qualitative analysis, Mosher, Auge and Hebb (n.d.) demonstrate that specific training regarding the nature of sexually abusive behaviour in ID men led to a significant decrease in the amount of negative expressed emotion direct-care staff disclosed regarding those in their care. This intervention was brief in duration, lasting only one day, but the effects were still present three months after training. Given the likelihood that negative feelings about service users will affect the quality of care they will receive, such findings, while limited and not consistent (see Tierney, Quinlan & Hastings, 2007), are nevertheless encouraging.

Taylor, Keddie and Lee (2003) evaluated an introductory workshop for direct-care staff working with ID sex offenders. They found a significant improvement in staff knowledge and attitudes regarding this offending group. The length of worker experience did not reduce the impact or positive evaluation of this intervention. While other training programmes have been published (Briggs, 1994; Cox-Lindembaum, 1990), they have not been empirically validated.

Although the evidence supporting the efficacy of staff training on ID sex offending is limited, staff tend to appreciate education in this area (Briggs, 1994; Taylor, Keddie & Lee, 2003). While there are commercial training packages available to assist staff working with ID and general sexuality, such as Sex and Staff Training (McCarthy & Thompson, 1994), none are widely available for the more specific area of training regarding sex offending or sexually abusive behaviour.

Despite this apparent lack of resources, a specific training package incorporating the latest in theoretical and research insights should be provided for all staff who work with this population regardless of their grade or profession. This should include the following:

- pre- and post-training measurement of staff attitudes and attributions
- discussion about appropriate and inappropriate expressions of sexuality generally
- sexuality and intellectual disability, including means of sexual expression and the limits ID could place on this
- discussion of the Good Lives model (Ward & Hudson, 1998) as well as other models of offending
- exposition of how the models can be applied to LD offenders
- work on possible reasons for sex offending, including mention of triggering mechanisms and cognitive distortions
- pharmacological and psychological treatment options for ID sex offenders
- effective management techniques tailored to the setting in which the people being trained are working

Training, no matter what its content, needs to be delivered using a variety of methods of instruction. A combination of teaching, discussion and experiential exercises should be used in order to maximise participant's assimilation and recall of the material presented. Didactic teaching, in which an 'expert' lectures participants about a topic or skill, does increase knowledge on the topic but not necessarily the implementation of what has been taught (Milne, 1986). As mentioned earlier, distance learning (so-called e-learning) packages can be effective for geographically isolated sites and are also useful for sharing knowledge, as well as for assessing the learner's understanding of it. In common with the shortcomings of didactic instruction, however, implementation of the knowledge *in situ* cannot be offered or assessed.

Interactional staff training (Corrigan, 1998; Corrigan & McCracken, 1997) is considered to be the most effective method of training. As the name implies, it involves the entire team in participating in the training, including members of management. This inclusion can reinforce the importance of training as well as ensuring that all members of a care team share common knowledge and the same caring ethos. Since everyone is being taught the same set of skills at the same time and in the same manner, consistency across the team – which can be a difficulty – is promoted. Considerable evidence points to the value of interactional training (Corrigan & McCracken, 1995; Gentry, Iceton & Milne, 2001; Tierney, Quinlan & Hastings, 2007). This form of training can be enhanced further by the use of extensive role plays and experiential exercises. Many learners can be intimidated by having to engage in role plays and group discussions, but feedback following such sessions generally supports the view that doing such things improves the quality of the learning experience. This form of training is also considered to maintain knowledge over time, although any such work will need regular refreshing.

ONGOING SUPPORT

Induction and training, while undoubtedly important in supporting good quality, motivated staff, are nevertheless usually time limited and are generally 'one off' exercises. Staff morale and skills can be developed and, crucially, maintained through a programme of ongoing support. This can take the form of regular continuous professional development (CPD) opportunities for professional staff. This is generally required by various professional regulatory bodies, but positive support of this requirement not only enables staff to keep up to date with emergent thought and research but is an opportunity for them to feel valued. CPD is easier to arrange for some professionals, such as psychiatrists and psychologists, but may be more difficult for nurses because of changing shift patterns and regulatory or registration requirements to maintain minimum numbers at all times. Also, 'unqualified' frontline care workers, who usually have the most service user contact, have similar issues to nurses and may be seen as less of a CPD priority than more costly professionals.

These can be in part ameliorated by the provision of things such as on site learning and training facilities, including e-learning and Internet connections. While electronic learning can greatly increase compliance with mandatory training components such as food hygiene (Lipe, Reeds, Prokop, Menousek & Bryant, 1994), its use remains restricted. Access to electronic databases would also be beneficial, however limitations of finance and space possibly restrict the practicality of such suggestions. In addition, care workers are often neglected where CPD is concerned and may therefore require a different type of support.

There is an important role for CPD in supporting staff who work with ID sex offenders. Additionally, supervision is often a requirement of various professional bodies in order for individuals to retain their registration. Often this supervision must take specific forms. Organisations tend to be effective at offering this form of supervision owing to its statutory requirement. However, unqualified support workers are often reliant on line management arrangements and on adherence to policies and procedures (Perini, 2004). This is important, but it does not allow the level of personal, individualised support that is often required for people working at the 'coal face' of sexually abusive intervention. It can be very demoralising to work for long period of time with a challenging client group that responds only slowly to intervention. A sense of optimism and of feeling valued is extremely important but at the same time can be difficult to achieve with some of the core staff.

One way of offering this affirmation could be through 'Circles of Support'. This concept, developed in Canada in the 1980s, is usually applied to ID service users as a means of allowing them to express their wishes and views regarding their care and, through doing this, to meet their goals in life. The circle involves some of the people who are important in the focal person's life (the person in the centre of the circle). The focus person is in charge of the circle, but this group is generally facilitated by another member. While the focal person's goals are the main concern of the circle, each member can also bring their interests and talents to the group so that all members enrich, support and inform the others. Considerable research points to the support and positive change such circles can offer (Byers, 2006; Jay, 2007).

A similar form of support could be devised for staff. This could be either informal or created and facilitated more formally by the organisation, although the members of the circle will have to be approved of by the focal person. A series of interlocking circles could in theory be set up so that members of staff all feel that they have a support network that is focused on their frustrations, hopes and concerns. As an additional benefit, the person who is supported in one circle would be able to in turn support others in their colleagues' circles. Circles of support are seen as a means of allowing participants to take more control over their lives, something that dovetails with research suggesting that staff who have an internal locus of control tend to have greater job satisfaction when working with persons with ID (Schmitz, Neumann & Opperman, 2000; Snow, Langdon & Reynolds, 2007).

Regardless of the form that support may take, workers need a space to be able to acknowledge their feelings and share them in a non-judgemental setting. This is easier to facilitate for members of professional bodies, such as psychologists and psychiatrists, than it is for direct care workers, for whom availability and opportunity to take part in such work are much more restricted. Nevertheless, efforts to ensure that this opportunity is available will go a considerable way to allowing an employee to feel valued.

More generally, organisations could ensure that support is there to clarify policies and procedures and to communicate changes in the organisational structure or in its expectations clearly. Many large services undergo frequent reconfigurations – as is common in the National Health Service – (Perini, 2004), legislation can change and working practices may alter. These developments could serve the unintended purpose of making employees feel confused, devalued or that they are 'pawns' in the larger organisational structure. Uncertainty and change within organisations can negatively impact the performance of employees as well as their sense of well-being (Stolte, 1994; Sylvester & Chapman, 1997). This is important for all workers but perhaps especially for direct-care staff (Dychawy-Rosner, Eklund Isacksson, 2000), who may feel that they have little control over their workplace.

It is accordingly important to manage the organisational culture, perhaps especially so given the difficulties inherent in working with ID sex offenders. Many settings for this work are specialist and are therefore set apart both physically and philosophically from other services. Goffman (1961) points out that organisations can be at risk of developing a separate and distinct culture. This can be problematic if not managed effectively. Perini (2004) describes how easily a culture and its attendant value systems can drift in the absence of effective leadership, supervision and training. Implied within this, as well, is accountability. Management must ensure that all members of staff from directors to unskilled ancillary workers are aware of their responsibilities and professional obligations. Workers must also feel free to be able to 'whistle blow' and to point out examples of poor care so as to ensure that all staff have mutual responsibility to the people they work with. Isolation can breed complacency and lack of risk awareness, both of which can be avoided if staff are adequately supported and empowered.

There are many ways that organisations and, within organisations, management can support care staff. However, these must be done proactively. Changes that only occur following critical incidents or considerable staff unrest may lead workers to believe that their welfare is not of primary concern to their employer. It is an often repeated phrase that employees are any organisation's most valuable resource but it is crucial that workers feel that this is more than just a cliché. Good two-way communication and effective, sensitive managing can be buttressed by active monitoring of employee wellbeing and morale. This not only allows staff to communicate their concerns but also makes it possible for remedial action to be taken before systems break down.

Studies have demonstrated the positive impact ongoing managerial and organisational support can have on the mental health and well-bring of staff. Ito, Kurita and Shiiya (1999) found that direct-care workers have higher burnout and stress rates than staff who have less or only indirect contact, but they reported that these difficulties significantly abated when support was available to discuss work and personal problems. Burnout has also been found to be lessened when people feel they have more control over their work environment (Schmitz, Neumann & Opperman, 2000). Some organisations have recognised this issue and have developed dedicated staff support departments or have arranged for staff support via external, impartial organisations. It will be important that these provisions are advertised widely and that their confidential nature be strictly enforced.

ISSUES OF SECURITY

Most ID services are provided in setting of limited security, either in nursing homes, independent hospitals or community settings. Indeed, many people who have sexually inappropriate or offending behaviour are managed in such settings. This could be because offending behaviour has not attracted official attention or, if it has been reported to the police, has not led to prosecution and conviction. Also, some behaviours may have occurred sufficiently long ago to no longer been deemed an immediate risk of relapse. However, regardless of the setting in which ID sex offenders are managed or the reason the service user is in that setting, issues of security are important to allow staff to feel supported and safe.

There is a certain degree of conflict between therapy and security (Perini, 2004). While there should always be a proportional balance between the two, members of staff have the difficult task of trying to maintain this balance on a daily basis and in different settings (such as on a unit and during community access). This is at its most acute in secure services and special hospitals but also exists to a lesser extent in any setting where staff exert a degree of control over the lives of the people using the service. It is imperative that staff feel comfortable in their duties and supported in their decision making in this regard.

Kingsley (1998) provides a useful framework for dividing security into typologies. The first is *relational security*, which encompasses the detailed professional knowledge and under-standing of the client. This is derived from the therapeutic relationship between worker and client and will accordingly be different for different relationships. A direct-care worker, for example, may know a service user on a far more personal level than a psychiatrist or psychologist who sees him only occasionally. At the same time, these professionals may have a better grasp of the client's risk history than the care worker. Regardless of the nature of the relationship, all staff must be sufficiently trained in risk assessment and security. This is especially important in forensic settings (Perini, 2004) but is applicable to other settings as well. Management can ensure that staff are protected by installing appropriate training and regular refresher courses as they are required, by maintaining appropriate numbers of staff and by ensuring staff do not work an excessive number of hours.

Procedural security is encompassed by cogently written and effective policies and procedures. Clear management guidance on how various aspects of service-user care is to be managed will reduce stress and increase staff confidence in dealing with even difficult situations. This could include

- up-to-date risk assessments for the activities the service user is likely to engage in;
- effective policies for the management of aggression, including verbal de-escalation techniques and the use of physical restraint as required;
- a hierarchy of steps to be taken leading up to restraint, and a clear chain of command regarding how such incidents are dealt with;
- search policies regarding service users and, if residential, their living quarters;
- policies on matters such as mobile telephone usage, Internet access, and family visiting, especially by small children;
- policies on investigation of alleged staff misconduct, including clear means of effectively supporting the employee(s) under investigation.

It is perhaps with *physical security* that the interplay between therapy and security is most clearly felt. Treatment or therapeutic intervention must be balanced with the requirement to maintain the safety of the public as well as of the service user. Errors on the side of lenient security could endanger innocent people but excessive restriction could seriously hamper interventions. It is generally the case that the more secure the treatment facility is the more relaxed the internal environment can become as the possibility of inappropriate or unintended interaction with the public is small (Perini, 2004). This internal relaxation is inevitably counterbalanced by restricted access to the wider community, therefore hampering the possibility of meeting the person's 'human goods' requirements (Ward & Hudson, 1998). As with the other forms of security, it can be challenging and stressful to get this balance right. However, it is almost inevitable that sometimes, despite workers' best efforts, things can go wrong in day-to-day risk management, and it is this element of uncertainty that must be addressed by supportive management through careful staff selection, training and ongoing, proactive support.

CONCLUSIONS

Work with persons with an ID can be highly challenging but ultimately very rewarding employment. A large component of job satisfaction and success in this field is the amount of support and relevant development staff members feel they receive from the organisation for which they are employed. Effective support of service users relies on staff feeling confident, knowledgeable and important to the organisation. This chapter has discussed several ways in which workers can be empowered to be good at their jobs, confident in their decisions and able to build up a therapeutic and supportive rapport with the people they support.

This necessarily requires considerable investment in recruitment, training and ongoing staff development. Such investment in staff will have the effect of being an investment in the people with an ID the organisation cares for. It is difficult to separate the effectiveness with which an organisation supports its employees from the effectiveness with which it supports its service users. Such investment in staff will reduce turnover, stress and burnout and will encourage work of the highest clinical and ethical standards.

REFERENCES

Ager, J. & Littler, J. (1998). Sexual health for people with learning disabilities. *Nursing Standard*, *13* (2), 34–9.

Aitken, C.J. & Schloss, J.A. (1994). Occupational stress and burnout amongst staff working with people with an intellectual disability. *Behavioral Interventions*, *9*, 225–34.

Allen, D. & Tynan, H. (2000). Responding to aggressive behaviour: Impact of training on staff members' knowledge and confidence. *Mental Retardation*, *38*, 97–104.

Blumenthal, S., Lavender, T. & Hewson, S. (1998). Role clarity, perception of the organization, and burnout amongst support workers in residential homes for people with intellectual disability: A comparison between an national health service trust and a charitable company. *Journal of Intellectual Disability Research*, *42*, 409–17.

Bond, F.W. & Bunce, D. (2000). Mediators of change in emotion-focused and problem-focused worksite stress management interventions. *Journal of Occupational Health Psychology*, *5*, 156–63.

Briggs, D. (1994). The management of sex offenders in institutions. In, T. Morrison, M. Erooga, & R.C. Beckett (Eds), *Sex offending against children* (pp. 129–45). London: Routledge.

Brown, H. & Brown, V. (1997). *Understanding and responding to difficult behaviour*. Brighton: Pavilion.

Byers, R. (2006). *CREDO East evaluation report*. Cambridge: University of Cambridge, Faculty of Education.

Carr, L.T. (1995). Sexuality and people with learning disabilities. *British Journal of Nursing*, *4* (19), 1135–41.

Chatterton, S. (1999). Communication skills workshops in learning disability nursing. *British Journal of Nursing*, *8* (2), 90–6.

Christian, L., Stinson, J. & Dotson, L.A. (2002). Staff values regarding the sexual expression of women with developmental disabilities. *Sexuality and Disability*, *19* (4), 283–91.

Chung, M.C., Corbett, J. & Cumella, S. (1996). Relating staff burnout to clients with challenging behaviour in people with a learning disability: Pilot study 2. *European Journal of Psychiatry*, *10*, 155–65.

Corrigan, P.W. & McCracken, S.G. (1997). *Interactive Staff Training*. Plenum Press: New York.

Corrigan, P.W. (1998). Building teams and programs for effective rehabilitation. *Psychiatric Quarterly*, *69* (3), 193–209.

Corrigan, P.W. & McCracken, S.G. (1995). Psychiatric rehabilitation and staff development: Educational and organisational models. *Clinical Psychology Review*, *15*, 699–719.

Cox-Lindembaum, D. (1990). A model for staff training and clinical treatment for the mentally retarded sex offender. A. Dosen, A. Van Gennep & G.J. Zwanikken (Eds), *Treatment of mental illness and behavioural disorder in the mentally retarded*. Proceedings of the International Congress, Amsterdam, 3–4 May. Amsterdam: Logon Publications.

Craft, A. (1987). *Mental Handicap and Sexuality, Issues and Perspectives*. Kent: Costello.

Dagnan, D. & Cairns, M. (2005). Staff judgements of responsibility for the challenging behaviour of adults with intellectual disabilities. *Journal of Intellectual Disability Research*, *49*, 95–101.

Day, K. (2001). Service provision and staff training: An overview. In A. Dosen & Day, K. (Eds), *Treating mental illness and behavior disorders in children and adults with mental retardation*. Washington DC: American Psychiatric Press.

Department of Health (2001). *Valuing people – government white paper*. London: Department of Health.

Dowey, A., Toogood, S., Hastings, R.P. & Nash, S. (2007). Can brief workshop interventions change care staff understanding of challenging behaviours? *Journal of Applied Research in Intellectual Disabilities*, *20*, 52–7.

Dychawy-Rosner, I., Eklund, M. & Isacksson, A. (2000). Direct care staff's need for support in their perceived work role in day activity units. *Journal of Nursing Management*, *8* (1), 39–48.

Dyer, S. & Quine, L. (1998). Predictors of job satisfaction and burnout among the direct care staff of a community learning disability service. *Journal of Applied Research in Intellectual Disabilities*, *11*, 320–32.

Epps, K. (2003). Time to grow: A comprehensive programme for people working with young offenders and young people at risk. *Journal of Sexual Aggression*, *9*, 151–2.

Gardener, B., Rose, J., Mason, O., Tyler, P. & Cushaway, D. (2005). Cognitive therapy and behavioural coping in the management of work-related stress: An intervention study. *Work and Stress*, *19*, 137–52.

Gentry, M., Iceton, J. & Milne, D. (2001). Managing challenging behaviour in the community: Methods and results of interactive staff training. *Health and Social Care in the Community*, *9* (3), 143–50.

Gill-Monte, P.R. & Peiro, J.M. (1998). A study on the significant sources of the 'burnout syndrome' in workers at occupational centres for the mentally disabled. *Psychology in Spain*, *1*, 55–62.

Goffman, E. (1961). *Asylums*. London: Penguin.

Hames, A. (1996). Parenting under pressure: Mothers and fathers with learning difficulties. *Child Care, Health, and Development*, *22* (2), 140–1.

Hastings, R. (2002). Do challenging behaviors affect staff psychological well-being? Issues in causality and mechanism. *American Journal on Mental Retardation*, *6*, 455–67.

Hatton, C. & Emerson, E. (1998). Organisational predictors of actual staff turnover in a service for people with multiple disabilities. *Journal of Applied Research in Intellectual Disabilities*, *11* (2), 116–71.

Hatton, C., Rivers, M., Emerson, E., Kiernan, C., Reeves, D., Alborz, A, Mason, H. & Mason, L. (1999a). Staff characteristics, working conditions, and outcomes amongst staff in services for people with intellectual disabilities. *Journal of Applied Research in Intellectual Disabilities*, *12*, 340–7.

Hertzburg, F. (1966). Work and the Nature of Man. New York: World Publishing.

Hogg, J., Campbell, M., Cullen, C. & Hudson, W. (2001). Evaluation of the effect of an open learning course on staff attitudes towards the sexual abuse of adults with learning disabilities. *Journal of Applied Research in Intellectual Disabilities*, *14*, 12–29.

Holmstrom, P. & Elf, H. (2004). Staff retention and job satisfaction in a hospital clinic: A case study. Paper presented at the Twenty-second International Conference of the System Dynamics Society, Stockholm, July 25–9.

Ito, H., Kurita, H. & Shiiya, J. (1999). Burnout among direct care staff members of facilities for persons with Mental Retardation in Japan. *Mental Retardation*, *37* (6), 477–81.

Jay, N. (2007). Peer Mentorship: Promoting advocacy and friendship between young people. *Learning Disability Today*, *7* (3), 18–21.

Jones, C. & Hastings, R.P. (2003). Staff reactions to self-injurious behaviours in learning disability services: Attributions, emotional responses, and helping. *British Journal of Clinical Psychology*, *42*, 189–203.

Jewell, T.C., Corry, R., Snyder, S., Kulju, K., Stewart, D.A. & Silverstein, S.M. (2001). A new initiative to enhance services for people with severe mental illness. *New Psychologist*, *13* (1), 25–30.

Kalsy, S., Heath, R., Adams, D. & Oliver, C. (2007). Effects of training on controllability attributions of behavioural excesses and deficits shown by adults with Down's Syndrome and dementia. *Journal of Applied Research in Intellectual Disabilities*, *20*, 64–8.

Kingsley, J. (1998). Security and therapy. C. Kaye & A. Franey (Eds), *Managing High Security Psychiatric Care*. London & Philadelphia: Jessica Kingsley.

Langdon, P.E., Yaguez, L. & Kuipers, E. (2007). Staff working with people who have intellectual disabilities within secure hospitals. *Journal of Intellectual Disabilities*, *11* (4), 343–57.

Lipe, D.M., Reeds, L.B., Prokop, J.A., Menousek, L.F. & Bryant, M.M. (1994). Mandatory in-service programs using self-learning modules. *Journal of Nursing Staff Development, 10*, 167–72.

McCarthy, M. & Thompson, D. (1994). *Sex and staff training: Sexuality, sexual abuse and safer sex.* Brighton: Pavilion.

McConkey, R. & Ryan, D. (2001). Experiences of staff in dealing with client sexuality in services for teenagers and adults with intellectual disability. *Journal of Intellectual Disability Research, 45*, 83–7.

Milne, D.L. (1986). *Training behaviour therapists: Methods, evaluation, and implementation with parents, nurses and teachers.* London: Croom-Helm.

Money, D. (1997). A comparison of three approaches to delivering a speech and language service to people with learning disabilities. *European Journal of Disorders of Communication, 32* (4), 449–66.

Mosher, S.W., Auge, S. & Hebb, J.(n.d.). The effect of brief staff training on levels of expressed emotion. Unpublished manuscript.

Mossman, D.A., Hastings, R.P. & Brown, T. (2002). Mediators responses to self-injurious behaviour: An experimental study. *Journal on Mental Retardation, 107*, 252–60.

Murray, J.J. & Minnes, P.M. (1994). Staff attitudes towards the sexuality of persons with intellectual disability. *Australian and New Zealand Journal of Developmental Disability, 19*, 45–52.

Perini, A.F. (2004). Staff support and development. In W.R. Lindsay, J.L. Taylor & P. Sturmey (Eds), *Offenders with developmental disabilities* (pp. 307–26). London: Wiley.

Purcell, M., McConkey, R. & Morris, I. (2000). Staff communication with people with intellectual disabilities: The impact of a work based training programme. *Journal of Language and Communication Disorders, 35* (1), 147–58.

Rose, J.L. & Cleary, A. (2007). Care staff perceptions of challenging behaviour and fear of assault. *Journal of Intellectual and Developmental Disability, 32* (2), 153–61.

Rose, J.L., Jones, F. & Fletcher, C.B. (1998). The impact of a stress management programme on staff well-being and performance at work. *Work and Stress, 12*, 112–24.

Roundy, L.M. & Horton, A.L. (1990). Professional and treatment issues for clinicians who intervene with incest perpetrators. In *The incest perpetrator: A family member no-one wants to treat.* Newbury Park: Sage.

Schmitz, N., Neumann, W. & Oppermann, R. (2000). Stress, burnout, and locus of control in German nurses. *International Journal of Nursing Studies, 37* (2), 95–9.

Skirrow, P. & Hatton, S. (2007). 'Burnout' amongst direct care workers in services for adults with intellectual disabilities: A systematic review of research findings and normative data. *Journal of Applied Research in Intellectual Disabilities, 20*, 131–44.

Snow, E., Langdon, P.E. & Reynolds, S. (2007). Care staff attributions towards self-injurious behaviour exhibited by adults with intellectual disabilities. *Journal of Intellectual Disabilities, 11* (1), 47–63.

Stolte, K. (1994). Adjustment to change: Basic strategies. *Nursing Management, 25* (4), 90–2.

Sturmey, P. (1996). *Functional analysis in clinical psychology.* Chichester: John Wiley & Sons.

Sylvester, J. & Chapman, A.J. (1997). Asking 'why' in the workplace: Causal contributions and organisational behaviour. C.L. Cooper & D.M. Rousseau (Eds), *Trends in organisational behaviour, 4* (pp. 1–14). New York: John Wiley & Sons.

Taylor, J.L., Keddie, T. & Lee, S. (2003). Working with sex offenders with intellectual disability: Evaluation of an introductory workshop for direct care staff. *Journal of Intellectual Disability research, 47* (3), 203–9.

Tierney, E., Quinlan, D. & Hastings, R.P. (2007). Impact of a 3-day training course on challenging behaviour on staff cognitive and emotional responses. *Journal of Applied Research in Intellectual Disabilities, 20*, 58–63.

Ward, T. & Hudson, S.M. (1998). A model of the relapse process in sexual offenders. *Journal of Interpersonal Violence, 13* (6), 700–25.

Yool, L., Langdon, P.E. & Garner, K. (2003). The attitudes of medium-secure unit staff toward the sexuality of adults with learning disabilities. *Sexuality and Disability, 21* (3), 137–50.

15

Community-Based Treatment Programmes for Sex Offenders with Intellectual Disabilities

WILLIAM R. LINDSAY, AMANDA M. MICHIE AND FRANK LAMBRICK

INTRODUCTION

In the last three decades of the twentieth century there were extensive policies of deinstitutionalisation for people with intellectual disability (ID) throughout North America, Europe, parts of Asia and Australia and New Zealand. These policies have had a profound and positive influence in that many people with ID now have greater access to community services, greater individual choice and opportunity, a better quality of life and fewer of the restrictions associated with institutional care. One of the less easily predicted consequences was that while individuals with ID would have access to the general community services and facilities in the same way as the rest of us, a few such individuals would commit antisocial behaviour and criminal acts and would have access to the police and criminal justice processes. For this reason, research on offenders with ID in the community has increased significantly since the early 1990s (Lindsay, 2009; Lindsay, Taylor and Sturmey, 2004; Taylor & Novaco, 2005) so that in 2010 most offenders with ID live in the community and may receive services such as housing, support, supervision, monitoring, counselling and treatment in community settings.

A clear example was presented by McGrath, Livingston and Falk (2007) when they described the development of services for people with ID in Vermont, USA. In 1993 the authorities in Vermont closed their institutions for people with ID and instituted a complete community-based system of services. The implications of this policy were that offenders with ID would have to be catered for in the community since there were no longer any institutional services. The authors described the way in which services for sexual offenders were then set up in the community including housing, supervision and treatment arrangements. The process also provided the opportunity for a major evaluation of the success and outcome of these

Assessment and Treatment of Sexual Offenders with Intellectual Disabilities: A Handbook
Edited by Leam A. Craig, William R. Lindsay and Kevin D. Browne
© 2010 John Wiley & Sons, Ltd.

organisational and treatment developments. Services have responded to these major social policy initiatives with the development of assessment and treatment procedures that can cater for offenders with ID who are living in these community settings.

OPPORTUNITIES AND ADVANTAGES OF TREATMENT IN THE COMMUNITY

At first blush, it may seem that the setting in which the offender lives makes little difference to the delivery of the sex offender treatment. Often such treatments are programme-based and the sex offender group will work through a series of linked modules dealing with the relevant aspects of the sex offence process. Since this is generally the case, the setting might make little difference as to the way in which the treatment is delivered and received by individual group members. However, Lindsay (2005) outlined a model for the treatment of sex offenders with ID which incorporates both treatment of offence-related issues and the importance of integration and identification with the community. By drawing on theories of the development of criminal behaviour and a wealth of data from studies on the development of criminal careers, he concluded that community integration and identification with the values of the community are as important as the sex offender treatment programme in addressing inappropriate sexual behaviour and recidivism. At the same time, Ward and colleagues (Ward & Gannon, 2006; Ward & Marshall, 2004; Ward & Stewart, 2003), writing on mainstream sexual offenders, proposed the Good Lives Model (GLM), which stressed the importance of constructing a balanced, pro-social personal identity in offenders. This is achieved through the fulfilment of human needs through pro-social and adaptive strategies and improving the quality of relationships and quality of life in sex offenders. We will explain below the way in which these issues pertain to sex offenders with ID.

The theoretical relationship between crime and developmental experiences in society was outlined by Cohen (1955) when he hypothesised that boys began committing crime because they were identifying with the delinquent subculture and conforming to its expectations. This theory suggested that some boys from lower socio-economic groups were disadvantaged in achieving pro-social goals because they had not had the developmental experience and learning opportunities to establish pro-social skills in the way that boys from less disadvantaged sections of society might.

The hypothesis was criticised on a number of bases, most notably that it assumed that middle-class aspirations and the skills to fulfil these aspirations were at its core. However, there is subsequent research which supports some of these basic tenets regarding family interaction, development experiences and pro-social problem-solving skills. For example, Patterson and colleagues (Patterson, 1986; Patterson, Reid & Dishion, 1992) produced a major developmental model to explain the onset of delinquency and criminal behaviour. In their studies they found that some families may encourage antisocial behaviour such as temper tantrums and aggression because these behaviours are reinforced. They found that in these families these behaviours brought an end to arguments and conflict and so they acquired functional value. On the other hand, in other families, children learned interactions that were quite distinct from those learned in distressed families. In this case, more adaptive, pro-social behaviours were reinforced and the child learns that interaction such as talking and negotiating can reduce conflict. In this way, these authors demonstrated that while in some families boys had repeated developmental experiences which promoted pro-social behaviour, in others, the repeated developmental experiences did not include problem-solving and language skills but rather included antisocial and confrontational skills. As an inadvertent result, these boys develop coercive and antisocial problem-solving styles for the termination of conflict.

Palmer (2003) has written that two basic 'world views' typify poor social problem-solving in offenders. Firstly, the offender tends towards an egocentric view of interpersonal and other problem-solving situations, and secondly, he may view the world as a hostile place. It is fairly logical to see that repeated developmental experiences reinforcing the success of antisocial behaviour will promote the development of a schema that the world is a hostile environment. It also follows that a lack of developmental experience in negotiating and language skills will not encourage the individual to adopt a position which encourages the understanding of the perspective of others. While all of this may seem somewhat esoteric in the consideration of community treatment for sex offenders, it is a powerful area of applied research which establishes the importance of interpersonal experience in families and communities for the development of criminality.

In a separate series of studies, Farrington (1995, 2005) has demonstrated that delinquency in early adolescence is significantly associated with developmental experiences. In a prospective study, they found that interpersonal variables when a boy is 8 years of age are important in the prediction of delinquency and criminality in later years. Troublesome behaviour, an un-cooperative family, poor parental behaviour and low IQ are all associated with delinquency in adolescence. Therefore, already at the age of 8–10 years, delinquent behaviour is associated with uncooperative families, poor housing and poor parental behaviour. These developmental experiences continue to exert an influence on delinquent and criminal behaviour throughout teenage years and young adulthood. This research reinforces the importance of developmental, family and community experiences in the development of criminal careers.

Prior to this extensive body of research, Hirschi (1969) developed Control Theory, which paid attention to both the positive learning of criminal behaviours through association with criminal subcultures and also the development of self-control through appropriate social learning, the adoption of law-abiding behaviour and the adoption of the views of society. Hirschi felt that the success of social learning was dependent on four factors: attachment, commitment, involvement and belief. Attachment referred to the extent to which the individual identified with the expectations and values of others within society, such as teachers and parents. Commitment invokes a rational element in criminality in that individuals make subjective evaluations about the loss they will experience following arrest and conviction. Involvement refers to the fact that many individuals are engaged in ordinary activities such as work, education and other occupational activities and have little opportunity to consider delinquency. The less involved individuals are with the day-to-day activities of society, the more likely they are to engage in criminal activity. Belief referred to the extent to which individuals accepted the laws of society as reasonable framework for community cohesion. Elliot, Huizinga and Ageton (1985) reported a great deal of evidence supporting this hypothesis. They found that negative attitudes to schoolwork and authority were associated with delinquent and antisocial activity. The disruption of attachments between children and authority figures such as parents and teachers resulted in a failure to internalise parental values, promote social conformity and identify with society. Therefore, community engagement and community identification have become core concepts in the consideration of mainstream criminality.

These various sociological theories of criminal behaviour suggest that we should promote methods that will increase attachment, commitment and engagement to society and its social values as a major strand for the treatment of all offenders including sex offenders. Therefore, as we have mentioned above, it is not only important to promote sex offender treatment programmes, it is also important to promote greater commitment to, and engagement with, society. Because of the processes of deinstitutionalisation and the corresponding emphasis and extensive amount of research on the promotion of quality of life, these practices are common-place in the field of ID. There is a wealth of literature on varying levels of support, the development of leisure opportunities and the organisation of supported employment for this client group. We are able to take advantage of this favourable situation of being able to focus on social engagement as a specific theoretical and practical method for the treatment of offenders. We are in the position of incorporating the vast amount of experience and research on quality of life into our treatment and management regimes for sexual offenders with ID. In mainstream work on sex offenders, it is clear that the theoretical importance of human values and quality of life has been made explicit in the form of the GLM. Because of the extent of community services for people with ID, we are in a very strong position to incorporate these procedures into treatment for sex offenders with ID.

One study on offenders with ID was particularly relevant to these theories and hypotheses. Steptoe, Lindsay, Forrest and Power (2006) compared a group of 28 sex offenders with ID and 28 members of a control group. They assessed quality of life and relationships in both groups. These measures included scales on community engagement, relationships with family and friends and the quality of home and living arrangements. They found that although the sex offender group participants reported the same opportunities as other participants they seemed to choose to take advantage of these opportunities less often than the control participants. Their scores on the quality of life scales were consistent with the control group but they reported less engagement with these opportunities. This suggested a higher level of isolation in the sex offender group. Turning to the assessment of relationships, they appeared to have more impoverished relationships than the control group but reported being quite content with this more restricted range of relationships. This led to the conclusion that while sex offenders as a group might appear lonelier and more isolated than other groups of individuals with ID this may reflect a more self-contained way of life. Therefore, they are fulfilling human needs in a more self-contained, relatively independent manner.

Clearly, this was a group study (Steptoe, Lindsay, Forrest & Power, 2006), and these findings will not pertain to all sexual offenders. We are all aware of certain individuals who are persistent and frequent in the way they strive for interpersonal contact. However, as a group, they appeared relatively less integrated with the community but quite content with their lower levels of contact. This research is consistent with the GLM in that a greater number of these sex offenders with ID are likely to be achieving their various human needs, whether they are interpersonal, spiritual, work or leisure related, in the context of relative isolation rather than integration with the community. Integration with the community would promote and en-courage a greater level of pro-social values and attitudes that is clearly more difficult in situations where the individual has less contact with others.

The corollary of these considerations is that sex offender treatment should promote community integration and contact with others. In this way, any cognitive distortions and antisocial attitudes will be frequently challenged through the normal processes of human interaction. It is also the case that the fulfilment of human relationship and interpersonal needs will be fulfilled through normal everyday pro-social contact rather than in situations which might be conducive to sexual offending. All of these considerations are possible when treatment is conducted in community settings. They are clearly more difficult in secure or restricted settings.

A further advantage of treatment in the community is that at a very practical level, behavioural skills and strategies and cognitive strategies that are developed during treatment sessions can be practised in real community settings. Skills for approaching appropriate friends and partners and attitudes and strategies for developing appropriate relationships can be practised in ordinary environments. This is especially true if staff members who may be involved with the client at other times during the week are informed about treatment or even incorporated into the treatment sessions (Lambrick & Glasser 2004). Ways of including staff members into treatment sessions will be discussed later.

These are some of the simple, fundamental principles on which the community forensic service described and evaluated by Lindsay, Steele, Smith, Quinn and Allan (2006) is based. There is an extensive literature on community engagement outlining the reasons why people with ID tend to have lower rates of employment, increased levels of social deprivation and greater disengagement with the general aspects of society (Emerson, 2007). While for the vast majority of individuals with ID these obstacles to involvement do not produce antisocial and criminal behaviour, when lack of engagement is allied to other factors such as sexual drive, developmental disruption, poor relationship skills and antisocial behaviour, it is likely to become an even more important factor. At a very simple level, people will do things during the day. If they are not engaged in pro-social activities then they may well engage in antisocial activities. Lindsay, Steele, Smith, Quinn and Allan (2006) described the way in which the forensic ID service provides clients with activities and encouragement to engage. These may be supported occupation, day service activities, educational placements and other pro-social activities, and all conform to the basic principle of community integration that we have outlined above. Therefore, the fact that ID services stress the importance of community living and community integration provides ample opportunity for the fulfilment of human needs and the promotion of the GLM and quality of life.

RISKS AND OBSTACLES TO TREATMENT IN THE COMMUNITY

It is the case that in contemporary society most individuals with ID live in the community and most people with ID who have committed inappropriate sexual behaviour or sexual offending also live in the community. It is therefore important that services address the treatment needs of these individuals, but it is also undoubtedly true that there are significant risks and obstacles to such treatment. The first is public perception of sexual offenders as opposed to other types of offenders. Hogue, Daniels, Henderson and Leeming-Sykes (2008) reported that public fear of sexual offending is far higher than public fear of violent offending. This is true despite the fact that sexual offences are significantly less frequent than violent offences and re-offending in sexual cases is much lower than re-offending in violent cases (Hanson & Bussière, 1998). It is axiomatic that if an individual is living in the community rather than any kind of secure environment then their access to victims will be greater. Access to victims is one of the major risk factors in any dynamic risk assessment, and in various workshops Lindsay (e.g., 2004, 2009) has noted adverse community reactions to sex offender services.

In a major comparison of offenders with ID across levels of security, Hogue *et al.* (2006) compared participants in maximum security services, low/medium secure services and community forensic services. Interestingly, there were no significant differences between the groups in relation to sexual offences. The main differences between groups in terms of offence history were in relation to violence. Indeed, although it was not a significant difference, the community forensic service had slightly higher rates of sexual offending as the index problem. The secure services had significantly higher rates of violent offending and weapon use. Therefore, it was clear that a significant number of men with ID who have committed inappropriate sexual behaviour or sexual offences are managed and treated in the community. Working with the same samples, Taylor *et al.* (2008) analysed the use of the Historical Clinical Risk (HCR-20) (Webster, Eaves, D., Douglas, K. S. & Wintrup, 1995) with this client group. They found that, in general, the HCR-20 was reliable and valid in that the historical items had high correlations with other risk measures which rely on historical items. An interesting point to emerge from the study was that the community sample were rated as having a higher risk score than the medium secure sample. In addition, again analysing the same sample, Lindsay *et al.* (2008) found that using a standardised assessment of dynamic risk, the community sample had a higher score than the low/medium secure sample. While there were no significant differences between groups in these studies, it is clear that the community group is considered to be as much at risk of immediate re-offending as are those individuals who have been placed in secure settings. The conclusion from this argument is that those of us who are treating sex offenders with ID in the community are likely to have risk of re-offending as a major consideration throughout the process.

This will have two major consequences. Firstly, self-regulation, self-restraint and issues related to risk are likely to be a major theme for most, if not all, group sessions. Even when the topic is something entirely different, such as understanding the feelings and reactions of victims, some part of the session may be given over to reinforcing the importance of self-restraint over the coming week. This is not least because any incidents of inappropriate sexual behaviour during treatment are inevitably a reflection on the treatment process. It is unfortunate, but it is a simple fact of life that relapse in sex offender treatment may be perceived as much more important than relapse in other psychological therapies. If a therapist is treating an anxiety disorder and the patient has some form of relapse then it is unlikely to be as public or as highlighted as an incidence of inappropriate sexual behaviour. Therefore, as therapists, we are always aware of the public nature of any re-offending.

This leads on to the effect on staff of treatment in the community. The nature of sex offender treatment can be draining for some therapists. In workshops, the authors have repeatedly made the point that many therapists may feel that going over accounts of sexual abuse, analysing incidents of sexual offending, dealing with inappropriate and aberrant sexual preference and considering effects on victims is too emotionally arduous for them to cope with. This is fine, and there should be no pressure put on individuals to be therapists in a sex offender group in these cases. It is simply not for them and that fact holds no criticism whatever. On the other hand, those who are comfortable running sex offender treatment groups in the community will still have to deal with the knowledge that group members will have a fairly constant access to situations where they can engage in inappropriate sexual behaviour. As we shall see later in this chapter, the recidivism rates are likely to be low and the number of incidents is massively reduced during and after treatment but it is still the case that there will be further incidents. Coping with the knowledge of this risk, in addition to the difficulties already mentioned concerning sex offender treatment, can be unsettling for staff, and it is important that staff are supported in dealing with these issues. (This is dealt with in greater detail in Chapter 14 of this volume.)

In terms of the evaluation of outcomes, another difficulty is illustrated by a treatment study of six sex offenders with ID by Craig, Stringer and Moss (2006). They conducted a seven-month treatment programme incorporating sex education, addressing cognitive distortions, reviewing the offence cycle and promoting relapse prevention, and they found no significant improvements on any measure including assessment of sexual knowledge. However, in a follow-up period of 12 months they reported no further incidents of sexual offending but also noted that all participants received 24-hour supervision. Where individuals are continually supervised in the community they presumably have little opportunity to engage in any inappropriate behaviour including sexual behaviour. Therefore, the value of outcome data in these studies is limited. The most important information to be reported in terms of social policy is the extent and seriousness of any further incidents following treatment. Indeed, Quinsey (1998) has argued that recidivism data may be the only data of interest to social policy makers. Therefore, the effects of treatment should be evaluated in the absence of other major variables such as supervision and escort. In fact there are a number of studies which report recidivism data on sex offenders who have been treated in community settings where participants have access to the community and these will be reviewed later.

THE TREATMENT OF SEX OFFENDERS WITH INTELLECTUAL DISABILITY IN COMMUNITY SETTINGS

It has been pointed out that most sex offenders are treated in community settings. This is true for mainstream offenders and those with ID. A great deal of work has been conducted in mainstream settings, with most offenders being treated in conjunction with probation orders. Hanson *et al.* (2002) conducted a meta-analysis of 43 studies (combined n = 9,454). They found that the sexual offence recidivism rate for the treatment group combined was 12.3 per cent compared to 16.8 per cent for the comparison (non-treatment) groups combined. A similar pattern was recorded for non-sexual recidivism with overall rates lower for the treatment groups (29 per cent) than for the comparison groups (39.2 per cent). Cognitive behavioural treatments were associated with higher reductions in both sexual recidivism (9.9 per cent for the treatment groups, 17.4 per cent for the comparison, non-treatment, groups) and general recidivism (32 per cent for the treatment groups, 51 per cent for the comparison groups). Behavioural treatments (older forms of treatment), seen more commonly in studies prior to 1980, seemed to have little effect on recidivism. The authors reported that 'current treatments [any treatment currently offered and cognitive behaviour treatments offered since 1980] were associated with significant reductions in both sexual and general recidivism whereas the older treatments were not' (ibid., p. 187).

In another contemporaneous review which concentrated on the same studies, Rice, Harris and Quinsey (2001) came to different conclusions. They meticulously reviewed the methodology of all the studies they gathered.[1] Following their analysis, they concluded that all but three of the studies reviewed were suspect in terms of methodological design. Of the three studies, one employing psychodynamic group psychotherapy found a significant increase in the re-arrest rate for the treated group (Romero & Williams, 1983), another found a significant decrease in the treatment of adolescent sex offenders (Borduin *et al.*, 1990) and a third found no significant positive effects of treatment (Marques, 1999). These three studies, which employed the highest standards of experimental design, had equivocal outcomes, with the best showing no effects of treatment. Rice, Harris and Quinsey (2001) were, therefore, less optimistic in their conclusions than Hanson *et al.* (2002). However, they gave a number of recommendations to promote investigation into treatment effectiveness which were consistent with the conclusions of Hanson *et al.* (2002). These included employing skill building, directive approaches and straightforward treatment with high face validity. This is quite consistent with those treatments employing cognitive behavioural methods and these treatments have become the method of choice for mainstream sexual offenders.

There are now a number of sex offender treatment programmes and most employ, more or less, the same approaches, methods, topics and treatment modules. For example, the Community Sex Offender Group Programme (CSOGP) (Leyland & Bain, 2007) is employed reasonably widely in probation services across the UK. It is a relapse prevention programme based on cognitive behavioural methods and has seven modules: induction, analysing cycles of offending and cognitive distortions, working on relationships and attachment styles, dealing with self-management and interpersonal skills, reviewing the personal role of sexual fantasy in offending, promoting victim empathy and developing a lifestyle change and relapse prevention plan. The recommendation is that eight to ten offenders are included in each group. It is designed to build on previously completed sex offender treatment programmes although it can stand alone with the introduction of modules on disclosure and intensive work on the cycle of previous offending.

In relation to community offenders with ID, Lindsay (2009) has described a detailed programme which includes the following:

- an introduction and induction
- offence disclosure and personal accounts of offending
- analysing pathways and cycles of offending
- dealing with cognitive distortions and maladaptive attitudes towards victims
- dealing with personal physical and sexual abuse
- promoting victim awareness and empathy
- understanding the role of pornography and sexual fantasy in personal offending
- promoting future appropriate relationships and attachments
- developing a lifestyle change and relapse prevention plan

As can be seen from these outline descriptions of two highly disparate programmes for different client groups, the topics and modules are essentially similar. Indeed, all mainstream programmes will employ the same format, which falls into three broad categories. The first general

---

[1] As an important aside, while this is common practice for sex offender treatment reviews it is less prevalent for other psychological problems. Because of this, the debate surrounding the effectiveness of sex offender treatment is robust and closely argued.

category is the nature of the offence which the individual has committed. In these sessions treatment will consider details of the offence, disclosure about the victim, the personal pathway that the individual has taken in committing the offence (see Chapter 3), and the personal needs which have been fulfilled through offending behaviour. The second broad category is related to the individual's personal emotional state, their thoughts and feelings related to the offence, their attitudes and views and understanding of the experience of being a victim, the way in which their personal sexuality (including pornography and sexual fantasy) is involved in their offending and personality variables such as feelings of entitlement or ways of dealing with confrontation. The final broad category incorporates these previous sessions into a plan for the future which will make alterations in lifestyle, consider all relevant risk factors, attempt to promote personal control in relation to sexuality, place protective factors into the context of personal risk factors and develop a comprehensive relapse prevention plan for the individual.

It is important to remember, however, the recommendations of Lindsay (2009) which are based on the repeated findings of sociological research over the years. These theories and findings attest to the fact that treatment of criminogenic issues should be done in conjunction with the promotion of an appropriate lifestyle and appropriate relationships. Integration with the community and identification with society's attitudes and conventions are as important as dealing with personal issues related to the inappropriate sexual behaviour.

THE PROCESS AND OUTCOME OF COMMUNITY TREATMENT FOR SEX OFFENDERS WITH INTELLECTUAL DISABILITY

The most significant developments in the field of sex offender treatment have been based on problem solving and CBT techniques. The application of these techniques to sex offenders with ID came somewhat later than in mainstream sex offender research and one of the first studies was published by O'Conner (1996). She developed a problem solving intervention for 13 adult male sex offenders. This involved consideration of a range of risky situations in which offenders had to develop safe solutions for both themselves and the potential victims. This seems to be an early application of relapse prevention techniques which analyse risk situations and provide alternative, protective ways of coping with them. She reported positive results from the intervention with most subjects having achieved increased community access. However, as noted with the Craig, Stringer and Moss (2006) study, the extent to which this increased community access was supervised is not mentioned in the report.

In a series of case studies, Lindsay and colleagues (Lindsay, Marshall, Neilson, Quinn & Smith 1998a; Lindsay, Neilson, Morrison & Smith 1998b; Lindsay, Olley, Bailie & Smith 1999; Lindsay, Olley, Jack, Morrison & Smith, 1998c) reported the development of treatment based on cognitive principles in which various forms of denial and mitigation of the offence were challenged over treatment periods of up to three years. They noted several aspects of treatment which adapted the basic principles from mainstream treatment to work with offenders with ID and these principles and adaptations are still in place in 2010 (Lindsay, 2009; Rose, Anderson, Hawkins & Rose, 2007). The first aspect was simplifying the rules of the group and the induction. Most agencies that have programmes for sex offenders with ID have a number of rules. Because of the intellectual limitations of the individuals involved, the information given to group members should be as simple as possible. Therefore, induction and group rules were confined to the important aspects of attendance and confidentiality.

Attendance

Attendance was compulsory and very few excuses were accepted for not attending. Any absence had to be planned and agreed upon. One of the clear messages given to offenders was that people who commit a sex offence have restrictions on their freedom. This restriction may not be as severe as incarceration, but it does mean that treatment for offending behaviour, beliefs and attitudes consistent with offending takes precedence over many other activities. Therefore, while group members are living in the community and are integrated into it, changes and restrictions will be imposed on their routines which they will be required to abide by and which some will see as an assault on their freedom. Many offenders are indeed dismayed when they find that attendance takes precedence over sports and other activities. This does not negate the importance of the development of social, occupational and physical skills. As we have made clear, these aspects of community integration remain crucial to treatment. The rule was made simply to emphasise that there is a cost to the offender and that treatment is extremely serious. It was made clear that breaches of this attendance rule would be reported to the court or other referral agencies.

Confidentiality

The second rule was that for group members and to some extent for facilitators, nothing would be said outside the group about what happens during sessions. This rule was made for two reasons. The first is the typical nature of group treatment activity. We emphasised that the personal material divulged by each group member during sessions should be treated confidentially. Group members should feel safe in divulging information about themselves in that it would not become general knowledge to other service users outside the group. This is a normal convention in group psychotherapy. A second important reason is safety. Group members were aware of the vindictiveness of society in relation to sex offenders. If it became known that certain groups of sex offenders were meeting regularly at a certain venue, then members of the local community might wait for and 'punish' them. Therefore, we believed it was crucial that the nature and venue of sessions did not become generally known. It is certainly the case that some group members will have had experience of vigilante activity to a greater or lesser degree, and this can be discussed within group sessions to emphasise the importance of confidentiality for each individual's safety. It is somewhat surprising that Lindsay (2009) has reported that attendance at his group sessions for around 150 sexual offenders over 25 years has been over 95 per cent.

Motivation

For sex offenders with ID, it will be the case that very few referrals will show any motivation to address the issues of offending or to change their behaviour. Rather, most will seek to deny that the problem has occurred at all and avoid discussing or addressing the important issues. Therefore, motivation will be a crucial and constant issue for treatment in any community sex offender treatment service. Lindsay and colleagues (Lindsay, Marshall, Neilson, Quinn &

Smith 1998a; Lindsay, Neilson, Morrison & Smith 1998b; Lindsay, Olley, Bailie & Smith 1999; Lindsay, Olley, Jack, Morrison & Smith, 1998c) described several methods to increase levels of motivation. They made attempts to ensure that legal processes would take their course so that the offender would realise that his behaviour was totally unacceptable to society as reflected in the legal system and that society had a very high expectation that he would change. The offenders themselves were often very aware that society was extremely vindictive towards them. As has been mentioned, many participants have experienced vigilante activity. These authors reported physical threats to certain men, physical threats to their relatives, attacks on property and family members and verbal threats and intimidation. The attitude of community members and the need for group participants to change in order to avoid this vindictiveness and vigilante activity was stressed.

It is also the case that participants themselves are fascinated by news on television and radio about inappropriate sexual behaviour and sex offenders. They brought information to the group concerning government policy, publications, societal attitudes towards sex offenders and newspaper reports about offenders themselves. These topics were discussed openly, with emphasis on the need for group members to change in order to avoid the results of various modifications in the law, more stringent sentencing of offenders and some of the consequences reported in newspapers for individual sex offenders.

These groups were set up in such a way that there were periods of time that were extremely enjoyable and reinforcing. Group members were very supportive towards each other if they had a problem and problem-solving exercises were designed to help individuals find solutions to any difficulties they were experiencing. It became a convention that from time to time the group went out to lunch after the formal session. At first, Lindsay, Marshall, Neilson, Quinn and Smith (1998a) reported that this was felt to be a minor treat, but it soon became clear that for the group members it was a major event. Group members would talk about the next lunch for several weeks in advance, deciding where they would like to go, what they would like to eat, what they would have to drink and so on. What appeared as a routine treat was in fact a much more important event in the lives of these men. It was one of the first indications that many of these men have very little in their lives and the prospect of a formal lunch in a restaurant or pub took on a greater importance than it did for group facilitators.

A great deal of group pressure was brought to bear when certain individuals were engaging in behaviour consistent with sexual offending. Therefore, if someone had been seen outside a school watching children in the playground, the others would be highly critical of this behaviour and be very clear about the consequences that would occur if the behaviour continued. Often group members would be inventive about the way in which police, neighbours, school teachers or other members of the public would observe the individual in such situations and report it. The consequences would then be discussed or role played graphically with the offender being apprehended and taken to the police station. Therefore group pressure was used as a highly motivating factor during sessions. Although these methods were the formal ways in which motivation was manipulated, Lindsay (2009) has noted that facilitators should always be aware of any possibly motivating opportunities during group sessions.

Dealing with Cognitive Distortions and Denial

There is a long history of sociological research in which investigators have elucidated the form and development of denial by various groups of offenders. In the theory of delinquency,

Sykes and Matza (1957) mentioned several types of denial as techniques that 'neutralise' the offending act for the offender. Scott and Lyman (1968) classified accounts into excuses and justifications in an erudite analysis of denial. Kennedy and Grubin (1992) outlined several types of denial exhibited by offenders. They identified four categories of denial that any harm was done to the victim, shifting blame onto the victim, invoking significant others such as spouses as the reason that they behaved in a manner which resulted in a sexual offence and attributing the action to a temporary aberration in behaviour or an aberration in mental state out of keeping with normal character. Lakey (1994) described these various types of denial as 'thinking errors' and classified them as denial that an offence took place, denial of any intent to offend, denial of responsibility for the offence (shifting responsibility onto others), denial of harm to the victim and denial of a typical state (consistent with Kennedy & Grubin, 1992).

In subsequent years, cognitive distortions, attitudes which justify sexual offences, attitudes which are consistent with sexual offences, attitudes which consider that victims are complicit in the sexual offending act and so on have become central to considerations regarding the cycle of abuse and pathways to sexual offending. Ward, Hudson, Johnston and Marshall (1997) reviewed the importance of cognitive distortions, the nature of cognitive distortions and the way in which they support the sex offending process. Ward and colleagues (Ward, Hudson & Keenan, 1998; Ward & Hudson, 1998) made hypotheses about the way in which cognitive distortions might change depending on the pathway to sex offending pursued by each individual offender. Because cognitive distortions and attitudes towards sexuality have become so central both in considerations of ways in which the offence is perpetrated and in the relapse prevention process, we will outline them in more detail.

Denial of the Offence

It is not unusual for sex offenders with ID to deny even the fact that an offence took place. This is true even when they have been tried and convicted of the offence. For this reason, it is important to document for each offender that the incident has occurred. At the initial stages of treatment, group members should be encouraged to describe the incident, reviewing in detail the various actions that took place. Several weeks of treatment may be necessary to get over these initial aspects of denial. In one example described by Lindsay, Neilson, Morrison and Smith (1998b) one individual continued denying that an offence took place for eight months. While this is an unusually long time, it is not uncommon for men to deny that an offence took place for two or three months. This can be so despite the fact that there has been witness evidence and a conviction. These initial months of denial are likely to be typified by evasion, lack of engagement and lack of acknowledgement of any reason for being in group sessions. Lindsay (2009) has written that in an open group where there are members who have been engaged for two and three years this process is considerably shortened. Group members who have been through these processes will be both confrontational and supportive with statements such as 'There is no point in trying to avoid it, you'll have to speak about it anyway so you might as well get it over with'; 'We've all been through it and it's better when it's over with'; 'It's really hard but you'll feel better when it's done.' In these instances, group members will continue to be reluctant, embarrassed, angry with themselves, angry with others and refractory in engaging with the process. However, it is important to begin to establish the disclosure accounts and an acceptance that an offence has taken place.

Denial of Intent to Offend

In some cases, the offender will accept that an incident has taken place but continue to maintain that his intent was misunderstood as a sexual offence. In these cases, a sex offender against children may maintain that he was simply trying to help or control the children and his actions have been misconstrued by others as sexually motivated. Examples of this might be that the offender was in bed with the children in the evening because he was trying to calm them down and get them to go to sleep rather than running around the house and that his actions have been misunderstood as sexually motivated. Alternatively, he might maintain that he was trying to help a child he found in an isolated spot and that, again, his actions have been misunderstood as inappropriate sexual behaviour.

Denial or Mitigation of Responsibility for the Offence

Many sex offenders with ID blame the victim's behaviour to deny the extent of their own responsibility for the offence. It is one of the most important issues during treatment to establish that the individual himself is responsible for the offence that took place. Any substantive work on this set of cognitions can only take place once the subject has accepted that the focus of the session is on the sex offence or inappropriate sexual behaviour that has taken place. Most of the men seen for sex offender treatment will argue that there are mitigating circumstances and many will invoke the victim's behaviour as being responsible for the incident. They are likely to assert that the victims encouraged them, that the victims are lying about the offence, that the victims are to blame because they did not need to respond to the perpetrator's behaviour in the way they did. Group members may further argue that because the victims responded to the incident in a certain way, they were encouraged to repeat the offence. This can be particularly true for incidents of indecent exposure. These cognitions indicate complicity on the part of the victim in that they enjoy the incident, that they pretend to be shocked in cases of indecent exposure, that they are sexually stimulated by the incident or that it afforded them a degree of comfort and even nurturance. All of these cognitions move some responsibility onto the behaviour of the victim.

Denial or Minimisation of Harm to the Victim

Related to denial of responsibility is a degree of denial that any harm was done to the victim. If the offender argues that the victim's behaviour was, to some extent, responsible for the incident, then it follows that in some instances they were expecting or encouraging the sexual behaviour and so would not be subsequently surprised or harmed. Therefore, the offender may accept that the incident took place, accept that he was to some extent responsible but deny that any harm was done to the victim. Group members may hold a strong belief that since a particular victim has been abused on repeated occasions, they must have enjoyed, or at the very least not been harmed by the repeated incidents. We have known cases of incest or long-term babysitting arrangements where children have been sexually abused many times before the incidents have come to the attention of the child's carers. In these cases, group members often argue that the lack of protest from the victim is an indication of both the mutuality of the sexual contact and the lack of harm done on a week-to-week basis.

Denial of a 'Normal State'

Kennedy and Grubin (1992) stated that a number of sex offenders accept that the offence occurred but say that they had a temporary aberration of mental state. On this basis they argue that they would never have offended if they had not been in a state of depression, anxiety and so on. Over the years, we have seen a number of sex offenders with ID who have invoked such cognitive distortions, although probably not as often as they are seen in mainstream sexual offenders. The most common aberration of mental state mentioned is intoxication through alcohol or drugs. A few sex offenders with ID have mentioned such cognitive distortions saying 'I was really high that night and that must have been why I did it'; or 'I would never have done that if I hadn't been so drunk.' The clear implication of these statements is that the offender behaved in such a way because of the mental state and disinhibition invoked by substance abuse. They might go on to argue that there is no requirement for treatment or group attendance because they will never use alcohol or substances to that degree again.

In the case studies reported by Lindsay and colleagues (Lindsay, Marshall, Neilson, Quinn & Smith 1998a; Lindsay, Neilson, Morrison & Smith 1998b; Lindsay, Olley, Bailie & Smith 1999; Lindsay, Olley, Jack, Morrison & Smith, 1998c) treatment was developed on the basis of intervention for these cognitive distortions. There were three fairly distinctive aspects of these reports. The first of these features was that, after each session, client attitudes were measured in relation to their specific offence. This was done using an early version of the Questionnaire on Attitudes Consistent with Sexual Offences (Lindsay, Whitefield & Carson, 2007). Therefore, it was possible to link the content of the session to the impact on specific cognitive distortions. The second distinctive aspect, central to this chapter, was that all participants lived in the community and had unsupervised access to their usual community routines such as leisure facilities, occupation, transport, shops, entertainment and so on. These reports did not, therefore, have the drawback noted earlier of continued close supervision which is a difficulty in studies which employ follow-up over periods of months. The third distinctive feature was the extent of the follow-up. These authors reported follow-up periods of four to seven years which, at the time, was an extensive follow-up period. The length of follow-up was determined by the writing of Marshall, Jones, Ward, Johnston and Barbaree (1991) when they reported an analysis of recidivism data across a number of studies and made the important point that re-offending rates of sex offenders increase as the length of follow-up increases up to four years. Thereafter it seemed more stable, and they recommended that reports should include follow-up data of at least four years. Taken together, the studies by Lindsay and colleagues (Lindsay, Marshall, Neilson, Quinn & Smith 1998a; Lindsay, Neilson, Morrison & Smith 1998b; Lindsay, Olley, Jack, Morrison & Smith, 1998c) reported on 17 sex offenders with ID reporting one documented incident of re-offending and one case in which they suspected that inappropriate sexual behaviour had once again taken place although there was no documented evidence of it.

Skills Teaching

Teaching appropriate social skills and establishing appropriate knowledge of sexual behaviour has been an important aspect of the treatment of sex offenders with ID since its inception.

The first comprehensive treatment regime for sex offenders with ID was reported by Griffiths, Quinsey and Hingsburger (1989). They felt that their referrals may have had restricted social and sexual opportunities, which caused them to develop inappropriate sexual choices. They developed a rehabilitation programme with a wide-ranging social and sexual focus, including the promotion of interpersonal skills to maintain relationships and sex education. Interventions included social skills training including role play, sex education courses and an emphasis on increasing personal and social skills to address issues of relationships and sexuality. They also developed a treatment plan which reviewed risk situations for individuals and their environment. Where it was felt necessary, they also introduced intervention for inappropriate sexual preference, which included aversion therapy in imagination and measures to promote appropriate masturbation.

Lindsay, Olley, Jack, Morrison and Smith (1998c) also described the promotion of social and interpersonal skills through frequent role plays of typical interactions. In this way, sessions will be given over to role playing appropriate social interaction with people in clubs and other places where clients might meet others with whom they can establish appropriate relationships. Problem-solving discussions would then follow concerning the way in which these relationships might develop. Similarly, sex education techniques have been widely described in the literature on work with people with ID and, where appropriate, sex education sessions might be included in the sex offender treatment. It is the experience of the authors and is reasonably well established in the research literature (Lunsky, Frijters, Griffiths, Watson & Williston, 2007; Michie, Lindsay, Martin & Grieve, 2006) that sex offenders with ID have a level of sexual knowledge as high or higher than non-sexual offenders with ID. However, while their level of sexual knowledge may be better than others in the client group, it does not necessarily follow that they have an optimum level of knowledge. In addition, isolated aspects of their sexual knowledge may be particularly deficient, especially in areas which are related to their specific offence. As an example, Lindsay, Neilson, Morrison & Smith (1998b) described a man who had committed non-penetrative offences against two girls whom he knew well. In this case, it was possible to address a number of the cognitive distortions which he held regarding sexuality with children. However, he continued to express the view that children would be more likely to be abused by strangers than by people they knew. This was clearly relevant to his own case where he abused two girls with whom he was very familiar. Therefore, the specific aspect of his sexual knowledge and cognitive distortions which were important to address were germane to his own inappropriate sexual behaviour.

These earlier reports, which focused on skills training and sex education, did report positive results. Griffiths, Quinsey and Hingsburger (1989) described a series of 30 cases to illustrate their methods and recorded no re-offending. Haaven, Little and Petre-Miller (1990) described a wide-ranging series of treatments, including social skills training, sex education and promotion of self-control, in a comprehensive programme which addressed sexual offending under a behavioural management regime. The report was related to a secure in-patient treatment unit and associated treatment programme and so participants were supervised constantly through the follow-up period and had little opportunity to re-offend. However, these programmes included comprehensive approaches for skills training and knowledge acquisition and indicate that, from early on, treatment for sex offenders with ID has included skills acquisition and sex education.

CHARACTERISTICS AND OUTCOME OF SEX OFFENDERS TREATED IN THE COMMUNITY

Two fairly large-scale studies have appeared recently which describe the characteristics of sex offenders who are living in the community, their treatment and the outcome of these treatment processes. Following a total deinstitutionalisation programme in Vermont, USA, McGrath, Livingston and Falk (2007) reviewed the treatment and management regimes for 103 adult sexual offenders with ID. They reported that the mean age of the sample was 34.6 years while the mean IQ was 61.8. Almost a quarter of their participants fell into the IQ band 45–56 and so a number were of more limited ability and would not have been considered able to stand trial for the incidents perpetrated. The rest fell into the IQ band 57–74, which is the range of mild intellectual disability if one includes the appropriate standard error of the test at an IQ of 70.

A mental illness was diagnosed in 44.7 percent of the sample and 36.9 per cent were known to have been sexually abused in childhood. All participants lived in a staffed or private home of between one and three people with paid care givers. Social and daily living skills were taught to the participants, they were encouraged to participate in the community and there were treatments to promote skills for managing risk. Just over half (53.4 per cent) of the offenders had a history of committing more than one type of sexual offence. For example, of ten who had sexually assaulted an adult male, four had also assaulted an adult female and one had assaulted a male child. In an 11-year follow-up period, with an average of 5.8 years, they reported 10.7 per cent re-offending. The 11 individuals who re-offended committed 20 new sexual offences. As a comparison, they reported 195 treated and untreated adult male sexual offenders without ID who had been followed up for an average period of 5.72 years. These individuals had had prison sentences and 23.1 per cent were charged with a new sexual offence at some point in the follow-up period. In a further comparison they reported 122 treated and untreated male sex offenders who had received probation orders and in a follow-up of 5.24 years, 6.5 per cent were charged with a new sexual offence.

As with other studies, one of the difficulties in the sex offenders with ID cohort was that 62.1 per cent had received 24-hour supervision, which limited their access to potential victims. However, they also considered that this level of supervision resulted in a more comprehensive identification of future incidents when compared to the other two cohorts who had been, of course, unsupervised. They also reported a considerable amount of harm reduction in that 83 per cent of the participants were classified as contact sexual offenders while only 45 per cent of the re-offences were contact offences. The rest were typified by exhibitionism and public masturbation.

Lindsay, Steele, Smith, Quinn and Allan (2006) published a second, similarly comprehensive, report. The sample in their community forensic ID service consisted of 247 consecutive referrals of whom 121 were referred for sexual offending or inappropriate sexual behaviour, 105 were referred for other types of offending, such as assault or alcohol related offences, and 21 were women, of whom 5 were referred for sexual offences. The male sex offender cohort had an average age of 36.3 years and an average IQ of 64.9, both of which are slightly higher than that reported in the McGrath, Livingston and Falk (2007) study. In this case, the sex offender cohort was significantly older than the other offenders but there was no significant difference between groups on IQ. More detailed analysis of the cohort revealed that 46.3 per cent of the male sex offenders were in the age band 35–54 while there were only 26.8 per cent of the other male offenders in this age band. They reported that 37.7 per cent of the sex offenders had been sexually abused in childhood, which is essentially the same figure as that of McGrath, Livingston and Falk (ibid.). In addition, 17.2 per cent had experienced physical abuse in childhood and 31.4 per cent had a recorded mental illness. This latter figure is somewhat lower than the 44.7 per cent reported by McGrath and colleagues (ibid.).

In the Lindsay, Steele, Smith, Quinn and Allan (2006) report, 48.2 per cent of the sexual offenders and 28.3 per cent of the other male offenders had been referred from the courts. In a more detailed analysis of referral patterns, they found that a significantly greater percentage of sexual offenders were referred from court (55.7 per cent) between 1997 and 2003 than in the earlier period of 1990–6 (30.3 per cent referred from court). There was therefore a significant trend for the court to deal with a higher proportion of sexual offences committed by men with ID as the years progressed. The authors felt that this was an adjustment to deinstitutionalisation policies in the 1980s whereby individuals who had committed sexual offences would be dealt with by community services such as criminal justice and court services. As these services became more familiar and experienced in dealing with people with ID living in the community they would be able to liaise with appropriate treatment agencies in relation to disposal. In fact, 42.8 per cent of the male sexual offenders had formal disposal from court while only 29 per cent of the other types of offenders had such a disposal.

Further assessment of the problems evidenced by participants at the time of referral revealed that in comparison with other types of offenders with ID, fewer of the male sex offenders were recorded as having problems with anger and aggression (25.8 per cent versus 55.3 per cent), fewer had problems with alcohol or substance abuse (12 per cent versus 30.6 per cent) and fewer had recorded problems with anxiety (11 per cent versus 19.4 per cent). As might be expected, the sexual offender cohort were assessed as having greater difficulties with social and sexual relationships (54.5 per cent versus 24.1 per cent).

Perhaps because the follow-up period was 13 years, re-offending rates were higher at 23.9 per cent for the sex offender cohort in comparison to the 10.7 per cent re-offending reported by McGrath, Livingston and Falk (2007). However, it should be noted that in the Lindsay, Steele, Smith, Quinn and Allan (2006) study all but a handful of participants had full access to the community and were not supervised. The authors also reported (ibid.) that the sex offender cohort had a lower re-offending rate than the 59 per cent re-offending recorded in the other types of male offenders. These authors also recorded the number of incidents perpetrated by participants over the follow-up period. This was possible because the study was conducted in a circumscribed region where incidents were gathered routinely. Six-monthly case reviews were held on each client for as long as any agent dealing with the client wished them to continue. The service on which the study was based was well known within the region and any incident of recidivism was reported routinely by community nursing staff, social workers and other agencies. Therefore it was relatively likely that if any incident came to light it would be reported to the researchers. They found that, for re-offenders only, there was a significant reduction in the number of offences committed when comparing figures from two years prior to referral and up to twelve years after referral. In conducting this exercise, they also biased the data against finding a positive result for harm reduction by using a cut-off of 15 offences prior to referral. They argued that some individuals had committed dozens of offences prior to referral and these participants would have significantly biased the analysis in favour of a harm reduction hypothesis. The highest number of offences committed by an individual after referral was 13. For the sex offender cohort, the 23.9 per cent of individuals who had recidivated committed 235 sexual offences prior to referral and 68 after referral. This represented around a 70 per cent reduction in the number of incidents and a significant amount of harm reduction in those individuals who did commit further offences. Therefore, it would appear that for the sexual offenders, there was a significant, positive outcome to treatment in a considerable amount of harm reduction even when comparing the re-offenders only.

Several other studies have reviewed the outcome of sex offender treatment in this client group, both when they have been treated in community settings and when they have been released from prison into community settings. Keeling, Rose and Beech (2007) conducted a comparison of convenience between 11 'special needs' offenders and 11 mainstream offenders matched on level of risk, victim's sex, offence type and age. The authors noted a number of limitations including the fact that 'special needs' was not synonymous with ID and as a result they were unable to verify the intellectual difference between mainstream and special needs populations. 'Special needs' included individuals who had significant numeracy and literacy deficits and one individual with brain damage, some of whom did not fall into the category of ID. All of the participants had been released from prison into the community with an average length of time since release of 16 months. There were no further recorded convictions for sexual offending for any of the 'special needs' participants. Murphy and Sinclair (2006) reported on the cognitive behavioural treatment of 52 men who had sexually abusive behaviour and mild ID. All of the men were living in community settings and treatment groups ran over a period of one year. There were significant improvements in sexual knowledge, victim empathy and cognitive distortions at post-treatment assessment. There were also reductions in sexually abusive behaviour at six-month follow-up. However, although the study was designed to include control participants, it was not possible to recruit controls for a range of unforeseen circumstances.

In another comparison of convenience, Lindsay and Smith (1998) employed seven individuals who had been in treatment for two or more years with another group of seven who had been in treatment for less than one year. The comparisons were serendipitous in that time in treatment reflected the probation sentences delivered by the court. Those individuals who had been in treatment for less than one year showed significantly poorer progress and were more likely to re-offend than those treated for at least two years. They concluded that shorter treatment periods may be of limited value for this client group. However, once again all of the individuals in their study were living in the community at the time and had unlimited free access to community facilities and services. In a further study on sex offenders who live in the community with free access to community services, Rose, Anderson, Hawkins and Rose (2007) conducted a group treatment with seven participants who had been in contact with the criminal justice system for at least one sexual offence. Although these authors did not have a control group, they did follow-up participants for 12–16 months after the completion of treatment and recorded no re-offending despite the fact that these individuals lived in family and group homes and had unescorted access to the community.

Clearly, these various studies have been conducted in circumstances which fall well short of the standards required for experimental rigour. Three have not included control comparisons, and in the other three, the control comparisons have not been randomised and have been controls of convenience. However, taken together they provide some evidence that treatment of sex offenders in the community is likely to have a highly significant and positive impact on the number of offences committed by participants following treatment.

CONCLUSIONS

This chapter has reviewed the opportunities and obstacles to the treatment of sex offenders with ID in community settings. The major opportunity is that treatment in the community affords access to an ordinary life and there are ample resources for fulfilling the human needs of participants in a socially appropriate manner rather than an offending manner. There is also a range of situations in which the offender is able to practice pro-social and acceptable interpersonal skills. However, with access to community settings, there is the obvious risk that there are greater chances of committing further offences. This can be difficult for service providers in that their service is at risk of becoming highlighted as a result of a public incident. Having said that, the outcomes of various studies which have reviewed treatment and management services over lengthy periods of up to 13 years suggests that these arrangements can provide low re-offending rates and significant amounts of harm reduction to the community. In addition, they are likely to represent relatively low-cost services with less recourse to expensive court facilities. A number of outcome studies have reported low rates of re-offending up to 13 years follow-up or no re-offending up to 16 month follow-up. The longer the follow-up, the higher the rates of re-offending, but even these long follow-up studies report significant amounts of harm reduction.

The chapter also reviewed the processes of sex offender treatment, which include the normal treatment sections of offence disclosure, reviewing the cycle and pathways of offending, addressing the issue of cognitive distortions and thinking errors, promoting an awareness of the effect on victims, considering personal sexuality, pornography and sexual fantasy and finally promoting lifestyle change and relapse prevention plans. Cognitive distortions are central to the process of sex offender treatment and these have also been reviewed in detail in the description of the treatment process.

REFERENCES

Borduin, C.M., Henggeler, S.W., Blaske, D.M. & Stein, R.J. (1990). Multi-systemic treatment of adolescent sexual offenders. *International Journal of Offender Therapy & Comparative Criminology*, *34*, 105–13.

Cohen, A.K. (1955). *Delinquent boys: The culture of the gang*. Glencoe, IL: Free Press.

Craig, L.A., Stringer, I. & Moss, T. (2006). Treating sexual offenders with learning disabilities in the community. *International Journal of Offender Therapy & Comparative Criminology*, *50*, 111–22.

Elliot, D.S., Huizinga, D. & Ageton, S.S. (1985). *Explaining delinquency and drug use*. Beverley Hills, CA: Sage.

Emerson, E. (2007). Poverty and people with intellectual disabilities. *Mental Retardation & Developmental Disabilities Research Reviews*, *13*, 107–13.

Farrington, D.P. (1995). The development of offending and antisocial behaviour from childhood: Key findings from the Cambridge study in delinquent development. *Journal of Child Psychology & Psychiatry*, *36*, 929–64.

Farrington D.P. (2005) Childhood origin of antisocial behaviour. *Clinical psychology and Psychotherapy*, *12*, 177–89.

Griffiths, D.M., Quinsey, V.L. & Hingsburger, D. (1989). *Changing inappropriate sexual behaviour: A community based approach for persons with developmental disabilities*. Baltimore: Paul Brooks Publishing.

Haaven, J., Little, R. & Petre-Miller, D. (1990). *Treating intellectually disabled sex offenders: A model residential programme*. Safer Society Press: Orwell, VT.

Hanson, R.K. & Bussière, M.T. (1998). Predicting relapse: A meta analysis of sexual offender recidivism studies. *Journal of Consulting & Clinical Psychology, 66*, 348–62.

Hanson, R.K., Gordon, A., Harris, A. J. R., Marques, J.K., Murphy, W., Quinsey, V.L. & Seto, M.C. (2002). First report of the collaborative outcome data project on the effectiveness of psychological treatment for sex offenders. *Sexual Abuse: A Journal of Research & Treatment, 14*, 169–94.

Hirschi, T. (1969). *Causes of delinquency*. Barclay: University of California Press.

Hogue, T. Daniels, R., Henderson, F. & Leeming-Sykes, J. (2008) Attitudes, Judgements and Sentencing of Mentally Disordered Sex Offenders. Paper presented to the British Psychological Society DFP Annual Conference, Edinburgh.

Hogue, T.E., Steptoe, L., Taylor, J.L., Lindsay, W.R., Mooney, P., Pinkney, L., Johnston, S., Smith, A. H. W. & O'Brien, G. (2006). A comparison of offenders with intellectual disability across three levels of security. *Criminal Behaviour & Mental Health, 16*, 13–28.

Keeling, J.A., Rose, J.L. & Beech, A.R. (2007). Comparing sexual offender treatment efficacy: Mainstream sexual offenders and sexual offenders with special needs. *Journal of Intellectual & Developmental Disability, 32*, 117–24.

Kennedy, H.G. & Grubin, D.H. (1992). Patterns of denial in sex offenders. *Psychological Medicine, 22*, 191–6.

Lakey, J. (1994). The profile and treatment of male adolescent sex offenders. *Adolescence, 29*, 755–61.

Lambrick, F. & Glaser, W. (2004). Sex offenders with an intellectual disability. *Sexual Abuse: A Journal of Research & Treatment, 16*, 381–92.

Leyland, M. & Baim, C. (2007). C-SOGP 50 hour relapse prevention programme. National Probation Service - West Midlands Area.

Lindsay, W.R. (2004). *Working with sex offenders with intellectual disability in the community*. Workshop presented to the Centre for Developmental Disability, Sydney, Australia.

Lindsay, W.R. (2005). Model underpinning treatment for sex offenders with mild intellectual disability: Current theories of sex offending. *Mental Retardation, 43*, 428–41.

Lindsay, W.R. (2009). *A treatment programme for sex offenders with intellectual disability*. Chichester: John Wiley.

Lindsay, W.R., Hogue, T., Taylor, J.L., Steptoe, L., Mooney, P., Johnston, S., O'Brien, G. & Smith, A. H. W. (2008). Risk assessment in offenders with intellectual disabilities: A comparison across three levels of security. *International Journal of Offender Therapy & Comparative Criminology, 52*, 90–111.

Lindsay, W.R., Marshall, I., Neilson, C.Q., Quinn, K. & Smith, A. H. W. (1998a). The treatment of men with a learning disability convicted of exhibitionism. *Research on Developmental Disabilities, 19*, 295–316.

Lindsay, W.R., Neilson, C.Q., Morrison, F. & Smith, A. H. W. (1998b). The treatment of six men with a learning disability convicted of sex offences with children. *British Journal of Clinical Psychology, 37*, 83–98.

Lindsay, W.R., Olley, S., Baillie, N. & Smith, A. H. W. (1999). The treatment of adolescent sex offenders with intellectual disability. *Mental Retardation, 37*, 320–33.

Lindsay, W.R., Olley, S., Jack, C., Morrison, F. & Smith, A. H. W. (1998c). The treatment of two stalkers with intellectual disabilities using a cognitive approach. *Journal of Applied Research in Intellectual Disabilities, 11*, 333–44.

Lindsay, W.R. & Smith, A. H. W. (1998). Responses to treatment for sex offenders with intellectual disability: A comparison of men with 1 and 2 year probation sentences. *Journal of Intellectual Disability Research, 42*, 346–53.

Lindsay, W.R., Steele, L., Smith, A. H. W., Quinn, K. & Allan, R. (2006). A community forensic intellectual disability service: Twelve-year follow-up of referrals, analysis of referral patterns and assessment of harm reduction. *Legal & Criminological Psychology, 11*, 113–30.

Lindsay, W.R., Taylor, J.L. & Sturmey, P. (2004). *Offenders with developmental disabilities*. Chichester: John Wiley.

Lindsay, W.R., Whitefield, E. & Carson, D. (2007). An assessment for attitudes consistent with sexual offending for use with offenders with intellectual disability. *Legal & Criminological Psychology, 12*, 55–68.

Lunsky, Y., Frijters, J., Griffiths, D.M., Watson, S.L. & Williston, S. (2007). Sexual knowledge and attitudes of men with intellectual disabilities who sexually offend. *Journal of Intellectual & Developmental Disability, 32*, 74–81.

McGrath, R.J., Livingston, J.A., and Falk, G. (2007) Community management of sex offenders with intellectual disability: Characteristics, services and outcome of a Statewide programme. *Intellectual and Developmental Disabilities, 45*, 391–8.

Marques, J.K. (1999). How to answer the question, 'Does sex offender treatment work?' *Journal of Interpersonal Violence, 14*, 437–451.

Marshall, W.L., Jones, R., Ward, T., Johnston, P. & Barbaree, H. (1991). Treatment outcome with sex offenders. *Clinical Psychology Review, 13*, 465–85.

Michie, A.M., Lindsay, W.R., Martin, V. & Grieve, A. (2006). A test of counterfeit deviance: A comparison of sexual knowledge in groups of sex offenders with intellectual disability and controls. *Sexual Abuse: A Journal of Research & Treatment, 18*, 271–9.

Murphy, G. & Sinclair, N. (2006). Group cognitive behaviour treatment for men with sexually abusive behaviour. Paper presented to 6th Seattle Club Conference on Research and People with Intellectual Disabilities.

O'Conner, W. (1996). A problem solving intervention for sex offenders with intellectual disability. *Journal of Intellectual & Developmental Disability, 21*, 219–35.

Palmer, E.J. (2003) *Offending behaviour, moral reasoning, criminal conduct and the rehabilitation of offenders*. Cullompton, Devon: Willan Publishing.

Patterson, G.R. (1986). Performance models for antisocial boys. *American Psychologist, 41*, 432–44.

Patterson, G.R., Reid, J.B. & Dishion, T.J. (1992). *A social interactional approach, vol 4: Antisocial boys*. Eugene, OR: Castalia.

Quinsey, V.L. (1998). Comments on Marshal's 'Monster, victim or everyman'. *Sexual Abuse: A Journal of Research & Treatment, 10*, 65–70.

Rice, M.E., Harris, G.T. & Quinsey, V.L. (2001). Research on the treatment of adult sex offenders. In J.B. Ashford, B.D. Sales & W.H. Reid (Eds), *Treating adults and juvenile offenders with special needs* (pp. 291–312). Washington, DC: American Psychological Association.

Romero, J.J. & Williams, L.M. (1983). Group psychotherapy and intensive probation supervision with sex offenders. *Federal Probation, 47*, 36–42.

Rose, J., Anderson, C., Hawkins, C. & Rose, D. (2007). A community based sex offender treatment group for adults with intellectual disabilities. Paper presented to the World Congress of Behavioural and Cognitive Psychotherapy, Barcelona.

Scott, M.B. & Lyman, S.N. (1968). Accounts. *American Sociological Review, 33*, 46–62.

Steptoe, L., Lindsay, W.R., Forrest, D. & Power, M. (2006). Quality of life and relationships in sex offenders with intellectual disability. *Journal of Intellectual & Developmental Disabilities, 31*, 13–19.

Sykes G.M. & Matza, D. (1957) Techniques of neutralisation: A theory of delinquency. *American Sociological Review, 22*, 67–9.

Taylor, J.L., Lindsay, W.R., Hogue, T.E., Mooney, P., Steptoe, L., Johnston, S. & O'Brien, G. (2008). Use of the HCR-20 in offenders with intellectual disability. Paper presented to the Annual Conference of the Forensic Division of the British Psychological Society, Edinburgh.

Taylor, J.L. & Novaco, R.W. (2005). *Anger treatment for people with developmental disabilities: A theory, evidence and manual based approach*. Chichester: Wiley & Son.

Ward, T. & Gannon, T.A. (2006). Rehabilitation, etiology and self-regulation: The comprehensive good lives model of treatment for sexual offenders. *Aggression & Violent Behaviour, 11*, 214–23.

Ward, T. & Hudson, S.M. (1998). A model of the relapse process in sexual offenders. *Journal of Interpersonal Violence, 13*, 700–25.

Ward, T., Hudson, S.M., Johnston, L. & Marshall, W.L. (1997). Cognitive distortions in sex offenders: An integrative review. *Clinical Psychology Review, 17*, 479–507.

Ward, T., Hudson, S.M. & Keenan, T. (1998). A self-regulation model of the sexual offence process. *Sexual Abuse: A Journal of Research & Treatment, 10*, 141–57.

Ward, T. & Marshall, W.L. (2004). Good lives, aetiology and the rehabilitation of sex offenders: A bridging theory. *Journal of Sexual Aggression, 10*, 153–69.

Ward, T. & Stewart, C.A. (2003). The treatment of sex offenders: Risk management and good lives. *Professional Psychology, Research & Practice, 34*, 353–60.

Webster, C.D., Eaves, D., Douglas, K.S. & Wintrup, A. (1995). *The HCR-20: The assessment of dangerousness and risk*. Vancouver, Canada: Simon Fraser University and British Colombia Forensic Psychiatric Services Commission.

16

The Treatment of Intellectually Disabled Sexual Offenders in the National Offender Management Service: The Adapted Sex Offender Treatment Programmes

FIONA WILLIAMS AND RUTH E. MANN

INTRODUCTION

Historically, initiatives to carry out offence-focussed work with sexual offenders have been developed separately in the prison and probation services. In 1991, HM Prison Service launched its national initiative to carry out offence-focussed work with sexual offenders during their imprisonment (Grubin & Thornton, 1994; Mann & Thornton, 1998; Thornton & Hogue, 1993). The Sex Offender Treatment Programme (SOTP) was designed in accordance with findings from research into effective programmes elsewhere in the world (Mann & Thornton, 1998, 2000). The central element of the SOTP is the Core Programme (for those who are of medium or high risk), which was first accredited by the Prison Service's independent accreditation panel in 1994 and has been re-accredited on several occasions as the programme has been refined. The Core Programme has been found to reduce sexual and violent reconviction rates significantly, especially for medium-risk sexual offenders (Friendship, Mann & Beech, 2003). However, it depends heavily on verbal and written skills, making participation more difficult for a lower ability offender.

Somewhat more recently, the English and Welsh Probation Service also began to offer accredited group work programmes for sex offenders. Three programmes were developed out of existing treatment provision between 1999 and 2001 and received accreditation from the reformed and renamed Correctional Services Accreditation Panel. The difference in the name and structure of the programmes reflects their original design in the West

Assessment and Treatment of Sexual Offenders with Intellectual Disabilities: A Handbook
Edited by Leam A. Craig, William R. Lindsay and Kevin D. Browne
© 2010 John Wiley & Sons, Ltd.

Midlands (C-SOGP), Thames Valley (TV-SOGP) and Northumbria (N-SOGP). Each has been designed to meet the needs of sex offenders living in the community who are subject to supervision either as a non-custodial sentence or on licence following release from a prison sentence.

Across the prison and probation services there is therefore a range of treatment options for sexual offenders. However, one of the limitations of all of the programmes is that they are only available to 'average ability offenders' (those with IQs above 80).

The need to provide specialised treatment to those with borderline intellectual disability (ID) has been highlighted elsewhere in the literature (Keeling, Rose & Beech, 2006; Lambrick, 2003). The Adapted Sex Offender Treatment Programme (ASOTP) was therefore developed in order to address the treatment needs of intellectually disabled sexual offenders. It was accredited for use in prisons in 1997 and has been running successfully across 13 Prison sites since this date (Williams, Wakeling and Webster, 2007). Following advice received from the Correctional Services Accreditation Panel in July 2006, the prison and probation services decided to jointly improve the treatment options for sex offenders with ID for both custodial and community settings. The proposed new ASOTPs provide a suite of four treatment programmes to target the needs of ID sex offenders. The four proposed programmes are summarised briefly as follows:

Becoming New Me (BNM). This is the main treatment programme targeted at criminogenic needs. It consists of 89 sessions divided into 12 blocks of treatment. Each session lasts between 2 and 2.5 hours, to be delivered at a minimum of 2 sessions per week. This programme is the equivalent of the ASOTP and the mainstream Core SOTP or Probation C-SOGP, TV-SOGP or N-SOGP. BNM is suitable for ID sex offenders assessed as medium, high or very high risk. In prison sites the BNM has been supplemented with a maintenance programme, based in part on Ward's Good Lives Model (GLM) of offender rehabilitation (Ward, Mann & Gannon, 2007): the Adapted Better Lives Booster programme (ABLB).

New Me Coping (NMC). The literature suggests that many areas of coping are likely to be more problematic for this client group than for mainstream sexual offenders. ID sexual offenders are likely to have problems with a range of socio-affective functioning areas, which may exacerbate their propensity to sexually offend. New Me Coping comprises a programme of modules that will include Communication Skills; Sex in Relationships; Managing my Relationships; Problem Solving; Managing my Feelings; Managing Anger; Drugs and Alcohol; and Feeling Better about Myself. This programme will be available for all risk groups (including the lower risk men). Relevant modules should be selected, according to identified need.

Healthy sex and relationships (HSR). In order to address the needs of high-risk men with a current sexual deviant interest, an individual treatment programme specifically targeting this issue is proposed.

Staying Strong Support group (SSS). The SSS group would be an ongoing rolling programme run once per week by a facilitator for maintenance and support of those who have completed other Adapted Programmes. The programme will offer opportunities to revisit the main learning points from BNM and also NMC and HSR according to need. A flexible treatment component which allows for individual needs will be incorporated.

As of 2010, the BNM is the only programme that has been written. The BNM is therefore, the focus of this chapter. The BNM was provisionally accredited by the Correctional Services Accreditation Panel in May 2009 and is now being rolled out across prison sites and probation areas. The BNM, like its forerunner, was designed to meet the needs of lower-ability sex offenders, defined as those who have an IQ of between 60 and 80. While this definition includes some individuals who would not technically be classed as learning disabled (LD), many of these individuals may not receive the level of support given to those with classified LD, although their needs may be just as significant.

DEVELOPING THE BECOMING NEW ME SEX OFFENDER TREATMENT PROGRAMME

Research suggests that for treatment of sexual offenders to be effective it must target the risk of the individual, the needs of the individual, and it must be delivered in a manner that is appropriate for the individual (Andrews & Bonta, 2003). The most effective treatment approach for non-ID sexual offenders, according to meta-analytic studies, is the cognitive-behavioural approach (Hall, 1995; Hanson *et al.*, 2002; Marshall, Anderson & Fernandez, 1999). Specialised programmes for ID offenders are comparatively rare and, in what is likely to be the continued absence of strongly designed evaluations of these programmes, Courtney, Rose and Mason (2006) proposed that 'similarities between these men and non disabled offenders give some validity to the use of programmes adapted from mainstream sex offender programmes' (p. 189). There is, at present, no randomised controlled trial based evidence to suggest the effectiveness of any intervention with ID sexual offenders (Ashman & Duggan, 2003). As Craig, Stringer and Moss (2006) suggested, 'until such time as randomized controlled trial evidence demonstrates the effectiveness of treatment interventions for sexual offenders with learning disabilities, clinicians will have to continue to base practice on clinical experience and evidence from non learning disabled populations' (p. 387).

Historically, it was considered that cognitive-behavioural techniques were inapplicable to those with cognitive and social deficits. However, more recently this view has changed (Kroese, Dagnan & Loumidis, 1997; Lambrick & Glaser, 2004). In recent years some studies have reported treatment success with ID sexual offenders (Charman & Clare, 1992; Lindsay, Neilson & Morrison, 1998; Lindsay, 2002; Lindsay & Smith, 1998; Murphy *et al.*, 2004). At the time of writing, group cognitive-behavioural treatment is generally recognized as the most effective treatment approach for ID offenders (Rose, Jenkins, O'Connor, Jones & Felce, 2002; Lambrick and Glaser, 2004).

Lambrick and Glaser (2004) suggested that the specific needs of the ID client group need to be taken into account when adapting mainstream treatment approaches. More specifically, they advocated the simplification of concepts; use of visual imagery; emphasis on the generalisation of skills from treatment into daily life; and the use of assessment and intervention methods historically used in the field of ID.

Our aim with the BNM was to combine the treatment targets and service delivery standards of the mainstream 'Core' SOTP with the treatment techniques and communication styles recommended in the ID literature. In particular, we aimed to create a programme that fully met the three essential principles of offender rehabilitation: risk, need and responsivity (Andrews &

Bonta, 2003). That is, we needed to ensure that treatment dosage took risk into account sufficiently; that treatment targets reflected known risk factors (or criminogenic needs) of ID sexual offenders; and that the delivery of treatment was fully tailored to the learning styles and potential of the ID population.

Risk Principle

An effective programme for sexual offenders should take account of the risk level of its clients, providing a greater dose of treatment to higher risk offenders. Little has been written about appropriate dose of treatment for sexual offenders. Beech, Beckett and Fisher (1999) found that low-risk sexual offenders seemed to benefit as much from a short, 80-hour, programme as from a longer, 180 hour, programme. However, Friendship, Mann and Beech (2003) found that 180 hours of treatment was insufficient for high-risk men and it is thought that a dose of about 300 hours may be necessary for the riskiest offenders (Mann & Fernandez, 2006). Lindsay (2002) commented that, while there was no empirical evidence as to the dose required for a reduction in reconvictions, it appeared that ID men generally needed longer in treatment to achieve treatment targets.

Added to this is the fact that most actuarial risk assessment tools have not been specifically validated on ID offenders. Relatively recent comprehensive research studies have identified the variables which are most important in the risk assessment of sexual offenders in general (Hanson & Bussière, 1998; Hanson & Harris, 2000; Hanson & Morton-Bourgon, 2004; Beech, Friendship, Erikson & Hanson, 2002; Mann, Hanson & Thornton, 2010). However, studies tend not to differentiate sexual offenders with ID from others within their sample (Lambrick, 2003). There is little empirical research on the relevance of established risk scales to ID sex offenders (Lindsay, 2002). Lambrick and Glaser (2004) reported that they were not aware of any established measures of risk that take into account specific issues relating to this population. Yet, as Lambrick and Glaser pointed out, ID is often included as a static risk factor in assessments (Boer, Hart, Kropp & Webster, 1997; Lambrick, 2003; Quinsey, Harris, Rice & Cormier, 1998). Craig and Hutchinson (2005) commented on the inapplicability of risk assessment scales to individuals with characteristics that differ from the original sample on which the research was based. Grubin and Wingate (1996) argued that empirical evidence from one population does not necessarily translate to another. However, Harris and Tough (2004) reported 'there is no scientific reason to believe that static and stable factors that reliably predict risk for a normal offender will not reliably predict risk for offenders from the intellectually disabled population. Indeed, what data exists ... suggests that these same factors predict quite well within the intellectually disabled population' (p. 237).

Given the lack of validation of static tools to date, the focus has instead tended to be on a clinical formulation approach, identifying known stable dynamic risk factors where possible. Boer (2003) suggested that individual risk assessments should be considered in terms of importance in relation to the particular characteristics of the client. Monahan et al. (2001) suggested that clinical judgement should be aided by empirical knowledge of the risk literature. Boer, Tough and Haaven (2004) outlined a risk assessment approach which uses the information provided by static actuarial instruments and relevant dynamic factors as an introduction to the formation of a risk management instrument for this client group. They suggested 30 items split into four categories relating to chronic and acute factors for staff, environment and the offender.

Some have proposed that, in comparing ID sexual offenders with non-ID sexual offenders, there are more similarities than differences (Coleman & Haaven, 1998). For this reason, it is often assumed that the risk factors pertaining to mainstream sexual offenders also apply to men with cognitive and social deficits. HM Prison and Probation Services use Risk Matrix 2000 (Thornton *et al.*, 2003) to describe the level of risk of sexual offending based on historical static factors. This tool is also used with the BNM group.

Our aim with the new proposed suite of treatment options for ID sex offenders is to provide different treatment options for individuals according to risk level, in accordance with the Risk Principle. Low-risk men will complete NMC only, and ideally this will be delivered one-to-one or in small groups separate from higher-risk men. This is to avoid contamination and the over-treatment of low-risk men (who, by definition, are statistically very unlikely to reconvict). Medium- and higher-risk men will firstly complete BNM. Additionally, depending on need, they may also complete NMC, HSR and SSS. Treatment dosage will therefore be significantly higher for those with the greatest risk and needs.

Need Principle

The Need Principle states that if an intervention is to reduce rates of sexual recidivism it must target factors that have been proven to raise recidivism likelihood, otherwise known as dynamic risk factors. Thanks to Hanson and Morton-Bourgon's (2004) large-scale meta-analysis of sexual offender recidivism, some of which has been updated in Mann, Hanson and Thornton (2010), sex offender treatment providers now have a sound base of knowledge about dynamic risk factors for sexual offending. However, once more there is no certainty about how closely this literature applies to ID offenders. Lindsay and Taylor (2005) suggest that similar variables to those found in relation to risk prediction with mainstream offenders are now being found with those with ID (Lindsay, Elliot & Astell, 2004). Craig, Stringer and Moss (2006), in a review of treatment provision for this group, noted that treatment components usually include 'challenging denial and restructuring cognitive distortions, enhancing victim empathy, social skills, offending awareness, sex education, relationship skills, law and offending behaviour, self-control and fostering self-reliance skills, appropriate arousal, insight into the effects on victims, self-control procedures and methods of avoiding risk situations, and treating sexual dysfunction using multimodal interventions' (p. 372). There is some overlap here with the criminogenic needs identified by Mann, Hanson and Thornton (2010), which are proposed to be the most appropriate targets for sex offender treatment. For instance, criminogenic needs identified by this study included offence-supportive attitudes, intimacy deficits, problems with sexual self-regulation, problems with general self-regulation and level of positive social influence. Hanson, Harris, Scott and Helmus (2007) investigated a large community sample using a specially designed dynamic risk assessment framework, the STABLE 2000. As part of their analyses, they were able to assess the incremental validity of STABLE 2000 over and above Static-99 for a subgroup which combined offenders with a diagnosis of developmental delay and offenders who had a history of psychiatric hospitalisation. Interestingly, they found that Static-99 was significantly related to all types of recidivism, but consideration of the stable dynamic variables did not improve upon this prediction for the developmentally delayed offenders.

This was in contrast to other groups of sexual offenders, in which assessment of stable factors did make a significant incremental contribution to recidivism prediction. Harris, Scott and Helmus concluded that these results should be replicated before any firm conclusions could be drawn. They speculated that either sexual offending was linked to different risk factors for this group or that the presentation of these offenders made it hard to determine which of their needs were criminogenic and which were not.

Although Harris, Scott and Helmus (2007) did not find that assessment of these variables added to recidivism prediction for developmentally delayed sex offenders, at present there is no other robust research from which to draw. Therefore, having reviewed published work into dynamic risk factors for both mainstream and ID sexual offenders, we selected the following targets for the BNM: to explore sexual interests, to modify offence-supportive attitudes, to improve skills relating to the management of relationships and to increase self-management skills.

HM Prison and Probation Services assess need using the Structured Assessment of Risk and Need (SARN), a close variant of Structured Risk Assessment (SRA) (Thornton, 2002), for both ID and non-ID sex offenders. The SARN framework organises psychological risk factors within four domains (sexual interests, pro-offending beliefs, socio-affective functioning and self-management). The framework was based on theoretical analysis, a review of the literature and preliminary studies that related psychological factors to having a history of repeated sexual offending (Thornton, 2002) The overall level of need is defined in terms of the number of domains in which the offender has major problems. The SRA/SARN framework has been shown to have predictive validity with offenders under community supervision (Craig, Thornton, Beech, & Browne, 2007), with prisoners participating in sexual offender treatment (Thornton, 2002) and with sexual offenders being assessed for an earlier generation of civil commitment programme (Knight & Thornton, 2007). As yet the applicability to sexual offenders with ID is assumed, not established; as such we use the framework with some caution.

Responsivity Principle

An effective treatment programme for offending behaviour ought to utilise treatment methods to which participants in the programme are responsive (Andrews & Bonta, 1998; Gendreau & Ross, 1980). Therefore the BNM was designed to appeal to the particular learning styles and needs of its participants. The first consideration is the willingness of the therapist to adapt their style to the ID offender's needs. Coleman and Haaven (2001) noted, 'an intellectually disabled person may be more hampered by the therapist's old fashioned and inept teaching methods than his own intellectual deficits' (p. 203). They observed that therapists tend to teach in the way they were taught, usually in large rooms with the teacher at some distance from the class using didactic methods and abstract formal lectures.

Secondly, ID sexual offenders, even more than mainstream offenders, need a lively and engaging experience in treatment. Haaven and Coleman (2000) noted that teaching ID sexual offenders requires more than just breaking skills down into small steps and rewards. Interventions with ID clients need to be multidimensional (Griffiths, Quinsey & Hinsburger, 1989). Courtney, Rose and Mason (2006) noted that successful interventions for people with ID are multimodal, involving a variety of components. Griffiths and colleagues observed that people learn more easily and effectively when emotion is linked with the learning process. Fun, dramatic and even bizarre techniques are recommended. Learning requires engagement (Ferguson & Haaven, 1990) and humour (Rieger, 2004). The BNM therefore adopted total communication strategies to enhance the effectiveness of learning (Ambalu, 1997). Multimodal communication strategies – for example, symbols, gestures, visual stimuli (pictures, drawings, photographs, videos) and the written word – are incorporated. The teaching style of the programme links emotion to the programme to emphasise the affective element of the learning process (Haaven, Little & Petre-Miller, 1990). To achieve this, BNM facilitators are encouraged to incorporate a range of interactive exercises into their therapeutic delivery: role plays, games, collage making and similar participatory devices.

PROGRAMME CONTENT AND STRUCTURE

The BNM's central framework is the Old Me/New Me model (Haaven, Little & Petre Miller, 1990). Using this framework, Old Me represents the thoughts, feelings and behaviours that are associated with offending behaviour. New Me is the non-offending self. Haaven and Schlank (2001) described how, by setting New Me goals, the individual is able to identify the person they want to become and the life they want to lead ('good life'). The good life represents various ways of living that provide life balance so that they are less likely to attempt to meet their needs in offending ways. In the BNM Programme we emphasise that Old Me and New Me coexist. In group, the concept of Old Me/New Me is likened to a tug of war that plays out in our heads. Old Me and New Me battle to direct the consequent behaviour. At the time of offending, Old Me was so strong that he overpowered New Me and a sexual offence took place. In treatment, offenders learn to identify Old Me and New Me thinking so that they are able to manage all aspects of Old Me and lead a more fulfilling and offence-free life. This model is similar to Ward's Good Lives Model (2002) because it is concerned with the enhancement of the offender's capabilities to improve their life. It is hypothesised that in so doing, the risk of the offender committing further crime is reduced.

The Old Me/New Me model has been widely used by clinicians with ID sexual offenders (as reported in Haaven, 2006aa). Indeed, following its success in the ASOTP, this model was integrated into HM Prison Service's treatment approach for mainstream sexual offenders. In an investigation of the approach with mainstream men, Mann, Webster and Schofield & Marshall (2004) found that the Old Me/New Me procedure, in comparison with more traditional relapse prevention techniques, led to equally clear knowledge of risk factors coupled with more engagement and participation in the process of change. Keeling, Rose and Beech (2006), in their review of the self-regulation model of the relapse process (Ward and Hudson, 2000), found that 'there is little to differentiate between mainstream sexual offenders and sexual offenders with special needs in terms of the relapse process' (p. 379).

The BNM Adapted programme is divided into 12 treatment blocks. Before starting treatment in many establishments, group members come together to complete group cohesion exercises. When BNM starts properly, therefore, the men are familiar and confident with each other.

Block 1: Getting Going

In Block 1 time is spent getting to know each other further, developing rapport with the facilitators and treatment manager and developing a set of group rules and expectations. The importance of group cohesion has been demonstrated by Beech and Fordham (1997). They found that successful sex offender groups (defined in terms of in-treatment change) were highly cohesive, well organised and well led. Group members were encouraged to be open in their expression of feelings. Treatment providers encouraged a sense of group responsibility and instilled a sense of hope in its members.

Block 2: New Me

In Block 2, group members present their life maps. They discuss their background and history, key life events, their families, interests and hobbies. Theories of sexual offending (e.g., Marshall & Barbaree, 1991) note that explanations for sexual offending usually begin during the offender's childhood. For instance, childhood experiences are thought to be related to the development of dysfunctional adult attachment styles (Ainsworth, Blehar, Waters & Walls, 1978; Bartholomew & Horowitz, 1991), which in turn may be part of the aetiology of sexual offending (Ward, Hudson, Marshall & Siegert, 1995). Ward and Hudson (2000) identified that some offender types (approach explicit offenders) may be influenced by their early developmental experiences that lead to maladaptive beliefs. The development of deviant sexuality probably follows from early pairing of deviant stimuli with sexual arousal (e.g., Laws & O'Donahue, 1998). It is thought that relating childhood experiences may assist group members and facilitators in understanding the aetiology of each individual's offending. In addition these disclosures of early life experiences may encourage the advancement of group cohesion as group members give each other support. Disclosure of childhood experiences tends to be accompanied by the expression of emotion, which was noted by Beech, Beckett & Fisher (1998) to be related to treatment success.

Through identifying their childhood experiences and problems, BNM participants are completing the groundwork for subsequent work on self-management and self-monitoring. Self-management is a difficult area for those with ID (Haaven, 2006aa). Numerous studies report that ID sexual offenders are characterised by poor coping skills and impulsivity (Glaser & Deane, 1999; Lane, 1991; Nezu, Nezu & Dudek, 1998). Coleman and Haaven (2001) and Haaven (2006b) suggested the importance of support systems to assist this client group in achieving an offence- free lifestyle in the community. On BNM, group members are encouraged to identify their personal supporters, often from family or friends. Sadly, however, in many cases group members are unable to obtain (appropriate) support so, in these circumstances, professionals are advocated (probation officers, religious leaders and so forth).

Men attending the programme in the community are supported by a complementary manualised intervention delivered by Offender Managers (case managers). The main aim of this work is to develop the group member's 'wrap-around support' network to enable him to manage changes in his life, support new me thinking and behaviour and provide motivation and encouragement to develop new skills. Dowden, Antonowiez and Andrews (2003) recognised that training significant others can help reduce recidivism.

In an attempt to develop and strengthen self-awareness/management skills, group members are also encouraged to self-monitor. Blasingame (2005) recognised the usefulness of self-monitoring in relation to the control of emotions. In the group, situations are enacted in role play and coping responses are discussed. Cortoni and Marshall (2001) suggest that sex offenders tend to use emotion-focussed coping and to over-use sex as a coping strategy for dealing with stress. Niedigh and Tomiko (1991) found that sex offenders made more use of self-denigration and avoidance techniques when dealing with stress in general and in dealing with urges to offend. Task-oriented (problem-focussed) coping is a more effective way of managing problems (Endler & Parker, 1990) than avoidance strategies or emotion-focussed strategies. It is also recognised that this client group tends to have particular problems with inhibition of impulses and the management of emotional states (Willner & Goodey, 2006). BNM group members are encouraged to adopt problem-focussed or 'OK' ways of coping. They work in the group to develop skills in this area. It is further recognised that this group tends to have difficulty generalising the skills learnt on treatment programmes to real-life situations (Griffiths, 2002). Throughout the programme, each participant completes a 'learning log'. This is, effectively, a diary, in which he is able to record his thoughts, feelings and behaviour in given situations. Group members are encouraged to record day-to-day problems/incidents and coping responses. In this, we are encouraging group members to think about their day-to-day behaviour and reaction to situations. We aim to highlight the importance of self-regulation, emotion regulation, self-control, appropriate coping and so forth. The learning logs provide a forum for discussing treatment aims within the day-to day-context.

Block 3: New Me and Sex

Coleman and Haaven (2001) report that clients generally have incorrect or inadequate knowledge of sexuality and hold rigid attitudes regarding gender roles. They suggest that the knowledge level resembles that held by children and adolescents. The aim of this block is to establish a common starting point and to give group members access to the same vocabulary and terminology for sexual terms and acts. Group members are taught to label body parts and functions. Crucially, they also learn to distinguish between 'ok' and 'not ok' sexual acts. To achieve this, the group discusses the meaning of consent and identify 'ok' and 'not ok' sexual encounters depending on the level of consent that was present. A set of specially developed pictures are used here to enable discussion. They also explore the topic of sexual fantasy and learn to differentiate between fantasy that is 'ok' and fantasy that is 'not ok'.

Block 4: My Feelings

Learning-disabled sexual offenders often have difficulties with emotional recognition and regulation (Haaven & Coleman, 2000). Problematic coping with emotions may impair an individual's ability to make healthy choices (Brown & Pond, 1999). For this reason there are two treatment blocks (Blocks 4 and 9) which aim to develop skills in this area.

Firstly, we aim to clarify the meanings of the words group members use to describe feelings. To increase their awareness of the physical states associated with feelings, and to become aware of the link between feelings, thoughts and behaviour. Blasingame (2005) notes the importance of this group being able to identify and express their emotions.

Block 5: Making it OK

In Block 5, group members are taught to understand the concept and purpose of excuses. Group members are encouraged to recognise the role excuses play in their lives and in their offending. With time, the emphasis played on this block of treatment has changed somewhat. When ASOTP first started, treatment practices were heavily influenced by the then prevailing belief that all sexual offenders' 'cognitive distortions' should be challenged (Salter, 1988). More recently, however, Maruna and Mann (2006) reviewed a large body of literature that indicates excuse-making is normal and probably healthy, and that behaviours frequently do have external causes. They suggested that just because many offenders seek to excuse their offending by appealing to external, unstable causes this does not justify the assumption that such a thinking style is automatically risky. They recommended that treatment providers should maintain more open, unbiased minds in regards to offender accounts and seek to avoid over-generalisation of labels such as 'cognitive distortion'. In treatment, it becomes important to identify which of the thoughts or explanations group members use are likely to increase their future risk and to differentiate these from post-offence justifications which may serve simply to protect someone's self-esteem.

Block 6: My Risky Things

Group members are introduced in block 6 to the risky areas that lead to offending. This is based on the SARN model of risk. Group members are taken through each area (domain). They work on creating symbols for each of the risk factors and are encouraged to sign up to the risky things that applied to their offending. This work is revisited throughout treatment.

Block 7: Old Me Versus New Me and Offending

At the start of this block, situations are examined in which Old Me was stronger than New Me and an offence took place. Group members disclose their offences to the group, identifying the decisions which Old Me made that led to their offending. New Me thinking that was not strong enough to prevent the offending is also explored. The aim is to obtain a relatively un-minimised account of events and behaviour from which criminogenic needs and risk factors can be identified in later sessions. Denial and minimisation are demonstrated by the majority of sexual offenders (Barbaree, 1991; Maletzky, 1991). However, they are not found to raise risk (Hanson & Bussière, 1998), and so are not viewed in our programme as a treatment target in themselves, rather as a stepping stone to the achievement of other targets. Times when New Me was strong enough to stop an offence happening are also described, so that the strengths of Old Me and New Me can be identified. Facilitators use specific role-play techniques to enable group members to give honest and accurate explanations of what happened. As group members often respond better to visual representation of material we developed the 'walk and talk' role-play method. An offender is encouraged 'to show' the group specific aspects of the lead-up to offending. The direction of the role play enables the offender to track his thoughts and feelings. (It should be noted that offenders never role play the offending behaviour itself.) New Me strengths (protective factors) are also identified for each group member. These factors have been described by Mann, Hanson and Thornton (2010) as the factors which 'protect' an offender from risk and enable a satisfying life without offending. The notion of protective factors is consistent with Haaven's description of the New Life and Ward's Good Lives Model (GLM) of offender rehabilitation, where needs are seen as obstacles that prevent someone from living a fulfilled life. On BNM group members develop New Me strengths posters, demonstrating currently possessed New Me strengths and those which they need to develop further.

Block 8: Mid-treatment Individual Interview

An individual session is provided in mid-treatment to further strengthen motivation and commitment to change. Each group member is encouraged to talk about their achievement in treatment to date. Their progress in relation to the risky things identified and any outstanding areas for development are discussed. Where possible, members from the group members' support networks are encouraged to attend this session.

Block 9: Other People's Feelings

This is the second of the blocks on emotion recognition and paves the way for the victim work.

Block 10: What My Offending Does To Victims

The enhancement of victim empathy is a treatment goal in the vast majority of programmes for sexual offenders (Knopp, Freeman-Longo & Stevenson, 1992; Marshall, Anderson & Fernandez, 1999). Haaven and Schlank (2001) report that ID sexual offenders have little capacity for empathy. They suggest that this group's ability to sense what others feel is compromised. For this reason, the BNM does not aim for group members to develop empathy with their victim, rather the aim is for group members to understand the harm that they are likely to have caused their victim. Facilitators make use of role play and game playing to achieve the aims of this block. Facilitators use specially created pictures depicting offending behaviour to stimulate discussion. Facilitators set up a role-play to depict the scene at various stages in relation to the offending, prior to and after the offence. The offending behaviour itself is not role played. Role-play directors enable discussion that focusses on the possible consequences in the short and longer term for the victim. These are presented as posters. Group members develop a personal poster relating to the possible consequences for their victim/s. The concept of thinking about other people's feelings is introduced within a concept of 'caring for others'.

Block 11: New Me Coping

Group members identify New Me tactics (problem-solving techniques) which will help them to control Old Me. Group members are introduced to a number of tactics that they can draw on to help them deal with risk. These include Stop and Think; What Happens to Me; Sticking at It; Better Life; Their Shoes; and Praise and Reward. In order to develop new behavioural skills, Craig, Stringer and Moss (2006) emphasised the need for new learning to be practice-based rather than theory-based. Research has indicated that skills training interventions have better proof to support them than traditional relapse prevention models. Marques, Nelson, Alarcon and Day (1999), in their reflections on the success of the Sex Offender Treatment and Evaluation Programme, note the importance of developing adequate coping skills for high-risk elements in the offending. They suggested that Relapse Prevention programmes should spend more time and energy practicing coping responses rather than simply identifying high-risk factors. They concluded that group members must be able to behave differently, not just grasp intellectually how they can behave differently. They recognised the importance of undertaking this work in institutions prior to release. Accordingly, in this treatment block group members are given the opportunity to practice New Me skills and coping. A role-play technique has been specifically developed for use in this stage of the programme to help identify the self-talk that takes place between Old Me and New Me. Using this methodology, New Me is firstly required to 'spot the risky thing'. He is asked to describe the risk and remember that he is required to 'stop and think'. The role-play director then encourages the offender as New Me to challenge his Old Me. New Me thinking, and ultimately New Me behaviour, is developed and reinforced. The chosen New Me behaviours are designed both to ensure offending is avoided and at the same time to lead to a 'good life' – that is, an offence-free, fulfilling life (Haaven & Coleman, 2000; Haaven & Schlank, 2001). Various role-play techniques to strengthen New Me have been developed to enhance this role-play process. It is important that role-play sessions conclude with New Me stronger than Old Me. Group members are encouraged to view their progress towards New Me as ongoing. In undertaking this work, Haaven (2006b) suggested that goals need to be realistic, broken down into small steps toward achievement, and that a learning orientation should be encouraged as opposed to an achievement orientation (Mann, 2000). That is, group members are encouraged to celebrate the achievement of each small sub-goal, rather than being instructed to focus only on achievement of long-term goals. Group members are encouraged to update their New Me strengths posters and take part in an exercise where they plan to receive a New Me letter from themselves in six-months' time.

Block 12: New Me Planning for the Future

To emphasise the need for striving towards New Me to be a continual process, group members in block 12 are encouraged to plan a New Me life line. This is what they hope that their future life will include. The final block of treatment ensures a healthy ending. The state of mind in which a sexual offender leaves treatment can be crucial in determining the quality of his self-management. It has even been suggested that very elaborate programmes, with extensive aftercare, can inadvertently 'convey the message to the participants that they are incapable of managing without a therapist or supervisor watching over them' (Eccles & Marshall, 1999). The intention of BNM, therefore, is to leave group members with a sense of optimism about the future (Beech & Fordham, 1997), with a commitment to keep working towards change and with a positive attitude towards support and group work, but not with a dependency on others.

THE BECOMING NEW ME ADAPTED SEX OFFENDER TREATMENT PROGRAMME FACILITATORS

The prison service SOTP was, from the beginning, designed to be delivered by lay therapists or 'para professionals' (Grubin & Thornton, 1994, Mann & Thornton, 1998). The personal qualities of the facilitators, rather than their professional qualifications, are the important factors in the delivery of treatment to sexual offenders (Mann & Thornton, 1998). Coleman and Haaven (1998) also suggested that clinicians should look for 'someone with the appropriate attitude and aptitude rather than a particular degree' when seeking therapists to work with this client group. They continue, 'working effectively with this intellectually disabled person requires someone who does not feel sorry for their client, but feels respect, is aware of limitations and is able to follow through on consequences' (p. 279). BNM facilitators are specifically selected from experienced SOTP facilitators who have expressed an interest in working in this area. They have passed a specialised selection process and successfully completed further training. Following a series of recent studies into effective therapeutic process with sexual offenders, BNM facilitators are taught during their training to adopt a Socratic non-confrontational style and to question offenders in a spirit of genuine inquiry. Our approach has carefully adhered to recommendations from research. For example, Beech and Fordham (1997) reported that therapists who adopt a non-confrontational but nevertheless challenging style produce greater benefit in their sexual offender clients than those who are aggressive and confrontational. Marshall *et al.* (2002) suggested that the therapist features that clearly facilitated change were displays of empathy and warmth by the therapist, encouragement and rewards for progress and some degree of directiveness. Frost (2004) noted the importance of creating a climate in which clients feel safe to disclose and work through issues. Blasingame (2005) suggested that therapists working with this client group need to have a good sense of humour. Stachen and Shevich (1999) noted the importance of being respectful and empathic with this group.

AUDITING TREATMENT DELIVERY

The Prison and Probation Service Sex Offender Treatment Programmes form a wide-scale treatment initiative, offering in excess of 2,000 treatment places per year. As such, to ensure consistency in treatment approach and delivery, all prison establishments running sex offender treatment have been audited annually. The auditing process measures the quality of delivery of programmes against a series of implementation quality criteria. These criteria relate to all aspects of treatment planning, delivery and continuity. Examples of criteria include institutional support (facilities, staff attitudes, environment); management of the treatment (supervision, training, assessment); continuity and resettlement factors (ensuring progress made in treatment is reinforced and taken forward during the remainder of the sentence and on release); and quality of treatment delivery (assessments of therapist skill via video monitoring, assessment of work produced by group members). This auditing process will be extended into the community during 2010 to ensure consistency of approach and delivery across all treatment sites. Adhering to these standards raises the likelihood that treatment will be effective.

ASSESSMENT OF TREATMENT NEED AND TREATMENT CHANGE

A number of authors have suggested areas that are relevant when assessing the dynamic risk factors of ID sex offenders (Caparulo, 1991; Clare, 1993; Seghorn & Ball, 2000). Lindsay (2002) discussed the paucity of available psychometric tools specifically designed for use with this client group. He noted that, 'it has to be recognized that there are few assessments which have been developed to be appropriate for individuals with intellectual disabilities'. We have therefore adapted and designed our own assessment tools to measure psychological factors or dynamic risk factors associated with sexual offending. These assessments are analysed to determine which are present in each individual case, and therefore which areas should be the focus of treatment. As noted above, the need assessment framework for non-disabled sexual offenders, the SARN (Thornton, 2002), divides risk factors into four domains: Inappropriate Sexual Interests, Offence-Supportive Attitudes, Relationships and Self-Management. It is obviously necessary first, however, to carry out a comprehensive assessment of intellectual and adaptive deficits in order to understand each individual's potential for learning.

Psychometric Assessment

The Weschler Abbreviated Intelligence Scales (WAIS III) (Weschler, 1997) are used to identify group members for BNM. A tailored, in-house procedure, The Adaptive Functioning Checklist (AFC, unpublished), is used to determine adaptive functioning skills. The AFC is a behaviour-monitoring tool designed to pick up on deficits in adaptive skills. Group members assessed from these tools as suitable for the adapted programmes then complete the BNM assessment battery. The following psychometric measures are administered, designed to represent dynamic risk areas which should improve through treatment.

Adapted Impulsivity Scale

This is a 13-item scale used to measure levels of impulsiveness. The scale reflects a tendency to act without thinking about long-term consequences. This scale is an adapted version of Eysenck & Eysenck's (1978) Impulsivity Scale.

Adapted Ruminations Scale

This is a 15-item scale used to measure a tendency to ruminate angrily and bear grudges. High scores reflect greater rumination. This questionnaire is an adapted version of Capara's (1986)

Dissipation–Rumination Scale. To create the Adapted Ruminations Scale the items were reworded using simpler phrasing. Following an in-house research study examining the psychometric properties of the adapted programmes assessment with the adapted prison population, the removal of a further four items improved the construct validity and internal consistency of the Adapted Ruminations Scale.

Adapted Relationships Style Questionnaire

The original RSQ is a 30-item questionnaire measuring four attachment patterns: Secure, Fearful, Pre-occupied and Dismissing. The RSQ was altered for the adapted client group by rewording the items using simpler phrasing, and changing the response format from a Likert scale to a dichotomous yes/no response format. Following an in-house research study examining the psychometric properties of the adapted programmes assessment with the adapted prison population, it was observed that the internal consistency of the original four subscales was poor, and furthermore a principal components analysis found a two-factor model to have better face validity with this population. Therefore a two-factor model is used to score the Adapted RSQ (ARSQ): Pre-occupied/Fearful and Dismissing. This questionnaire is an adapted version of Dutton, Saunders, Starzomski and Bartholomew's (1994) Relationship Style Questionnaire.

Adapted Openness to Women Scale

This is a nine-item scale used to measure openness or emotional congruence with women. High scores indicate that the respondent believes he is able to have and enjoys emotionally intimate relationships with women. This questionnaire is an adapted version of Underhill, Wakeling, Mann and Webster's (2008) Openness to Women scale. The items have been reworded slightly using simpler phrasing.

Adapted Openness to Men Scale

This is a nine-item scale used to measure openness or emotional congruence with men. Higher scores indicate that the respondent believes he is able to have and enjoys emotionally intimate relationships with men. This questionnaire is an adapted version of Underhill, Wakeling, Mann and Webster's (2008) Openness to Men scale. The items have been reworded slightly using simpler phrasing.

Sex Offenders' Opinion Test (SOOT)

The Sex Offenders Opinion Test (SOOT) is a 20-item instrument, which measures attitudes about victims of sexual offences. Items are summed to produce a total scale score, higher scores relating to higher distortions about victims of sexual offences. The SOOT comprises two sub-scales, 'Deceitful Women and Children' and 'Children, Sex and the Law'. This questionnaire originated from Bray (1996). This questionnaire has been slightly adapted from the original version, by omitting eight of the items and slightly rewording a couple of 'ambiguous' or 'complex' items.

My Private Interests Measure

This is a 54-item scale measuring sexual interests. The scale covers a variety of different areas of 'interests' and intends to provide an overall picture of participants' sexual interests. The scale has four subscales: Sexual preference for children, obsessed with sex, preferring sex to include violence or humiliation and other offence-related sexual interests. This scale was developed to use as part of the adapted assessment battery (Williams, 2005).

ENSURING PSYCHOMETRIC RESPONSIVITY

Clare (1993) discussed the difficulty that ID offenders have with complex language and concepts which are commonly inherent in sex offender assessments. She suggested that the discriminations involved in self-report questionnaires (such as those which use Likert scales) may prove problematic for ID clients to complete. Lindsay (2002) reported that many of the existing assessments for sex offenders are too linguistically complicated and so there is little likelihood that sex offenders with ID will have understood the requirements of the test and the items presented. He suggested that assessments need to be adapted to meet the needs of the ID group, but warned that in doing so the psychometric properties of the test will have to be re-established.

In designing the BNM assessment measures the limitations of the target population have been taken into consideration. All assessments are administered one-to-one with the client. The language used is as familiar as possible and has been simplified. Information is presented in 'easily digested chunks' (Hickey & Jones, 1996) in order to reduce the auditory memory load. We use concrete rather than abstract concepts and participative rather than didactic methodology. That is, the use of interviews and interactive response methods are preferred over paper and pencil tests. We also incorporate reliability checks to make sure that the offender understands what is required. Furthermore, where possible, information obtained from the offender is cross-referenced with file information. All the assessments include the repetition of instructions and the use of prompts to reword the instructions. The response scales use the minimum number of words possible. The use of symbols/gestures has also been incorporated where possible.

Validating the Psychometric Measures

Researchers stress the need to determine the psychometric properties of assessments that have been adapted for use with this group (Lindsay 2002). By adapting assessments, or creating new assessments, specifically to meet the needs of this client group, we are also changing the properties of the assessments. In order to ensure the new or adapted measures continue to be valid, the psychometric properties of some of the assessment battery have been examined (see Williams, Wakeling & Webster, 2007).

Measuring Change

It is important that treatment providers measure treatment effectiveness to evaluate the impact of treatment. Several good-quality studies of treatment efficacy among mainstream sexual offenders have been undertaken (Hanson, 1997). As noted earlier, there have been no such studies with ID offenders. Unfortunately, reconviction studies of prison-based programmes can take many years to complete because sentence lengths are such that programme completers are only slowly released back into the community. Therefore, it can take many years to achieve the sample size necessary for a decent outcome study. It is even more problematic to obtain a comparison or control group given that (in England and Wales, at least) there is no routine IQ testing or even screening of prison and probation offenders. In circumstances such as these, Hanson (1998) recommended measuring treatment change in relation to dynamic risk factors. We therefore undertook a clinical evaluation of treatment effect based on a sample of 211 ASOTP men by examining the pre- and post- treatment assessment measures. We found evidence of clinical change on all assessment measures (Williams, Wakeling & Webster, 2007). This was consistent for all risk categories and all offence types.

CONCLUSIONS

This chapter has described the development and refinement of a comprehensive programme for ID sexual offenders. Given the lack of robust, large-scale research into the criminogenic needs and treatment responsivity of this client group the programme was initially based on examples of practice found elsewhere. Over time, we have developed our own expertise in dealing with this client group, and the number of men who have completed treatment has reached a sufficient number for assessments to be validated. We are now exploring potential options for evaluating the impact of the programme on recidivism, bearing in mind the many obstacles to such research in forensic settings, and, particularly, the difficulties in defining an appropriate comparison group. Over the years, we have recognised the many rewards of working with this client group, which has resulted in a very stable and committed workforce in comparison with other areas of forensic work. We have also observed the many prejudices that learning disabled offenders face as they try to survive within a system that rarely understands, or even identifies, their particular needs (as is outlined in Talbot, 2007). The BNM-ASOTP is our attempt to target treatment in a responsive way to meet the needs of this client group.

REFERENCES

Ainsworth, M.S., Blehar, M.C., Waters, E. & Walls, S. (1978). *Patterns of attachment: A psychological study of the strange situation* (pp. xviii, p. 391). Lawrence Erlbaum, Oxford.

Ambalu, S. (1997). Communication. In J. O'Hara and A. Sperlinger (Eds), *Adults with learning disabilities: A practical approach for health professionals*. Chichester: John Wiley & Sons.

Andrews, D.A. & Bonta, J. (1998). *The psychology of criminal conduct*. Cincinnati, OH: Anderson Publishing Co.

Andrews, D.A. & Bonta, J. (2003). *The psychology of criminal conduct*, 3rd edn. Cincinnati, OH: Anderson Publishing Co.

Ashman, L. & Duggan, L. (2003). Interventions for learning disabled sex offenders. (Cochrane Review). In *The Cochrane Library*, Issue 1. Oxford. Update software.

Barbaree, A.G. (1991). Denial and minimisation among sex offenders: Assessment and treatment outcomes. *Forum on Corrections Research, 3*, 30–3.

Bartholomew, K., Horowitz, L.M. (1991). Attachment styles among young adults: A test of a four category model. *Journal of Personality and Social Psychology, 61*, 226–44.

Beech, A.R., Fisher, D. & Beckett, R.C. (1999). *An evaluation of the prison sex offender treatment programme*. UK Home Office Occasional Report. Available from Home Office Publications Unit, 50, Queen Anne's Gate, London, SW1 9AT, England. Available electronically from www.homeoffice.gov.uk/rds/pdfs/occ-step3.pdf.

Beech, A. & Fordham, A.S. (1997). Therapeutic climate of sexual offender treatment programs. *Sexual Abuse: A Journal of Research and Treatment, 9*, 219–37.

Beech, A., Friendship, C., Erikson, M. & Hanson, R.K. (2002). The relationship between static and dynamic risk factors and reconviction in a sample of UK child abusers. *Sexual Abuse: A Journal of Research and Treatment, 14*, 155–67.

Blasingame, G. (2005). *Developmentally disabled persons with sexual behaviour problems: treatment, management and supervision*, 2nd edn. Woods and Barnes Publishing, Oklahoma City.

Boer, D.P., Hart, S.J., Kropp, P.R. & Webster, C.D. (1997). *Manual for the sexual violence risk-20: Professional guidelines for assessing risk of sexual violence*. Vancouver BC: The Institute Against Family Violence.

Boer, D.P., Tough, S. & Haaven, J. (2004). Assessment of risk manageability of intellectually disabled sex offenders. *Journal of Applied Research in intellectual disabilities, 17*, 275–84.

Bray, D. (1996). The sex offender opinion test (SOOT). North Warwickshire NHS Trust. Unpublished.

Brown, J. & Pond, A. (1999). 'They just don't get it': Essentials of cognitive behavioural treatment for intellectually disabled sex offenders. *Journal of Applied Research in Intellectual disabilities, 17* (4), 1–9.

Capara, G.V. (1986). Indications of aggression: The Dissipation-Rumination Scale. *Personality and Individual Differences, 7*, 763–769.

Caparulo, F. (1991). Identifying the developmentally disabled sex offenders. *Sexuality and Disability, 9*, 311–22.

Charman, T. & Clare, I. (1992). Education about the laws and social rules relating to sexual behaviour. *Mental Handicap, 20*, 74–80.

Clare, I. C. H. (1993). Issues in the assessment and treatment of male sex offenders with mild learning difficulties. *Sexual and Marital Therapy, 8*, 167–79.

Coleman, E. & Haaven, J. (1998). Adult intellectually disabled sex offenders: Program considerations. In W.L. Marshall, Y.M. Fernandez, S.M. Hudson & T. Ward (Eds), *Sourcebook of treatment programs for sexual offenders*. New York: Plenum Press.

Coleman, E. & Haaven, J. (2001). Treatment of the intellectually disabled sex offender. In D.R. Laws, S. M. Hudson & T. Ward (Eds), *Remaking relapse prevention with sex offenders: A sourcebook*. Newbury Park, CA: Sage Publications.

Cortoni, F. & Marshall, W.L. (2001). Sex as a coping strategy and its relationship to juvenile sexual history and intimacy in sexual offenders. *Sexual Abuse: A Journal of Research and Treatment, 13* (1), 27–43.

Courtney, J., Rose, J. & Mason, O. (2006). The offence process of sex offenders with intellectual disabilities: A qualitative study. *Sexual Abuse: A Journal of Research and Treatment, 18,* 169–91.

Craig, L.A. & Hutchinson, R.B. (2005). Sexual offenders with learning disabilities: Risk, recidivism and treatment. *Journal of Sexual Aggression, 11,* 289–304.

Craig, L.A., Stringer, I. & Moss, T. (2006). Treating sexual offenders with learning disabilities in the community: A critical review. *International Journal of Offender Therapy and Comparative Criminology, 50,* 369–90.

Craig, L.A., Thornton, D., Beech, A. & Browne, K. (2007). The relationship of statistical and psychological risk markers to sexual reconviction in child molesters. *Criminal Justice and Behavior, 34* (3), 314–29.

Dowden, C., Antonowiez, D. & Andrews, D. (2003). The effectiveness of relapse prevention with offenders: A meta analysis. *International Journal of Offender Therapy and Comparative Criminology, 47,* 516–28.

Dutton, D.G., Saunders, K., Starzomski, A. & Bartholomew, K. (1994). Intimacy-anger and insecure attachment as precursors of abuse in intimate relationships. *Journal of Applied Social Psychology, 24,* 1367–87.

Eccles, A. & Marshall, W.L. (1999). Cognitive Behavioural treatment of sex offenders In V.B. Van Hasselt & M. Hersen (Eds), *Sourcebook of psychological treatment manuals for adult disorders.* New York: Plenum Press. pp. xii, 720.

Endler, N.S. & Parker, J.D. (1990). State and trait anxiety, depression and coping styles. *Australian Journal of Psychology, 42,* 207–20.

Eysenck, S. B. G. & Eysenck, H.J. (1978). Impulsivity and venturesomeness: Their place in a dimensional system of personality description. *Psychological Reports, 43,* 1247–55.

Ferguson, E.W. & Haaven, J. (1990). On the design of motivating learning environments for intellectually disabled offenders. *Journal of Correctional education, 41,* 32–4.

Friendship, C., Mann, R.E. & Beech, A.R. (2003). Evaluation of a national prison-based treatment program for sexual offenders in England and Wales. *Journal of Interpersonal Violence, 18,* 744–59.

Frost, A. (2004). Therapeutic engagement styles of child sexual offenders in a group treatment programme: A grounded theory study. *Sexual Abuse: A Journal of Research and Treatment, 16* (3), 191–208.

Gendreau, P. & Ross, R.R. (1980). Effective correctional treatment: Bibliotherapy for cynics. In Ross R.R. & Gendreau P. (Eds), *Effective correctional treatment.* Toronto: Butterworth and Co.

Glaser, W. & Deane, K. (1999). Normalisation in an abnormal world: A study of prisoners with intellectual disability. *Journal of Offender Therapy and Comparative Criminology, 43,* 338–50.

Green, G., Gray, N.S. & Willner, P. (2002). Factors associated with criminal convictions for sexually inappropriate behaviour in men with learning disabilities. *The Journal of Forensic Psychiatry, 13,* 578–607.

Griffiths, D. (2002). Sexual aggression. In W. Gardner (Ed.), *Aggression and other disruptive behavioural challenges.* Kingston, NY NADD. Available from www.thenadd.org

Griffiths, D.M., Quinsey, V.L. & Hingsburger, D. (1989). *Changing inappropriate sexual behaviour. A community based approach for persons with learning disabilities.* Baltimore, MD: Paul Brookes.

Grubin, D. & Thornton, D. (1994). A national programme for the assessment and treatment of sex offenders in the English prison system. *Criminal Justice and Behaviour, 21,* 55–71.

Grubin, D. & Wingate, S. (1996). Sexual offence recidivism: prediction versus understanding. *Criminal Behaviour and Mental Health, 6,* 349–59.

Haaven, J. (2006a). The evolution of the old me/new me model. In G. Blasingame (Ed.). *Practical treatment strategies for persons with intellectual disabilities*. Oklahoma city, Oklahoma. Wood 'n' Barnes.

Haaven, J. (2006). Suggested treatment outline using the old me/new me model. In G. Blasingame (Ed.), *Practical treatment strategies for persons with intellectual disabilities*. Oklahoma city, Oklahoma. Wood 'n' Barnes.

Haaven, J. & Coleman, E.M. (2000). Treatment of the developmentally disabled sex offender. In D.R. Laws, S.M. Hudson and T. Ward (Eds), *Remaking relapse prevention with sex offenders: A sourcebook*. London: Sage Publications.

Haaven, J., Little, R. & Petre-Miller, D. (1990). *Treating intellectually disabled sex offenders*. Orwell VT: Safer Society Press.

Haaven, J. & Schlank, A. (2001). The challenge of treating the sex offender with developmental disabilities. In A. Schlank (Ed.), *The sexual predator: Legal issues, clinical issues, special populations*, Vol 2. New York: Civic Research Institute.

Hall, G. C. N. (1995). Sexual offenders recidivism revisited: A meta-analysis of recent treatment studies. *Journal of Consulting and Clinical Psychology, 63*, 802–9.

Hanson, R.K. (1997). *The development of a brief actuarial risk scale for sexual offence recidivism* Department of the Solicitor General of Canada.

Hanson, R.K. (1998). What do we know about sex offender risk assessment? *Psychology, Public Policy and Law, 4*, 50–72.

Hanson, R.K. & Bussière, M.T. (1998). Predicting relapse: A meta-analysis of sexual offender recidivism studies. *Journal of Consulting and Clinical Psychology, 66*, 348–62.

Hanson, R.K., Gordon, A., Harris, A. J. R., Marques, J.K., Murphy, W., Quinsey, V.L. & Seto, M.C. (2002). First report of the collaborative data outcome project on the effectiveness of psychological treatment for sexual offenders. *Sexual Abuse: A Journal of Research and Treatment, 14*, 169–94.

Hanson, R.K. & Harris, A. J. R. (2000). *The sex offender need assessment rating (SONAR): A method for measuring change in risk levels*. (User Report). Ottawa: Department of the Solicitor General of Canada.

Hanson, R.K., Harris, A. J. R., Scott, T.L. & Helmus, L. (2007). *Assessing the risk of sexual offenders on community supervision: The dynamic supervision project*. Department of the Solicitor General of Canada.

Hanson, R.K. & Morton-Bourgon, K. (2004). *Predictors of sexual recidivism: An updated meta-analysis* (User Report 2004-02). Ottawa: Public Safety and Emergency Preparedness Canada.

Harris, A. & Tough, S. (2004). Should actuarial risk assessments be used with sex offenders who are intellectually disabled? *Journal of Applied Research in Intellectual Disabilities, 17*, 235–41.

Hickey, N. & Jones, J. (1996). The challenge of learning disabled sex offenders. Paper presented at the Division of Legal and Criminological Psychology Conference.

Keeling, J.A., Rose, J.L. & Beech, A.R. (2006). A comparison of the application of the Self Regulation Model of the Relapse Process for Mainstream and Special Needs Sexual Offenders. *Sexual Abuse: A Journal of Research and Treatment, 18* (4), 373–82.

Knight, R.A. & Thornton, D. (2007). *Evaluating and improving risk assessment schemes for sexual recidivism: A long-term follow-up of convicted sexual offenders*. US Dept of Justice National Institute of Justice United States Box 6000 Rockville, MD 20849 United States.

Kroese, B.S., Dagnan, D. & Loumidis, K. (1997). *Cognitive behaviour therapy for people with learning disabilities*. London: Routledge.

Lambrick, F. (2003). Issues surrounding the risk assessment of sexual offenders with an intellectual disability. *Psychiatry, Psychology and Law, 10*, 353–8.

Lambrick, F. & Glaser, W. (2004). Sex offenders with an intellectual disability. *Sexual Abuse: A Journal of Research and Treatment*, *16*, 381–92.

Lane, S.L. (1991). Special offender populations. In G.D. Ryan & S.L. Lane (Eds), *Juvenile sexual offending: Causes and consequences*. Lexington: Lexington Press.

Laws, D.R. & O'Donahue, W. (1998). *Sexual deviance: Theory, assessment and treatment*. New York: Guildford Press.

Lindsay, W.R. (2002). Research and literature on sex offenders with intellectual disabilities. *Journal of Intellectual Disability Research*, *46*, 74–85.

Lindsay, W.R., Elliot, S.F. & Astell, A. (2004). Predictors of sexual offence recidivism in offenders with intellectual disabilities. *Journal of Applied Research in Intellectual Disabilities*, *17*, 299–305.

Lindsay, W.R., Neilson, C.Q. & Morrison, F. (1998). The treatment of six men with a learning disability convicted of sex offences with children. *British Journal of Clinical Psychology*, *37*, 83–98.

Lindsay, W.R. & Smith, A. H. W. (1998). Response to treatment for sex offenders with intellectual disability: A comparison of men with 1- and 2- year probation sentences. *Journal of Intellectual Disabilities Research*, *42*, 346–53.

Lindsay, W.R., Taylor, H.L. & Sturmey, P. (2004). *Offenders with developmental disabilities*. Chichester: John Wiley & Sons Ltd.

Lindsay, W.R. & Taylor, J.L. (2005). A selective review of the research on offenders with developmental disabilities: Assessment and treatment. *Clinical Psychology and Psychotherapy*, *12*, 201–14.

Maletzky, B. (1991). *Treating the sexual offender*. Newbury Park, CA: Sage Publications.

Mann, R. (2000). Managing resistance and rebellion in relapse prevention. In D.R. Laws, S. Hudson and T. Ward (Eds), *Remaking relapse prevention with sex offenders*. Ventura, CA, Sage Press.

Mann, R.E. & Fernandez, Y. (2006). Sex offender programmes: Concept, theory and practice. In C.R. Hollin & E. Palmer (Eds), *Offending behaviour programmes: Development, application and controversies*. Chichester: John Wiley & Sons.

Mann, R.E., Hanson, R.K. & Thornton, D. (2010) Assessing risk for sexual recidivism: Some proposals on the nature of psychologically meaningful risk factors. Submitted for publication.

Mann, R.E. & Thornton, D. (1998). The evolution of a multi-site sex offender treatment programme. In W. L. Marshall, Y.M. Fernandez, S.H. Hudson & T. Ward (Eds), *Sourcebook of treatment programs for sexual offenders*. New York: Plenum Press.

Mann, R.E. & Thornton, D. (2000). An evidence-based relapse prevention programme. In D.R. Laws, S.M. Hudson & T. Ward (Eds), *Remaking relapse prevention with sex offenders*. Thousand Oaks, CA: Sage.

Mann, R.E., Webster, S.D., Schofield, C. & Marshall, W.L. (2004). Approach vs avoidance goals in relapse prevention with sexual offenders. *Sexual Abuse: A Journal of Research and Treatment*, *16*, 65–75.

Marques, J.K., Nelson, C., Alarcon, J. & Day, D. (1999). Preventing relapse in sex offenders: What we learned from the SOTEP's experimental treatment programme. In R. Laws, S. Hudson & T. Ward (Eds), *Remaking relapse prevention with sex offenders: A sourcebook*. Thousand Oaks, CA: Sage.

Marshall, W.L., Anderson, D. & Fernandez, Y. (1999). *Cognitive behavioural treatment of sexual offenders*. New York: John Wiley and Sons.

Marshall, W.L., Jones, R., Ward, T., Johnston, P. & Barbaree, H.E. (1991). Treatment outcome with sex offenders. *Clinical Psychology Review*, *11*, 465–85.

Marshall, W.L., Serran, G., Moulden, H., Mulloy, R., Fernandez, Y.M., Mann, R.E. & Thornton, D. (2002). Therapist features in sexual offender treatment: Their reliable identification and influence on behaviour change. *Clinical Psychology and Psychotherapy*, *9*, 395–405.

Maruna, S. & Mann, R.E. (2006). A fundamental attribution error? Rethinking cognitive distortions. *Legal and Criminological Psychology*, *11* (2), 155–77.

Monahan, J., Steadman, H.J., Silver, E., Appelbaum, P.S., Robbins, P.C., Mulvey, E.P., Roth, L.H., Grisso, T. & Banks, S. (2001). *Rethinking risk assessment: The McArthur study of mental disorder and violence*. Oxford University Press: New York.

Murphy, G.H., Sinclair, N., Hays, S., Offord, G., Langdon, P., Scott, J., Williams, J., Stagg, J., Tufnell, J., Lippold, T., Mercer, K. & Langheiet, G. (2004). Group cognitive behavioural treatment for men with intellectual disabilities at risk of sexually offending. *Journal of Intellectual Disability Research*, *48*, 467.

Nezu, C.M., Nezu, A.M. & Dudek, J.A. (1998). A cognitive behavioural model of assessment and treatment for intellectually disabled sexual offenders. *Cognitive and Behavioural Practice*, *5*, 25–64.

Niedigh, L.W. & Tomiko, R. (1991). The coping strategies of child sexual abusers. *Journal of Sex Education and Therapy*, *7*, 103–10.

Quinsey, V.L., Harris, G.T., Rice, M.E. & Cormier, C. (1998). *Violent offenders: Appraising and managing risk*. Washington, DC: American Psychological Association.

Rieger, A. (2004). Make it just as normal as possible with humour. *Mental retardation*, *42* (6), 427–44.

Rose, J., Jenkins, R., O'Conner, C., Jones, C. & Felce, D. (2002). A group treatment for men with intellectual disabilities who sexually offend or abuse. *Journal of Applied Research in Intellectual Disabilities*, *15*, 138–50.

Salter, A.C. (1988). *Treating child sex offenders and victims*. London: Sage.

Seghorn, T.H. & Ball, C.J. (2000). Assessment of sexual deviance in adults with developmental disabilities. *Mental Health Aspects of Developmental Disabilities*, *3*, 47–53.

Stachen, N.M. & Shevich, J. (1999). Working with the intellectually disabled/socially inadequate sex offender in a prison setting. In B. Schwarts (Ed.), *The sex offender: Theoretical advances, treating special populations, and legal developments*. Kingston, NJ: Civic Research Institute.

Talbot, J. (2007). *No one knows. Identifying and supporting prisoners with learning difficulties: The views of prison staff*. London: Prison Reform Trust.

Thompson, D. & Brown, H. (1997). Men with intellectual disabilities who sexually abuse: a review of the literature. *Journal of applied research in intellectual disabilities*, *10*, 140–158.

Thornton, D. (2002). Constructing and testing a framework for dynamic risk assessment. *Sexual Abuse: A Journal of Research & Treatment*, *14*, 139–53.

Thornton, D. & Hogue, T. (1993). The large scale provision of programmes for imprisoned sex offenders: Issues, dilemmas and progress. *Criminal Behaviour and Health*, *3*, 371–80.

Thornton, D., Mann, R., Webster, S., Blud, L., Travers, R., Friendship, C. & Erikson, M. (2003). Distinguishing and combining risks for sexual and violent recidivism. In: R. Prentky, E. Janus, M. Seto & A. W. Burgess (Eds), Understanding and managing sexually coercive behaviour. *Annals of New York Academy of Science*, *989*, 225–35.

Underhill, J., Wakeling, H.C., Mann, R.E. & Webster, S.D. (2008). Male sexual offenders' emotional openness with men and women. *Criminal Justice and Behavior*, *35*, 1156–173.

Ward, T. & Hudson, S.M. (2000). A self regulation model of relapse prevention. In D.R. Laws, S.M. Hudson & T. Ward (Eds), *Remaking relapse prevention with sex offenders*. Thousand Oaks, CA: Sage publications.

Ward, T., Hudson, S., Marshall, W.L. & Siegert, R. (1995). Attachment style and intimacy deficits in sexual offenders: A theoretical framework. *Sexual Abuse: A Journal of Research and Treatment*, *7*, 317–35.

Ward, T., Mann, R.E. & Gannon, T.A. (2007). The good lives model of offender rehabilitation: Clinical implications. *Aggression and violent behaviour*, *12* (1), 87–107.

Weschler, D. (1997). *WAIS III administration and scoring manual*. San Antonio, TX: The Psychological Corporation (www.pearsonassessments.com).

Williams, F. M. S. (2005). *My Private Interests Measure for Sexual Offenders with cognitive and/or social deficits*. Unpublished.

Williams, F. M. S., Wakeling, H. & Webster, S. (2007). A psychometric study of six self-report measures for use with sexual offenders with cognitive and social functioning deficits. *Psychology, Crime and Law*, *13* (5), 505–22.

Willner, P. & Goodey, R. (2006). Interaction of cognitive distortions and cognitive deficits in the formulation and treatment of obsessive-compulsive behaviours in a woman with an intellectual disability. *Journal of Applied Research in Intellectual Disabilities*, *19*, 67–73.

17

Journeying to Wise Mind: Dialectical Behaviour Therapy and Offenders with an Intellectual Disability

MARLEEN VERHOEVEN

INTRODUCTION

This chapter describes the complexities in the diagnosis of personality disorder (PD) for people with an intellectual disability (ID) and briefly describes psychological treatments for people who offend sexually. Dialectical Behaviour Therapy (DBT) and various adaptations, both for offenders and for people with an ID are discussed.

Personality disorders in people with an ID have a huge impact on behaviour, daily functioning and relationships. Successful treatment in residential and inpatient settings is hindered by the feelings of helplessness, confusion and hostility experienced by direct support staff responsible for treatment (Wilson, 2001). Many individuals are treatment resistant, which often results in team discord and burnout among providers (Lew, Matta, Tripp-Tebo & Watts, 2006). Sex offenders with an ID and personality disorder are at high risk for restrictive practises, ad hoc treatment, or rejection by providers, further contributing to their behaviour challenges and personality difficulties. The cost of medical, residential and psychiatric care for these individuals is significant. Sex offenders with an ID are commonly treated with behavioural therapy and cognitive behaviour therapy (CBT) (Barron, Hassiotis & Banes, 2002; Broxholme & Lindsay, 2003; Courtney & Rose, 2004; Craig & Hutchinson, 2005; Murphy, Sinclair, Hays & Heaton 2007; Tudway & Darmoody, 2005).

Based on the principle of normalisation, people with an ID are entitled to the same psychological therapy options that are available to the non-disabled population. An effective treatment for people with borderline personality disorder (BPD) is DBT (Linehan, 1993a).

Assessment and Treatment of Sexual Offenders with Intellectual Disabilities: A Handbook
Edited by Leam A. Craig, William R. Lindsay and Kevin D. Browne
© 2010 John Wiley & Sons, Ltd.

DBT offers an intensive treatment programme and opportunities for acceptance and validation of the person, at the same time drawing on behavioural change theory. DBT has been adapted for use with offenders in forensic services (McCann, Ball & Ivanoff, 2000; McCann, Ivanoff, Schmidt & Beach, 2007; Trupin, Stewart, Beach & Boesky, 2002) and for people with an ID (Dunn & Bolton, 2004; Esbensen & Benson, 2003; Lew, Matta, Tripp-Tebo & Watts, 2006; Mavromatis, 2000; Webb, Verhoeven & Eggleston, 2007; Wilson, 2001). The body of literature on interventions for people with an ID and PD is small and on the whole limited to single-case or small-sample-size studies. DBT lends itself well for use with individuals with an ID, and Lew, Matta, Tripp-Tebo and Watts (2006) identify the following features as reasons for this:

- DBT is a skills-based model that is consistent with psycho-educational and habilitative practice;
- DBT is fundamentally non-pejorative in its language and positive in its aspirations, without blaming the client;
- DBT has a strong focus on teaching individuals to advocate for themselves within the system of providers (the 'consultation to patients' model) that is decidedly consistent with values of assertiveness, independence, empowerment, and self-advocacy (p. 3).

Challenges with the use of DBT for people with an ID include the fact that it is strongly cognitively based. Individuals with poor or no reading skills, poor memory or limited insight will have difficulty with standard DBT. Adjustments to ensure its suitability for individuals with an ID are therefore common (Dunn & Bolton, 2004; Esbensen & Bensen, 2003; Lew, Matta, Tripp-Tebo & Watts, 2006; Webb, Verhoeven & Eggleston, 2007; Wilson, 2001).

Adapted DBT is a treatment programme for people with mild to moderate ID with minimal literacy skills that aims to treat the emotion dysregulation (e.g., mood disturbance, affective lability, uncontrolled anger) and behavioural dyscontrol (e.g., violence, self-inflicted injury, poor impulse control) that is commonly seen in persons with a PD. The model is useful for sex offenders with an ID for treatment of coexisting PD, impulsivity and, potentially, antisocial behaviour. DBT provides hope, structure, consistency and positive coping strategies for challenging behaviour, both for the client and the staff team. The result is a team approach and agreed goals on how to achieve a life worth living, as opposed to the more common dynamic of splitting, rejection and restrictive practises.

PERSONALITY DISORDER IN PERSONS WITH AN INTELLECTUAL DISABILITY

The diagnosis of PD in people with an ID may be important for service planning, management and appropriate treatment of the person. Research on PD and ID is limited. Torr (2003) and Alexander and Cooray (2003) reviewed publications and concluded that research has been hampered by methodological shortcomings, resulting in a huge range in figures for prevalence of PD in the ID population. The reviewers observe that existing diagnostic tools such as the Reiss screen (Reiss, 1994), the Psychopathology Inventory for Mentally Retarded Adults (PIMRA) (Matson, 1988) and the Standardised Assessment of Personality (SAP) (Mann, Jenkins, Cutting & Cowan, 1981) have limited data on reliability and validity. Furthermore, they note difficulties with diagnostic overshadowing, when a mental health presentation is explained as being caused by an ID or when features of the disability are explained as being symptomatic of a mental illness. For example, features of emotionally unstable (borderline) PD, such as self-injurious behaviour, impulsivity and affective lability are common in ID, specific syndromes and neurological impairment. The reviewers also report problems with distinguishing behavioural, psychiatric and personality features, especially in the more severely disabled. These problems are exacerbated by differences between ICD-10 (World Health Organization, 1992) and DSM-IV-TR (American Psychiatric Association, 2000) and different personality theories.

There appears to be a lack of clarity about the fundamental constructs of personality, psychiatric disorder and behavioural disorders in people with an ID. The diagnosis of PD in severe ID is extremely difficult to distinguish from the effects of the disability alone. The huge range of prevalence data indicates a lack of consistent criteria in the diagnosis of PD.

The Diagnostic Criteria in Learning Disability (DC-LD) (Royal College of Psychiatrists, 2001) is a major advance and offers a multi-axial approach to the diagnosis of psychiatric conditions in ID. The DC-LD is based on the ICD-10 (World Health Organization, 1992). Unlike the ICD-10, it tries to accommodate for the above-mentioned difficulties. The authors note, however, that the DC-LD diagnostic criteria have not primarily been designed for use with adults with an ID who offend. The DC-LD allows for an initial diagnosis of PD – unspecified if a distinction between subcategories cannot be made, indicating that different PDs may overlap when a person has an ID.

The diagnostic manual – intellectual disability (DM-ID) textbook and clinical guide (Fletcher, Loschen, Stavrakaki & First, 2007a, 2007b) are diagnostic manuals designed to facilitate an accurate DSM-IV-TR diagnosis in persons who have an ID. These manuals will hopefully contribute to overcoming the barriers in diagnosing PD in this population.

TREATMENT APPROACHES OF PERSONALITY DISORDERS IN INDIVIDUALS WITH AN INTELLECTUAL DISABILITY

A number of studies have described the high support needs of individuals with ID and PD. In a study by Naik, Gangadharan and Alexander (2002) individuals with PD required intensive accommodation and clinical input. The vast majority were on psychotropic drugs, although only a third had a coexisting psychiatric disorder. Coexisting affective disorder was common.

Flynn, Matthews and Hollins (2002) suggest treatment of PD in people with an ID needs to consider a combination of evidence-based psychotherapy (e.g., DBT, biological, behavioural and social models). Mavromatis (2000) described pharmacological and behavioural interventions in three individuals with BPD and ID. She concluded that pharmacological intervention must be tailored to the individual and directed at target symptoms of affective disorder and psychosis. Pharmacological intervention alone is rarely sufficient and must be combined with psychotherapeutic or behavioural strategies. In her treatment review, the most successful psychotherapy with BPD patients focussed on limit setting, structure, consistency, validation, empathy, challenging the person to develop new and more adaptive skills and behaviour and careful long-term structure of a positive therapeutic relationship.

SEXUAL OFFENDING AND INTELLECTUAL DISABILITY

The incidence of sex offending in offenders with an ID may be four to six times higher than in the general population (Barron, Hassiotis & Banes, 2002) (see Chapter 2). Compared to the general population, offenders with an ID have increased rates of coexisting mental illness and PDs (Lindsay et al., 2006; Lindsay et al., 2004) (see Chapter 6).

Day (1994) and Lindsay et al. (2002) reported that 32 per cent of sex offenders with ID had mental illness, excluding behavioural disorders. Lindsay et al. (2006) found that 39.3 per cent of offenders with an ID had a PD. The most common diagnosis was antisocial PD. They also found that the severity of PD was correlated with instruments predicting future violence and sexual offending. Alexander, Piachaud, Odebiyi and Gangadharan (2002) and Lindsay et al. (2004) researched patients referred to an inpatient forensic ID unit and found that women were significantly more likely to have exhibited physical violence towards self, physical violence towards others and have a diagnosis of PD. Lindsay et al. (2004) found that the two most frequent referral reasons for males were sexually abusive behaviour and aggressive behaviour. As only 9 per cent of referrals are female they concluded that fewer women are violent. They also found that females had a higher incidence of mental illness (67 per cent) and a lower incidence of re-offending than males.

TREATMENT OF SEX OFFENDERS WITH AN INTELLECTUAL DISABILITY

The sexual recidivism rate of offenders with ID is higher than that for non-disabled sexual offenders. They are also at greater risk of re-offending more quickly (Craig & Hutchinson, 2005).

Common treatment targets for sexual offenders are increasing motivation, sexual knowledge and attitudes, victim empathy, social and relationship skills, community engagement, confronting denial and self-control, improving relapse prevention and modifying cognitive distortions (Barron, Hassiotis & Banes, 2002; Broxholme & Lindsay, 2003; Craig & Hutchinson, 2005; Lindsay, 2005; Talbot & Langdon, 2006). Cognitive distortions are learnt beliefs that many sex offenders hold about behaviours such as child molestation and rape and are thought to be important in the offending process (Murphy, Sinclair, Hays & Heaton, 2007).

Assessment and treatment of adults with ID who commit sexual offences presents a number of challenges. Currently, there is little evidence to demonstrate the effectiveness or validity of the adaptation and application of mainstream models (Barron, Hassiotis & Banes, 2002; Broxholme & Lindsay, 2003; Courtney & Rose, 2004; Craig & Hutchinson, 2005; Tudway & Darmoody, 2005). In particular, the evidence for key factors such as cognitive distortions is weak. Methodological problems include inconsistencies in the definition of the group, the extent and nature of the offending, a lack of standardised methodology for assessment and comparison, failure to use a control group and small sample size. Some credible studies have found better and more durable attitudinal change with treatment lasting at least two years (Courtney & Rose, 2004). A series of small-scale group CBT interventions for sex offenders offered some evidence of success in reducing re-offending (Barron, Hassiotis & Banes, 2002). Craig and Hutchinson (2005) reviewed the evidence and found that cognitive behavioural techniques were most effective at reducing offending and sexual recidivism. They recommended modifying approaches to compensate for the specific difficulties of people with ID by strategies such as visual material in addition to verbal instructions, use of simple material and repetition of messages, concrete rather than abstract learning and allowing for a longer learning period.

Murphy, Sinclair, Hays and Heaton (2007) evaluated a group CBT for men in the ID and borderline range of functioning who had committed sexual offences. Of the 52 men, 94 per cent completed the treatment in a year, showing a high level of motivation. Over the period of treatment, the men showed increases in sexual knowledge and empathy and reductions in cognitive distortions which were maintained at six-months follow-up. Six men showed further sexually abusive behaviour during treatment and seven men sexually offended in the six-months follow-up period. Several predictive factors of the re-offending were investigated; however, only receipt of concurrent therapy and the presence of autistic spectrum disorders appeared to be positively related. It is likely that concurrent therapy was offered to men regarded at risk of continued offending, and the correlation does not appear useful as a predictor.

A closer match between specialist assessment and treatment targets appears a logical way forward. Keeling, Beech and Rose (2007) argue that treatment needs to be based on the assessments of risk, need and responsivity. They argue that a sexual offender who poses a high level of sexual recidivism should receive the most intensive treatment, which in current practice is not commonly the case. The assessment of need includes potentially treatment responsive dynamic risk factors like deviant sexual interest, pro-offending attitudes, socio-affective problems and self-management issues. The assessment of responsivity includes the assessment of intelligence, adaptive behaviour, literacy and comprehension. Offenders with an ID are not a homogenous group, and matching treatment to learning styles is important for effective treatment.

Dialectical Behaviour Therapy

DBT is a therapy designed for people with complex, multiple and severe mental disorders (Linehan, 1993a, Dimeff & Linehan, 2001). It focusses on behavioural dysregulation (self-inflicted injury, suicidality, impulsive behaviour) and emotional dysregulation (affective lability, problems with anger). It also addresses interpersonal dysregulation, self-dysregulation and cognitive dysregulation, as commonly seen in people with BPD.

DBT combines the strategies of behavioural therapy with Eastern mindfulness practices, within an overarching dialectical framework that acknowledges apparent opposites and works towards synthesis. The primary dialectical tension is between 'acceptance' and 'change'. A DBT therapist accepts a person non-judgementally (through therapeutic validation, mindfulness, focussing on effectiveness), while also benevolently demanding that they change (behavioural change theory). A therapist develops a collaborative relationship and acts as a coach in the development of behavioural change. In DBT, the therapist–client relationship is characterised by radical genuineness, equality within the relationship and the therapist observing their own limits, creating a somewhat different professional relationship to that which is typical in many therapeutic contexts.

Problem behaviour is defined as life-threatening behaviour (e.g., self- or other harm behaviour), therapy-interfering behaviour (e.g., non-compliance with therapy, behaviour that burns out the therapist) and quality-of-life threatening behaviour (e.g., issues related to money, housing, substance use, conflict). These behaviours are regarded as ineffective in getting a person's needs and goals met, as opposed to the more effective use of coping skills. Coping skills are mindfulness, interpersonal effectiveness, emotion regulation, distress tolerance and self-management.

Behaviour is modified through environmental intervention, chain analysis of problem behaviour with the client, correction and over-correction procedures ('repair'), exposure strategies, contingency management and cognitive modification. New coping skills are taught in group skills training. The use of coping skills is demonstrated by completion of a diary card and homework sheets.

A DBT therapist is usually engaged with a consultation team. How the therapist engages in consultation/supervision and who the community is depends on the work setting and borderline client load. The team is used to ensure adherence to DBT principles, observe the therapists' limits, and accepts that all therapists are fallible.

DBT Therapeutic Process

DBT starts with a commitment and agreement stage, in which pros and cons of therapy are discussed. Goals are targeted around the client's definition of a life worth living. The person agrees to reduce life-threatening and therapy-interfering behaviour and use more effective methods to solve problems. The person also agrees to attend therapy.

Standard DBT modalities are

- weekly individual therapy
- weekly group skills training
- as-needed consultation with the client by telephone
- weekly case consultation for providers
- other uncontrolled treatments like pharmacotherapy and acute inpatient care

The treatment focuses primarily on achieving emotional and behavioural control (Stage 1). The next three stages are less prescribed by the model. These stages help the client to feel better (Stage 2: 'emotional experiencing'), to resolve problems in living and residual disorders (Stage 3: 'ordinary (un)happiness') and to find joy (Stage 4: 'capacity for joy and freedom'). Therapy using trauma disclosure strategies is not commenced until the person has achieved emotional and behavioural control.

Biosocial Perspectives on Personality Development in Intellectual Disability

The biosocial model underpinning DBT argues that BPD is a result primarily of a dysfunction of the *emotion regulation system* (Linehan, 1993a). This theory proposes that emotion dysregulation develops from innate biological emotional sensitivity in combination with exposure to an invalidating environment in childhood. Emotion dysregulation causes significant behavioural dyscontrol, which is viewed as maladaptive attempts to manage extreme emotions.

Invalidating Environment

An invalidating environment is characterised by incompatibility between the needs of the child and environmental experiences, including abuse. The child learns to think that she or he is wrong in how they make sense of their emotions. They learn to rely on external agencies for understanding, rather than developing a sense of personal judgement. An invalidating environment also prevents the child from learning to label and modulate internal emotional experiences (Linehan, 1993a). Often the only means of provoking a helpful environmental response to internal distress is to produce an extreme reaction. For example, a child may learn that crying does not evoke sympathy from the family, but self-harm does. Learnt childhood patterns tend to be repeated in later life, often met by further invalidating responses from subsequent situations, leading to a vicious cycle between the person and their environment.

People with an ID may be invalidated through experiences of abuse, neglect and stigmatisation. A high percentage of ID individuals (25 per cent to 83 per cent) have been sexual abused (Lew, Matta, Tripp-Tebo & Watts, 2006). Invalidating experiences specific to the disability include institutionalisation, identity issues related to living with a disability, dependency needs, overprotection or overestimation of ability, limited opportunities and choices, the social consequences of dysmorphic features and parents with limited skills and resources to support their child with special needs.

Biological Emotional Sensitivity

Linehan (1993a) describes biological sensitivity as a pervasive deficit in a person's capacity to regulate emotions. The biosocial theory of BPD implies that genetic and biological factors inherent to ID may further contribute to the development of personality traits and disorder. Kojima and Ikeda (2001) identified specific personality traits in persons with Down's syndrome. Neurological dysregulation in persons with an ID is common (Mavromatis, 2000). This may include neurological and syndrome specific issues (e.g., frontal lobe dysfunction, perseveration and foetal alcohol syndrome). Lew, Matta, Tripp-Tebo and Watts (2006) argue that people with ID are vulnerable to developing psychiatric disorder because of brain damage, seizure disorders, sensory impairment and a range of genetic syndromes. This may present as PDs. Consistent with the vulnerability–stress model, it is also common for people with ID and severe emotion dysregulation in the absence of adaptive coping skills to suffer intermittent psychotic episodes (Nuechterlein & Dawson, 1984; Zubin & Spring, 1977).

Disability Related Factors

Poor coping skills as seen in people with a PD may be a function of the ID itself (Alexander & Cooray, 2003; Dunn & Bolton, 2004). For example, a history of early protective restrictions may influence whether a person with a disability learns the skills to negotiate the world independently or manage their anxiety in new situations. Medical fragility may reinforce somatic complaints and a dependent personality style. Cognitive and physical characteristics may affect social and intimate relationships and increase experiences of rejection. Specific learning disabilities may result in unrealistically high expectations in all areas of their life when they may have deficits in specific functioning (Lew, Matta, Tripp-Tebo & Watts, 2006).

Antisocial Personality Disorder

Despite being developed for people with BPD, McCann, Ball and Ivanoff (2000) and McCann, Ivanoff, Schmidt & Beach (2007) argue that the biosocial theory also applies to persons with antisocial personality disorder (ASPD). Consistent with the situation for BPD individuals, the environment of persons with ASPD is notable for invalidation with harsh and inconsistent discipline, little positive parental involvement and inadequate supervision. Individuals with ASPD appear emotionally insensitive, unlike individuals with BPD who are emotionally oversensitive. The biosocial theory of ASPD is therefore a combination of biological emotional *insensitivity* combined with an environment characterised by *disturbed caring* (caring acts were not validated or were even punished) and *positive reinforcement of antisocial behaviour* (e.g., reinforcement of using aversive behaviours to terminate aversive interactions).

Traumatic Life Events, Personality Disorder and Offending in Persons with an Intellectual Disability

Owing to high rates of co-ocurrence, it may be hypothesised that similar developmental pathways lead to PD and offending. A few preliminary studies show interesting results on the association of traumatic life experiences and inappropriate sexual behaviour, offending and PD in people with an ID. Flynn, Matthew and Hollins (2002) found a significant association between traumatic childhood experiences and a diagnosis of PD in adults with ID who are in specialist challenging behaviour inpatient services. Sequeira, Howlin and Hollins (2003) found that people with an ID with a proven or probable history of sexual abuse had higher rates of mental illness (post traumatic stress disorder, neurosis and depression) and behavioural problems (predominantly aggressive and agitated behaviour, temper outbursts and sudden changes in mood, social withdrawal and inappropriate sexual behaviour) compared to an ID control group. Similarly, Murphy, O'Callaghan and Clare (2007) found a relationship between alleged abuse in people with severe or profound disabilities and aggressive, non-compliant, stereotyped, sexualized, self-abusive, withdrawn and disturbed behaviour.

Alexander, Piachaud, Odebiyi and Gangadharan (2002) and Lindsay et al. (2004) researched patients referred to an inpatient forensic ID unit comparing men and women. Both studies had a similar outcome and found that the proportion of women who reported being victims of sexual or physical abuse was 60 per cent and 40 per cent respectively. Both sexual and physical abuse was significantly higher for females than for males, being 7 per cent and 10 per cent for males. Lindsay, Law, Quinn, Smart and Smith (2001) found a higher rate of history of sexual abuse among ID sexual offenders and a higher rate of history of physical abuse among ID non-sexual (predominantly violent) offenders. Lindsay (2005), in his review, concludes that in spite of these data, sexual and physical abuse is a factor for less than 50 per cent of offenders and would appear to be an insufficient aetiological explanation for sexual offending on its own.

ADAPTATIONS OF DIALECTICAL BEHAVIOUR THERAPY

DBT is an evidence-based treatment. The approach was originally designed and found to be effective in reducing self-inflicted injury and psychiatric inpatient stays and in increasing treatment retention in women diagnosed with BPD (Linehan, Armstrong, Suarez, Allmon & Heard, 1991). Randomised clinical trials have compared DBT to treatment-as-usual (TAU) for a number of different applications and adaptations of the model. DBT has been adapted to people with an additional diagnosis and in additional settings, such as drug dependence (Linehan *et al.*, 2002), suicidal adolescents (Rathus & Miller, 2002), male forensic inpatients

(McCann, Ball & Ivanoff, 2000; McCann, Ivanoff, Schmidt & Beach, 2007) and behavioural problems among inpatient juvenile female offenders (Trupin, Stewart, Beach & Boesky, 2002).

Dialectical Behaviour Therapy for People who Offend

The prevalence of emotion dysregulation in people who offend suggests that DBT may be an effective strategy for this population (Trupin, Stewart, Beach & Boesky, 2002; McCann, Ball & Ivanoff, 2000; McCann, Ivanoff, Schmidt & Beach, 2007). In spite of this, there are only a few published studies describing the effectiveness of DBT in forensic services, although pre-liminary information suggests DBT can be successful for this population. Different forensic treatments adapt DBT in different ways. Two examples are discussed here. Both programmes target impulsive and antisocial behaviour as well as staff attitudes and burn-out.

Treatment of Female Offenders Targeting Behaviours Sensitive to Dialectical Behaviour Therapy

Trupin, Stewart, Beach and Boesky (2002) applied an abbreviated DBT model with juvenile female offenders in a psychiatric inpatient unit. DBT was chosen because many in this population have serious mental health issues (e.g., affective disorder, conduct disorder and BPD), substance use disorder and emotional problems. They noted that the apparent conflicting responsibilities of the justice system, mainly security versus rehabilitation, created problematic staff attitudes, including the risk of punitive responses. DBT was implemented on two units with a third unit used as a TAU control. On one DBT unit female offenders demonstrated a significant reduction in serious behaviour problems and an increased participation in other services (e.g., alcohol and drug treatment, internal transfers and employment). Youths in the other DBT unit had fewer behavioural problems to start with and did not show a reduction. Youths in the control unit did not display any target behaviour. Staff's use of restrictive punishment was reduced in the first unit but increased in the other DBT unit because of a lack of adherence to the DBT model. The authors concluded that with intensive training, motivated staff and the targeting of specific behaviours sensitive to DBT (self-inflicted injury, suicidality, aggression and non-compliant behaviour), DBT intervention can be successful in reducing behavioural problems and increasing staff's use of therapeutic rather than restrictive and punitive responses.

Treatment of Male Offenders Targeting Impulsive and Antisocial Behaviour

McCann, Ball and Ivanoff (2000) and McCann, Ivanoff, Schmidt & Beach (2007) describe the use of DBT in a forensic inpatient setting for males with antisocial behaviours. Their issues included violent histories and multiple diagnoses (e.g., BPD, ASPD and coexisting psychotic or mood disorders). Similarly as with the previous study, DBT was chosen for its focus on life-threatening behaviours of clients and therapy-interfering behaviours of both clients and staff. They noted that, rather than is the case with outpatient DBT, clients and staff have limited choices and are confronted by the treatment versus security dialectic. Staff burn-out was common. They adapted DBT to suit the population (incarcerated, ASPD, males) and the environment (inpatient forensic, more involvement on the part of the team) by, for example, adding skills modules on victim empathy, developing a non-judgemental DBT chain analysis of their crime and writing an extensive relapse prevention plan. Staff were encouraged to increase their validation strategies.

The number of programmes using DBT components in correctional and forensic settings has increased, including 10 programmes in USA/Canada and several settings across the UK. In spite of attempts to evaluate the programmes and strong anecdotal evidence, reliable data were hard to obtain (McCann, Ivanoff, Schmidt & Beach, 2007). Reported difficulties were staff not being trained in mental health or behavioural therapy, staff motivation, adapting the standard outpatient treatment to highly restricted settings and adapting the treatment to address the needs of a male population (McCann, Ivanoff, Schmidt & Beach, 2007). Unpublished data suggests that, in comparison to TAU, people receiving DBT had a significant decrease in depressed and hostile mood, paranoia and psychotic behaviours. Furthermore, they had a significant decrease in several maladaptive interpersonal coping styles and an increase in adaptive coping in comparison to those receiving TAU. A trend towards reduction in staff burn-out was reported, again favouring DBT (McCann & Ball, 1996; McCann, Ball & Ivanoff, 1996).

Dialectical Behaviour Therapy and Sex Offenders with an Intellectual Disability

There are a number of arguments for why DBT offers an interesting alternative to existing therapeutic models for sex offenders with an ID. A person with an ID and challenging behaviour is traditionally treated with an Applied Behaviour Analysis informed behavioural management plan. Behavioural interventions alone, or in combination with other treatments, are generally seen as important aspects of a comprehensive therapeutic plan for offenders with an ID aimed at improving competencies in adaptive skills while decreasing undesirable behaviours (Barron, Hassiotis & Banes, 2002). In this treatment, the environment manipulates the contingencies of the target behaviour, which the offender may view as an invalidating experience. The person may or may not be aware of the existence of the plan and is unlikely to have participated in its development. The dialectic between 'acceptance' and 'change' leans heavily to the latter. DBT not only offers a treatment that is validating, it also builds on the strengths of behavioural approaches.

Treatments of sex offenders with an ID have also drawn on CBT approaches for sex offenders in mainstream forensic services. Unfortunately, there is no evidence base that cognitive distortions actually contribute to sex offending in people with an ID (Barron, Hassiotis & Banes, 2002). Limited cognitive abilities are more likely to cause distortions in perceptions and the likelihood of misunderstandings (Mavromatis, 2000). DBT is loosely based on CBT principles. DBT is based on the chain antecedent, emotion dysregulation, behaviour and consequences, making it easier to adapt for this population. Cognitions are considered part of this chain, but it is not essential to identify the specific cognitions.

Lindsay (2005) comments that research in the treatment of people with a PD has focussed on BPD, only a very little on ASPD or psychopathy and is merely anecdotal with regard to ID. Some work has been conducted on the persoality characteristic impulsivity. Craig and Hutchinson (2005) and Lindsay (2005) argue that sexual offenders with an ID are less impulsive than non-sexual offenders. Their offending behaviour may be opportunistic with delayed gratification if grooming behaviour is involved, rather than being based on impulsive behavioural acts. Lindsay (2005) further notes that different categories of sexual offenders may differ on impulsiveness; for example, offenders against children may have a greater ability to plan and delay gratification than offenders against adults, who act more impulsively. He also makes an important distinction between trait (static) and state (transitory) impulsivity and agitation. DBT may be a useful tool, to treat co-existing emotion and behavioural dysregulation, and to treat the sex offending and impulsivity itself by creating a stronger link between action and consequences.

The State Government Victoria Department of Justice (2007) describes ID in the Victorian prison system, Australia. On average, prisoners with an ID had a greater total number of incidents recorded against them than had prisoners in the non-disabled sample. Only 46 per cent did not have an incident recorded against them compared to 60 per cent of prisoners without a disability. Prisoners with an ID were involved in significantly more incidents involving assaults/fights, property damage and attempted suicide/self-harm than were non-disabled prisoners, and in significantly fewer incidents involving drugs and rule infractions (e.g., smoking, refusing directions). These statistics indicate that behavioural dysregulation is more common in ID prisoners. They also emphasise that models of offending and treatment need to cater for the specific emotional and behavioural characteristics of offenders with an ID.

ADAPTATIONS OF DBT FOR PEOPLE WITH AN INTELLECTUAL DISABILITY

The Journeying to Wise Mind programme is based on DBT principles and adapted for people with an ID. It has not been developed specifically for sexual offenders but has been used with this population and shows promise. The Journeying to Wise Mind programme will be described in detail below.

Journeying to Wise Mind

At the Dual Disability Service, a tertiary mental health service for people with an ID in Auckland, New Zealand, DBT has been adapted for use with people with an ID in the community or in a clinic setting. DBT provides a well-structured approach to the treatment of people with a moderate or mild ID. The therapy is offered to persons who struggle with emotion and behavioural dysregulation, with severe, multiple and complex issues, preferably those with some literacy skills. Experience shows that the treatment may be applied to a range of complex behavioural issues. People with an ID commonly struggle with poor coping skills and are likely to benefit from the programme. In addition to BPD, the treatment has been useful for people diagnosed with depression, psychosis, brain injury, autism and chronic schizophrenia. This section describes some of the modifications that have been made to make the DBT approach more usable by people with an ID.

Biosocial and Behavioural Formulation

The biosocial formulation addresses biological emotional sensitivity in the context of an invalidating environment. As described earlier, an invalidating environment may include experiences common to the general population, for example, traumatic life events as well as disability specific invalidation. The formulation of biological sensitivity needs to consider neurological dysregulation, syndrome specific issues and mental illness.

The behavioural formulation addresses the function and the meaning of the behaviour of concern, and the lack of more effective coping skills. Owing to their learning difficulties and high support needs, people with ID commonly have limited opportunities to learn effective coping skills. The behaviour of concern may have inadvertently been reinforced by family and staff and is maintained by the contingencies of the behaviour.

An example of a DBT formulation is provided by Dunn and Bolton (2004). They describe a man with a mild to borderline ID making escalating threats to stab people. In their formulation, predisposing factors include disturbed early relationships influencing attachment development. Additionally, behaviour and emotional problems were explained in terms of ID and managed externally, limiting opportunities to learn to regulate emotions and relationships. His ID label and bullying at school made him feel stupid and socially undesirable. His psychological vulnerabilities included a lack of skills to regulate relationships and emotions, lack of consistent positive self-image and lack of skills to make sense of the social world. His triggers were social rejection, loneliness, emotional distress at not being taken seriously and limited opportunities to gain interpersonal attention. His cognitions included that he was worthless and unlovable and (in defence) that he was dangerous, powerful and bad. He saw the world as a dangerous place that was out to get him. His poorly controlled emotions included anxiety, anger and sadness. His challenging behaviour, including threats to kill and carrying a knife, was positively maintained (shorter term) by emotion reduction, gaining interpersonal attention and going to hospital/prison, thus reinforcing his sense of being dangerous and powerful. His negative maintaining factors (longer term) were feeling bad and guilty, having freedom restricted and becoming isolated and rejected, thus reinforcing his negative self-image.

The treatment plan arising from this formulation included increased consistency in the management of his behaviours by minimising the impact of challenging behaviour and increasing attention for adaptive behaviours. Individual therapy allowed him to identify the functions and the short- and long-term consequences of his behaviour. Staff identified ways in which he could feel powerful, gain attention and manage internal experiences in a more effective manner. This included relaxation training, cognitive restructuring and increased reflection skills. The outcome of this intervention was a significant reduction in challenging behaviour and improvement in relationships on the unit. The person is being prepared for discharge.

Commitment and Agreement

For people with an ID, the commitment and agreement stage addresses the dialectic of acceptance and change. In my experience it is generally easy to achieve an agreement to participate in DBT (acceptance); it is harder to achieve and maintain commitment to active participation in the programme (change). Persons with an ID tend to have experiences of rejection and not fitting in, and they may crave attention and friendships. They commonly have a poor concept of relationships as most of their close companions are paid support workers. They have learnt that their support worker's role is not only to provide companionship but also to resolve their issues and problems. In addition they are commonly gullible and suggestible and may agree without understanding the implications of the decision to participate. A person with an ID may have the desire to off-load experiences and emotions and gain attention from a validating person who promotes equality in their relationship. They may lack motivation or insight to process and change their behaviour.

The commitment and agreement stage includes explaining the biosocial theory in basic terms. The client is given an opportunity to explore what a life worth living looks like for them and what stops them from achieving this, linking DBT goals with personal goals in a validating framework. The therapist points out that the therapy is hard work ('The Devil's Advocate' strategy), and what the pros and cons of making a real commitment are. If the person agrees, they are asked to sign a contract explaining the rules of treatment. This contract is also signed by the staff person and the service provider to ensure it is understood that we work cooperatively as a team. The contract may be referred to if commitment becomes an issue. A confidentiality clause in the contract allows the therapist to speak with the service provider. Confidentiality is guaranteed outside the 'team' with the usual provisos.

Service Milieu

A person with an ID is mutually dependent on their support milieu. In DBT, the service milieu provides resources, availability of support workers and a validating, supportive attitude. DBT in this population needs to be considered as a longer-term treatment requiring several repetitions. A strong administrative commitment to the use of the model is required, especially in light of frequent staff changes in services. An analysis of costs and benefits of the programme may be of help (Swenson, Torrey & Koerner, 2002), as is regular communication and cheerleading (focussing on the positives) of the efforts of the service. In the first instance residential services may agree and commit to DBT treatment of a client. Logistical and motivational changes may become a barrier to continuation – for example, staff availability and changes in management and staff. The complexities and challenges of keeping all stakeholders engaged are obvious and require as much attention to commitment and agreement with the service providers as with the client.

Staff working with people with an ID may be unskilled or have limited training opportunities. Training is required at the outset of the sessions to promote skills development in the model. An advantage is that this offers them a new set of skills they can use with other clients. Support workers have an important role in DBT and bring validation, contingency management, modelling of skilful behaviour, coaching, cheerleading and use of DBT vocabulary. Staff training addresses the biosocial theory, behavioural theory, the coping skills package as well as the skills of acceptance and validation. Staff formulate validating expressions based on examples of invalidation (see Table 17.1). However, staff have to find a balance between 'observing their limits' and validation of the client to ensure clients do not get the message that their target behaviour is acceptable.

As with Lew Matta, Tripp-Tebo and Watts (2006), staff participate in sessions with the client. This enhances their own learning, teaches them how to support the client, enhances collaboration with the programme and promotes non-judgemental provision of collateral information. Staff attending the sessions assists the client with the message that they take the coping skills package seriously and are willing to form a team with the client and the therapist. It also keeps the client honest about their target behaviour and use of skills. Staff commonly report that by attending the sessions they develop personal skills and cope better with their own circumstances.

Table 17.1 Examples of (in)validating expressions

Invalidating Expression (closing the person off)	Validating Expression (opening up the conversation)
Be happy!	*You don't look happy. Do you want to talk about it?*
I tried to help you …	*It sounds like what we tried did not work. What can we try next?*
I am sure she means well	*I can see she hurt your feelings. I do not think she intended to. What could she have done differently?*
Just use your coping skills	*Are you in feeling mind right now? What coping skill would you like to try?*
This is getting really old	*It must be important to you to keep bringing this up.*
Don't you ever think of anyone but yourself?	*What do you think could be the other person's point of view?*
Time heals all wounds	*I understand that you are hurting right now. I know from my own experience that the pain won't last and will get better over time.*

It is important for the treatment team to follow a client when they move residence, to ensure generalisation and monitoring of the behaviour. For example, a person treated in an inpatient setting may be treated for self-inflicted injury. Through increased opportunity, new behaviours may emerge once the person moves to a community setting. The person may feel overwhelmed and desire an institutionalised environment. Behaviours may aim to achieve this, for example increase in criminal behaviour.

Coping Skills Training

Both therapy and skills training are provided in weekly individual sessions, with additional group skills training. Like Lew and colleagues (2006), it is my experience that not all individuals are willing or able to participate in a group as low self-esteem makes them reluctant to expose their cognitive challenges. The result may be undue anxiety, dissociation or emotion dysregulation to the point that the individual and other group members are not participating in the learning experience. Individual adjustments may be required for specific cognitive and literacy abilities, further complicating group-based coping-skills training. Transport can also present practical and financial issues for clients.

The coping skills package is based on Linehan's skills training manual (Linehan, 1993b). It consists of handouts and homework sheets in easy-to-use language and simplified concepts using pictures, prompt cards and other aids to explain and simplify the concepts further. Modules are 'mindfulness', 'skills I can use when I am in feeling mind' and 'skills I can use to stay in wise mind'. An interpersonal effectiveness module is currently under review and is a particularly challenging module to modify as relationships for people with an ID are often dependent in nature (caregivers) and they often have to socialise with people they do not choose to live with and whose behaviour may be an understandable trigger. An example of 'skills I can use when I am in feeling mind' is 'good outcomes and bad outcomes' ('pros and cons'), see Table 17.2.

Table 17.2 Good outcomes and bad outcomes

Feeling Mind	Good Outcome	Bad Outcome
Describe acting out behaviour	feel in control visitors and attention	put self and others at risk staff frustrated 'nobody cares' loss of control
	Short-term gain	*Long-term loss*
Wise Mind	Good Outcome	Bad Ooutcome
Describe use of coping skills	proud of self fun, help, care, trust goals e.g., increased independence in living arrangement (flatting), friends, work	needs practise not instant hard work
	Long-term gain	*Short-term loss*

Individual Therapy

Sessions start with a mindfulness exercise, sometimes initiated by the client. Coping skills homework and diary cards are then reviewed (see Figure 17.1), followed by talking about the week. This reinforces skills that may have been used, even if the person is not aware of these ('cheerleading'). If an incident has occurred we complete a chain analysis. This is followed by discussing the next coping skills handouts. A new diary card and homework specific to the handouts are given. Consistent with Lew, Matta, Tripp-Tebo and Watts (2006), staff are generally encouraged to assist the person with practising the new skills and completing the daily homework.

Mindfulness

The concept of mindfulness is important but difficult to explain to a cognitively challenged person. Key concepts in the mindfulness module are wise mind, rational mind and emotion

My goals	Goal: Describe the person's goal to achieve a life worth living e.g., going flatting		Behaviour of concern: Define behaviour that interferes with the goal	
Day and date	Was I in feeling mind today?	Did I have behaviour of concern? Which one(s)?	Which feeling did I have when I was in feeling mind? (angry, sad, worried, frustrated, shame)	Which coping skills did I use? (sometimes divided in before and after the behaviour)

Figure 17.1 Adapted diary card

mind, with wise mind being the preferred mental state and the cooperation of the other two. Experience shows that people with an ID intuitively understand wise mind and feeling ('emotion') mind, which gives a framework to base the coping skills training on. Not surprisingly they have more difficulty with thinking ('rational') mind.

A good example of the use of mindfulness is described by Singh, Wahler, Adkins and Myers (2003). They treated an adult with mild ID, psychotic disorder not otherwise specified and high intensity aggressive behaviour with a mindfulness-based self-control strategy. He was taught a simple meditation technique that required him to shift his attention from the anger-producing situation to a neutral point on his body, the soles of his feet. He increased self-control over his aggressive behaviours. He had six months of aggression-free behaviour in the inpatient facility before being transitioned to the community. No aggressive behaviour was seen during the one-year follow-up after his community placement.

Chain Analysis

Chain analysis is the process of describing the chain of events leading up to and following an incident. While the person describes the events, questions are asked and the answers written up. In some cases, additional pictures are used for review in the next session, to assist memory and insight. The chain may include vulnerability factors, the prompting event and the links of behaviour, including actions, body sensations, cognitions, feelings and events. The consequences in the environment and the person are explored, both for the short- and long-term, sometimes using a 'good and bad outcomes' sheet. Prevention of future events (i.e., changing vulnerability factors) and use of coping skills are then talked about. The harm of the behaviour is discussed and a suitable repair chosen. To conclude, the person is asked what they have learnt from the experience. This self-reflection is very powerful in people with an ID, who in the past have often been judged for these behaviours without being afforded the opportunity to reflect or explain how this behaviour has worked for them. A chain analysis is a slightly aversive process, partly because the therapist withdraws warmth and stays on task until completed. The therapist targets the aspects that need to be focussed on to ensure the analysis takes part of a session only, before handouts and homework for the next coping skills session can be discussed.

Behaviour Management

'Consultation to the patient' is when the person is encouraged to resolve their own issues. This is opposed to 'environmental intervention', which is used in acceptance of where a person is at and acknowledges the need for external intervention. A behavioural management plan may either have the function of 'environmental intervention' or 'consultation to the client'. Environmental intervention serves the function of prevention, early intervention and safety in the case of dangerous impulsive behaviour. The behavioural management plan may include crisis management strategies, for example, non-violent crisis intervention (Crisis Prevention Institute, 2007). On occasion, a crisis plan is drafted for use by the local mental health crisis team, the police and/or the local accident and emergency clinic.

Table 17.3 The four-stage model

Stage 1	Stage 2	Stage 3	Stage 4
Optimal function	Antecedents/ Precursors	Crisis	Resolution
	Behaviour		
Individual is engaged in their daily activities	Early warning signs of escalating behaviour	Individual displays crisis behaviour	Individual is calm/ exhausted
	Goal		
Maintain function at this stage	Return to Stage 1	Maintain safety and move to Stage 4	Gradual return to Stage 1
	Interventions		
Reinforce and teach appropriate behaviour	Use coping skills	Ensure safety for all involved	Use coping skills
Maintain structure	Maintain structure	Observe for signs of Stage 4	Reinstate structure
Teach and practice coping skills			Validate feelings

Consultation to the client is preferred over environmental intervention. A behavioural management plan developed in consultation with the client is more likely to be informed by DBT strategies the client has learnt. The language used is validating and informed by the person. The plan may be used cooperatively by the client, their support workers and family. The purpose of the plan is to generalise skills over different environments and to maintain learnt skills. Wilson (2001) described a four-stage model for the management of BPD in people with ID, see Table 17.3.

Strategies tend to be simple and proactive and encourage the person to take responsibility for their own behaviour and become part of the treatment team. If prescribed, medication *pro re nata*, (according to need) is encouraged at Stage 2 or 4 rather than at Stage 3 to avoid inadvertently reinforcing unskilful behaviour. The model provides an opportunity for the person and therapist to educate staff. Staff learn to predict changes and plan and implement appropriate interventions at appropriate times, resulting in optimum consistency and staff feeling more empowered and positive.

Additional behavioural strategies may be used – for example, token economy system for skilful behaviour and avoiding undue attention for target behaviour. Therapists are likely to become a reinforcer themselves, and can use personal reinforcement within a validating stance to achieve behavioural change. Other strategies that may be used are shaping (gradually introducing a new behaviour by reinforcing progressive aspects of the behaviour) and exposure to emotions and situations to learn increasingly to tolerate these. People with disabilities are likely to have anxieties about academic work and homework, and gradual exposure to DBT materials may on occasion be required to allow them to learn to achieve rather than fail.

Telephone Consultation

As in DBT, telephone consultation for crisis situations is offered. However, as the caregivers are involved in the DBT training and sessions, they are commonly the first-line support for a distressed person. Calls are typically short and focus more on skills and natural supports they can use than on venting their distress. This is sometimes a challenging balance when the client, not understanding the purpose, perceives the therapist as non-caring and rejecting. Validation of emotions is an important aspect of these calls. I find that even after people have been discharged they sometimes continue to ring me when they want to, commonly in relation to a crisis situation. These calls help in long-term maintenance of their skills.

If a person rings frequently for no apparent reason the therapists explains the effect of the behaviour on their limits. Pros and cons are discussed for example their calls may not be taken seriously. The client is invited to assist in developing strategies including management of frequent calls. Strategies to limit calls are discussed (e.g. distraction) and how the person can more effectively keep the therapist engaged (e.g., putting flowers from the garden on their table, sending an occasional card or making a hot drink for their guest). When the person leaves frequent messages or texts the therapist observes their limits, for example only responds to wise mind texts at most once a day or have a scheduled warm telephone conversation contingent on absence of contacting behaviour by the client.

Therapist Consultation Team

As the only ID DBT therapist in the therapist consultation team at a community mental health centre, the focus on mental health versus ID has been difficult for me at times, especially when consultation was about individual clients. More consistent with the DBT model, the focus shifted to what the therapist rather than the client needs, including therapist skills and dialectical dilemmas. This shift allowed us to work across client populations and was felt to be more beneficial for all therapists involved.

DBT assumptions are repeated and regularly reviewed. For example, when tempted to blame a client or support person for target behaviour, the supposition that 'the person is doing the best they can' is revisited.

A Multi-Disciplinary Team Approach

As in Esbensen and Benson (2003), Flynn, Matthews and Hollins (2002) and Mavromatis (2000), experience shows it is important to integrate behavioural, psychological and pharmacological approaches in the DBT based treatment of persons with emotional and behavioural dysregulation.

Outcome

DBT may be effective in treating people with an ID with emotional and behavioural dysregulation with the aim of reducing violent and destructive behaviours (Dunn & Bolton, 2004; Singh, Wahler, Adkins & Myers, 2003). Like Wilson (2001) and Esbensen and Benson (2003), the most dramatic improvements I have seen are cases where serious self-injurious behaviour reduced from several times a month to none over a period of months. Lew,

Matta, Tripp-Tebo and Watts (2006) evaluated the treatment of eight women who presented with moderate risk issues at baseline. All were multi-problem individuals, five of whom were diagnosed with PD. A significant improvement in risk behaviour was measured at 12 and 18 months of treatment, in particular a decrease in self-inflicted injury.

DBT does not only treat impulsive behavioural acts, it also allows the person to become aware of and review the short- and long-term consequences of their target behaviour. This is achieved by the evaluation of good outcomes and bad outcomes, insight into how the target behaviour comes in the way of achieving long-term goals, chain analysis of the behaviour, repairing behavioural damage and the development of their own behavioural management plan. These approaches are likely to offer additional skills useful in a person with sexual offending behaviour if the antisocial behaviour is the agreed target behaviour. Of interest is offering these skills in a non-judgemental framework by allowing the person to discover and evaluate the consequences of the behaviour themselves. The commitment and agreement strategy 'highlighting freedom to choose and absence of alternatives' may be of use here.

Case Vignettes

A person with a mild ID lives in a service for people with high and complex needs. He has not sexually offended for some years. He is committed to achieving his goals of visiting relations overseas and becoming more independent. A contract is drawn up including pictures, outlining the expected behaviours to achieve his goals. Barriers to achieving his goals (target behaviour) include verbal abuse, threats, cutting himself and staying in bed after a perceived conflict. Behaviours to achieve his goals include attending sessions, work and resolving conflict with staff and peers. Modes of treatment that particularly work for him are cheerleading of effective strategies, chain analysis of target behaviour, identification of alternative behaviour and a 'repair'. Cognitions that are challenged are his belief that others are to blame for his negative emotions and behaviours. Coping skills including 'distraction' and 'using the five senses' allow him to act less on feeling mind and improve skills of wise mind. He has shown a commitment to the sessions and homework. His work attendance has improved and he has not cut himself. A referral has been made for a move to a more independent service. He has since visited his relations overseas. Another person with a mild ID and a history of sexual offending appeared well-adjusted in his emotion management. He already had adaptive coping skills and did not show signs of behavioural dysregulation such as self-harm or aggression. During a visit to a public place he re-offended sexually. A chain analysis was attempted; however, he continued to deny that the incident had taken place. This person is less suited to the programme in its current form. His supervision requirements remain high to ensure safety of the public.

CONCLUSIONS

Single case studies and a small-sample study suggest that there is merit in DBT for people with an ID in reducing emotional and behavioural dysregulation including violence, destructive behaviour and self-inflicted injury. DBT for sex offenders may effectively treat coexisting emotional and behavioural dysregulation. This may reduce sexual offending and antisocial behaviours. However, DBT is likely to require further adaptation and integration with CBT and other techniques specific for this population.

DBT may work with people with an ID because it is structured and solution-focussed and the skills are relatively simple. DBT avoids complex rational skills required to discuss traumatic events. Clients feel empowered by learning concepts and skills they recognise, and they have an opportunity to speak honestly about their target behaviours and how this stops them from achieving their long-term goals. DBT accepts and validates the person and at the same time offers alternatives to behaviour. The client is empowered to take part in their own treatment planning. DBT offers a team approach and has been effective in the prevention of staff splitting, staff burn-out and aversive practises. DBT offers a relatively new treatment and worthwhile approach. To be able to utilise the approach effectively and safely, it requires clinicians to seek training in DBT and DBT for people with an ID.

ACKNOWLEDGEMENTS

With thanks to the people with an ID and their support workers who have helped me on my journey to wise mind.

I wish to acknowledge Dr Malcolm Stewart for his encouragement and ongoing support.

REFERENCES

Alexander, R. & Cooray, S. (2003). Diagnosis of personality disorders in learning disability. *The British Journal of Psychiatry, 182*, 28–31.

Alexander, R.T., Piachaud, J., Odebiyi, L. & Gangadharan, S.K. (2002). Referrals to a forensic service in the psychiatry of learning disability. *British Journal of Forensic Practice, 4*, 29–33.

American Psychiatric Association (2000). *Diagnostic and statistical manual of mental disorders*, 4th edn, text revision. Washington, DC: American Psychiatric Association.

Barron, P., Hassiotis, A. & Banes, J. (2002). Offenders with intellectual disability: The size of the problem and therapeutic outcomes. *Journal of Intellectual Disability Research, 46* (6), 454–63.

Broxholme, S.L. & Lindsay, W.R. (2003). Development and preliminary evaluation of a questionnaire on cognitions related to sex offending for use with individuals who have mild intellectual disabilities. *Journal of Intellectual Disability Research, 47* (6), 472–82.

Courtney, J. & Rose, J. (2004). The effectiveness of treatment for male sex offenders with learning disabilities: A review of the literature. *Journal of Sexual Aggression, 10* (2), 215–36.

Craig, L.A. & Hutchinson, R.B. (2005). Sexual offenders with learning disabilities: risk, recidivism and treatment. *Journal of Sexual Aggression 11* (3), 289–304.

Crisis Prevention Institute (2007). *Non-violent crisis intervention*, Brookfield, WI: Crisis Prevention Institute. Retrieved October 17, 2007 from www.crisisprevention.com.

Day, K. (1994). Male mentally handicapped sex offenders. *British Journal of Psychiatry, 165*, 630–9.

Dimeff, L. & Linehan, M.M. (2001). Dialectical behaviour therapy in a nutshell. *The California Psychologist, 34*, 10–13.

Dunn, B.D. & Bolton, W. (2004). The impact of borderline personality traits on challenging behaviour: Implications for learning disability services. *The British Journal of Forensic Practice*, 6 (4), 3–9.

Esbensen, A.J. & Benson, B.A. (2003). Integrating behavioural, psychological and pharmacological treatment: A case study of an individual with borderline personality disorder and mental retardation. *Mental Health Aspects of Developmental Disabilities*, 6, 107–13.

Fletcher, R.J., Loschen, E., Stavrakaki, C. & First, M. (Eds). (2007a). *Diagnostic manual – intellectual disability (DM-ID): A clinical guide for diagnosis of mental disorders in persons with intellectual disability*. Kingston, New York: NADD Press.

Fletcher, R.J., Loschen, E., Stavrakaki, C. & First, M. (Eds). (2007b). *Diagnostic manual – intellectual disability (DM-ID): A textbook of diagnosis of mental disorders in persons with intellectual disability*. Kingston, New York: NADD Press.

Flynn, A., Matthews, H. & Hollins, S. (2002). Validity of the diagnosis of personality disorder in adults with learning disability and severe behavioural problems. *The British Journal of Psychiatry*, 180, 543–6.

Keeling, J.A., Beech, A.R. & Rose, J.L. (2007). Assessment of intellectually disabled sexual offenders: The current position. *Aggression and Violent Behavior*, 12, 229–41.

Kojima, M. & Ikeda, Y. (2001). Relationships between self-regulation and personality scores of persons with Down syndrome. *Perceptual and Motor Skills*, 93 (3), 705–8.

Lew, M., Matta, C., Tripp-Tebo, C. & Watts, D. (2006). Dialectical behavior therapy (DBT) for individuals with intellectual disabilities: A program description. *Mental Health Aspects of Developmental Disabilities*, 9, 1–12.

Linehan, M.M. (1993a). *Cognitive behavioral treatment of borderline personality disorder*. New York: Guilford Press.

Linehan, M.M. (1993b). *Skills training manual for treating borderline personality disorder*. New York: Guilford Press.

Linehan, M.M., Armstrong, H.E., Suarez, A., Allmon, D. & Heard. H.L. (1991). Cognitive-behavioral treatment of chronically parasuicidal borderline patients. *Archives of General Psychiatry*, 48, 1060–4.

Linehan, M.M., Dimeff, L.A., Reynolds, S.K., Comtois, K.A., Welch, S.S., Heagerty, P. & Kivlahan, D.R. (2002). Dialectical behaviour therapy versus comprehensive validation therapy plus 12-step for the treatment of opioid dependent women meeting criteria for borderline personality disorder. *Drug and Alcohol Dependence*, 67, 13–26.

Lindsay, W.R. (2005). Model underpinning treatment for sex offenders with mild intellectual disability: Current theories of sex offending. *Mental Retardation*, 43 (6), 428–41.

Lindsay, W.R., Hogue, T., Taylor, J.L., Mooney, P., Steptoe, L., Johnston, S., O'Brien G. & Smith A. H. W. (2006) Two studies on the prevalence and validity of personality disorder in three forensic intellectual disability samples. *Journal of Forensic Psychiatry*, 17 (3), 485–506.

Lindsay, W.R., Law, J., Quinn, K., Smart, N. & Smith, A. H. W. (2001) A comparison of physical and sexual abuse histories: Sexual and non-sexual offenders with intellectual disability. *Child Abuse and Neglect*, 25, 989–5.

Lindsay, W.R., Smith, A. H. W., Law, J., Quinn, L., Anderson, A., Smith, A., Overend, T. & Allan, R. (2002). A treatment service for sex offenders and abusers with learning disability: Characteristics of referral and evaluation. *Journal of Applied Research in Learning Disabilities*, 15, 166–74.

Lindsay, W.R., Smith, A. H. W., Quinn, K., Anderson, A., Smith, A., Allan, R. & Law, J. (2004). Women with intellectual disability who have offended: Characteristics and outcome. *Journal of Intellectual Disability Research*, 48 (6), 580–90.

McCann, R.A. & Ball, E.M. (1996). Using dialectical behavior therapy with an inpatient forensic population. Workshop presentation at the First Annual Meeting of the International Society for the Improvement and Teaching of Dialectic Behavior Therapy (ISITDBT). New York.

McCann, R.A., Ball, E.M. & Ivanoff, A. (1996). The effectiveness of dialectical behavior therapy in reducing burnout among forensic staff. Unpublished Manuscript.

McCann, R.A., Ball, E.M. & Ivanoff, A. (2000). DBT with an inpatient forensic population: The CMHIP forensic model. *Cognitive and Behavioral Practice, 7*, 447–56.

McCann, R.A., Ivanoff, A., Schmidt, H. & Beach, B. (2007). Implementing dialectical behaviour therapy in residential forensic settings with adults and juveniles. In L.A. Dimeff & K. Koerner (Eds), *Dialectical behavior therapy in clinical practice: Applications across disorders and settings* (pp. 112–38). New York: Guilford Press.

Mann, A.H., Jenkins, R., Cutting, J.C. & Cowan, P.J. (1981). The development and use of a standardized assessment of abnormal personality. *Psychological Medicine, 11*, 839–47.

Matson, J. (1988). *The psychopathology inventory for mentally retarded adults (PIMRA) manual*. Orland Park: International Diagnostic Systems.

Mavromatis, M. (2000). The diagnosis and treatment of borderline personality disorder in persons with developmental disorder: Three case reports. *Mental Health Aspects of Developmental Disability, 3*, 89–97.

Murphy, G.H., O'Callaghan, A.C. & Clare, I. C. H. (2007). The impact of alleged abuse on behaviour in adults with severe intellectual disabilities. *Journal of Intellectual Disability Research, 51* (10), 741–9.

Murphy, G.H., Sinclair, N., Hays, S. & Heaton, K. (2007). *Effectiveness of group cognitive-behavioural treatment for men with learning disabilities at risk of sexual offending*. Report to the Department of Health England. London: DOH.

Naik, B., Gangadharan, S. & Alexander, R. (2002). Personality disorders in learning disability: The clinical experience. *British Journal of Developmental Disability, 48*, 95–100.

Nuechterlein, K. & Dawson, M.E. (1984). A heuristic vulnerability–stress model of schizophrenia. *Schizophrenia Bulletin, 10*, 300–12.

Rathus, J.H. & Miller, A.L. (2002). Dialectical behavior therapy adapted for suicidal adolescents. *Suicide & Life - Threatening Behavior, 32* (2), 146–57.

Reiss, S. (1994). *Manual for the Reiss screen for maladaptive behaviour test*, 2nd edn. Chicago: University of Illinois.

Royal College of Psychiatrists (2001). *Diagnostic criteria for psychiatric disorders for use with adults with ID/mental retardation (DC-LD)*. London: Gaskell.

Sequeira, H., Howlin, P. & Hollins, S. (2003). Psychological disturbance associated with sexual abuse in people with learning disabilities. *The British Journal of Psychiatry, 183*, 451–6.

Singh, N.N., Wahler, R.G., Adkins, A.D. & Myers, R.E. (2003). Soles of the feet: A mindfulness-based self-control intervention for aggression by an individual with mild mental retardation and mental illness. *Research in Developmental Disabilities, 24*, 158–69.

State Government Victoria Department of Justice (2007). *Intellectual disability in the Victorian prison system. Characteristics of prisoners with an intellectual disability released from prison in 2003–2006. Corrections Research Paper Series, 02.* Melborne: Victoria Dept. of Justice.

Swenson, C.R., Torrey, W.C. & Koerner, K. (2002). Implementing dialectical behaviour therapy. *Psychiatric Services, 53* (2), 171–178.

Talbot, T.J. & Langdon, P.E. (2006). A revised sexual knowledge assessment tool for people with intellectual disabilities: Is sexual knowledge related to sexual offending behaviour? *Journal of Mental Deficiency Research, 50* (7), 523–31.

Torr, J. (2003). Personality disorder in intellectual disability. *Current Opinion in Psychiatry, 16* (5), 517–21.

Trupin, E.W., Stewart, D.G., Beach, B. & Boesky, L. (2002). Effectiveness of a dialectical behaviour therapy program for incarcerated female juvenile offenders. *Child and Adolescent Mental Health, 7* (3), 121–7.

Tudway, J.A. & Darmoody, M. (2005). Clinical assessment of adult sexual offenders with learning disabilities. *Journal of Sexual Aggression, 11* (3), 277–88.

Webb, O.J., Verhoeven, M. & Eggleston, E. (2007). Principles of psychological work with adults with intellectual disability. In: I.M. Evans, J.J. Rucklidge & M. O'Driscoll (Eds), *Professional practice of psychology in Aotearoa New Zealand* (pp. 445–65). Wellington: New Zealand Psychological Society.

Wilson, S.R. (2001). A four-stage model for management of borderline personality disorder in people with mental retardation. *Mental Health Aspects of Developmental Disabilities, 4,* 68–76.

World Health Organization (1992). *Tenth Revision of the International Classification of Diseases and Related Health Problems (ICD-10).* Geneva: WHO.

Zubin, J. & Spring, B. (1977). Vulnerability: A new view of schizophrenia. *Journal of Abnormal Psychology, 86,* 103–26.

PART SIX

Future Directions

18

Improving Service Provision for Intellectually Disabled Sexual Offenders

HANNAH FORD AND JOHN ROSE

INTRODUCTION

Considering responses to offending by those with intellectual disabilities (ID) is not a recent trend. As far back as the thirteenth century some crimes committed by those with ID in the UK were pardoned, and individuals could be sent to hospital rather than prison in the early twentieth century (Murphy & Mason, 1999), indicating some historical belief of a need to treat offenders with ID differently to those without. The response to ID offenders has become conflicted in recent history, perhaps partly as a consequence of suggestions by earlier researchers that the presence of ID made individuals more likely to commit offences (see McBrien & Murphy, 2006; Murphy & Mason, 1999). Aside from the (in)accuracy of this, linking offending and ID in this way potentially labelled the ID as a static factor which was not amenable to change (Jahoda, 2002) and which perhaps hindered the development of therapeutic interventions for this group. However, assuming associations between ID and offending perhaps also removed responsibility from individual offenders, particularly when considered alongside beliefs such as 'disability implies an innocence or lack of malicious intent' (ibid., p. 175). If responsibility or intention (*mens rea*) for criminal activity is removed from ID offenders, where do they fit in the criminal justice system (CJS), which is built on ideas of personal agency and punishment (Jahoda, 2002)? However, if we embrace the concept of normalisation and equality, is it a double standard to offer offenders with ID alternative treatment within the CJS (Petersilia, 2000)?

This chapter begins by reviewing possible pathways for ID offenders through the CJS, briefly comparing these components across the UK, USA and Australia, where the greatest quantity of research has been conducted. It moves on to outline programme content, delivery and outcome across different service models and to consider factors in intervening with ID

Assessment and Treatment of Sexual Offenders with Intellectual Disabilities: A Handbook
Edited by Leam A. Craig, William R. Lindsay and Kevin D. Browne
© 2010 John Wiley & Sons, Ltd.

offenders in these different settings. Although it has been necessary to review the literature selectively, the research presented clearly highlights the need for development and improvement at all stages, and recommendations for research and clinical practice are offered. This chapter concentrates on male offenders, primarily those in the mild-to-moderate ID range. Although beyond the scope of this chapter, further consideration should be given to offenders with more severe ID, as well as potential gender-specific needs of women with ID who offend, who, historically, have been under-researched (Cockram, 2005a).

THE INITIAL STAGES: FROM OFFENCE TO COURT APPEARANCE

Although it is not possible to address these issues here comprehensively, brief consideration is important. Initial responses to offending behaviour by those with ID clearly influence subsequent actions. If offences are not reported, help and services for the offender and the victim are limited. If the offences are reported to the police, but the ID is not recognised or appropriately dealt with, this may also have consequences for the offender and the help and services available to him or her. As these initial responses strongly influence those made at later stages, focussing only on decisions made when offenders reach the courts is inappropriate (Cockram, 2005b), and so a brief discussion of research findings is required.

Reporting of Offences

Some research from the UK has suggested a tendency to under-report offences by those with ID. Lyall, Holland and Collins (1995) found high tolerance for offending behaviour among care staff, even when the offending was serious, with less than one-quarter stating that they would always report sexually assaultive behaviour to the police. While these staff were asked to respond to hypothetical situations which do not necessarily indicate responses to real-life situations, any acceptance of such behaviours is concerning. Nor can such responses solely be explained as representing older attitudes, before awareness or consideration of offending by those with ID became greater. McBrien and Murphy's (2006) study, building upon that of Lyall *et al.* (1995), found that while care staff described greater willingness to report assaults and thefts by people with ID to the police, staff were less willing to report rape than they had been in the original study by Lyall *et al.* For all three offence types, McBrien and Murphy (2006) state, care staff's willingness to report was much lower than the police recommended. Although these two studies are not absolutely comparable, as they used different samples and staff grades, and explanations for the decisions made are not elucidated, they both clearly demonstrate how initial reporting decisions impact on subsequent CJS agency involvement. It may be important to investigate further whether the reporting of sexual offences is a particular area of difficulty and concern for staff, and how this could be addressed.

Police Investigation

If the police become involved in offending by someone with an ID, further factors can impact on the offender's experience and subsequent progress through or out of the CJS. Howard and Tyrer (1998) and Murphy and Mason (1999) summarise a number of these factors, including the offender's difficulty in understanding his legal rights, the police caution, the written 'Notice to Detained Persons' or the overall legal process, as well as the increased suggestibility and acquiescence of those with ID, which may lead to self-incrimination and even false confessions.

The Police and Criminal Evidence Act (PACE) 1984 introduced special provisions for vulnerable suspects but, as Murphy and Mason (1999) note, it is often difficult for the police to determine when an individual has an ID and requires these provisions. Assessment of such needs has relied on the judgement of individual officers (Barron, Hassiotis & Banes, 2002), who often had difficulty in distinguishing individuals with ID's from those who were simply poorly educated, relying primarily on the suspect's appearance or behaviour (Howard & Tyrer, 1998). Such difficulties may have been further compounded by individual's attempts to mask their ID, perhaps through embarrassment or fear (Noble & Conley, 1992).

Murphy and Mason (1999) suggest that with the advent of screening by custody sergeants to ensure that available protections are used for those who need them, the situation is changing. This has been aided by the development of tools such as the Hayes Ability Screening Index (HASI), which is being used in a variety of service settings and can be used by the police to identify whether a suspect requires special provisions while they are interviewed or in custody (Hayes, 2005a). As Hayes (2005b) notes, whether or not ID is accurately identified has important implications for the individual offender, for any subsequent court process and for those who must provide a service to the offender.

Sentencing

This stage will not apply to all ID offenders because, as described below, diversion from the CJS before reaching the courts is possible. However, the sentencing stage has important implications for offenders who do reach the courts. Analysing Dutch data, van den Bergh and Hoekman (2006) reported that whether or not an individual had an ID did not appear to be a major factor in furnishing proof or reaching a conviction in cases of sexual offences. Similarly, Cockram (2005b) found that in Western Australia there was little difference between the proportions of those with and without ID who were convicted. However, Cockram did note some major disparities in the types of sentences imposed. Individuals with ID were sent to prison more frequently than those without ID, and where sentencing was carried out, charges of sexual offences were the most likely of any offence committed by a person with ID to receive a custodial sentence. However, sexual offences were also the charges least likely to reach this stage as, among offences charged to those with ID, they were the most commonly dismissed/withdrawn or given a not guilty verdict. Therefore, sentencing of those with ID occurred disproportionately at either end of the penalty scale. Such patterns clearly indicate very divergent possibilities for ID offenders who have committed the same type of offence, from having to deal with prison life, but potentially receiving some form of intervention, to the possibility of receiving no service or support if charges are dismissed.

POSSIBLE DISPOSAL ROUTES FOR ID OFFENDERS

Possible disposal options are influenced by whether or not an individual's ID has been accurately identified. While Hayes (2005b) acknowledges potentially negative consequences from receiving a label of 'ID', she believes the consequences of incorrect or absent diagnosis of ID to be more serious, resulting in offenders being placed inappropriately in services or diverted to the mental health system when they have no mental health needs. Even if ID is accurately diagnosed, however, available options may be limited and attitudes towards this group may be problematic. Murphy (2000), for example, suggests that ID offenders are sometimes turned away from mainstream mental health services as they are believed to be a difficult group to treat. However, they may also be denied access to ID services as they are either thought too able or there are concerns about their risk to other service users.

The main disposal options are prison, probation, mental health services and specialist ID services.

Prison

There is some consensus in the literature that prison is not the most appropriate environment for ID offenders (e.g., Barron, Hassiotis & Banes, 2002; Murphy & Mason, 1999). This view has been shared by legislators; in the UK, the Reed Report (1992) stated that offenders with mental disorder or ID should be placed in community settings when possible (cited in Barron *et al.*, 2002). While diversion from prison is therefore available, the issue remains one of identifying those with ID, a task made more difficult by the fact that the mean IQ of prison inmates is lower than that of the general population (Hayes, 2005a). Although prevalence rates are uncertain, it is clear that the prison population contains offenders with ID, and they may be over-represented in prison populations when compared with the general population prevalence of ID (Cockram, 2005a). Murphy and Mason (1999) note that previous studies demonstrate a higher prevalence rate in US prison populations than in the UK, perhaps owing to the UK diversion policy. However, while Mason and Murphy (2002a) cite several studies from the mid-1990s indicating that few ID offenders go to prison, a recent study by Hayes, Shackell and Mottram (2006) suggested a 10 per cent prevalence rate in HMP Liverpool in the UK. This is compared to national estimates that suggest a rate of 2–3 per cent in the general population (Department of Health, 2001). These differing rates may also reflect variation in the measures used to diagnose ID, as well as potentially differing actual rates over time and between institutions. Petersilia (2000) states that in the USA diversion programmes and intermediate sanctions are not available in many states, and if ID offenders are sent to prison, they tend to remain there longer because of inability to participate in early-release programmes or develop appropriate pre-release plans or on account of their behavioural responses to the difficulties of prison life.

Probation

If offenders with ID are diverted away from the prison system what other disposals are available? Murphy and Mason (1999) hypothesise that, in the UK at least, ID offenders are increasingly receiving community sentences to be served under the supervision of the probation service rather than being sent to prison or hospital. Allam, Middleton and Browne (1997) reported that sex offenders with ID constituted 8 per cent of the West Midlands Probation Service Sex Offender Unit caseload. Mason and Murphy (2002a) reported that nearly 6 per cent of a sample from another UK probation service had ID, while 11 per cent fell into the bottom 5 per cent of the general population in terms of cognitive and social functioning.

Following a different model, Hayes (2004b) describes the permanently-staffed residential programmes in the USA, which focus on living skills, vocational training and individualised 'justice plans' that are monitored until the individual finishes their sentence.

Mental Health Services

The UK Mental Health Act enables individuals to be diverted from the CJS into hospitals if they can be shown to demonstrate 'mental disorder' or 'mental impairment'. Murphy and Mason (1999) suggest that the numbers of individuals detained under the 'mental impairment' category are decreasing. However, Hayes (2005a) contends that individuals with ID who are charged with offences still tend to be diverted into the mental health system, where they will not necessarily receive a finite sentence and may not have mental health needs, while McBrien and Murphy (2006) suggest that being subject to the Mental Health Act is fairly common for ID sex offenders. Part of the problem again lies in different definitions and assessments of ID between service systems, but the fact that the available systems for diverting offenders with mental disorders from the CJS are not clearly paralleled for those with ID (Hayes, 2004a) results in gaps in service provision. However, Green, Gray and Willner (2002) cite a personal communication from Lindsay suggesting that community sentences with conditions of treatment are increasingly being given as courts become more familiar with treatment provisions available in the community.

In the UK, then, some ID offenders are being diverted into mental health services, even if this is not appropriate to their needs. In Australia, meanwhile, diversion from the CJS into hospitals is not possible unless the individual is shown to have a diagnosable psychiatric illness (Hayes, 2004b). While these measures were implemented to prevent ID offenders from being detained indefinitely for a condition from which recovery was not possible, she states, the closure of the mental health route and lack of other specific services for ID offenders has inevitably tended to push them back into the correctional system.

Specialist ID Services

There is a general lack of specialist units and services for ID offenders, which limits the options available to sentencers. Hayes (2004b) notes that some community specialist units are operating in Australia, usually on the sites of former institutions, or within prisons. However, until recently there have been few outcome studies of such units and they tend to focus on managing difficult or vulnerable individuals rather than on treatment/rehabilitation per se. However, recent evaluation of a treatment facility for special needs offenders in the Australian prison system suggests that treatment in this context can be effective (Keeling, Rose & Beech, 2006b; Keeling, Rose & Beech, 2007). Unfortunately Hayes (2004b) notes that specialist units can have very long waiting lists, limiting the options of those required to provide services for ID offenders.

In the UK, the Mental Impairment Evaluation and Treatment Service (MIETS) (Xenitidis, Henry, Russell, Ward & Murphy, 1999) offers individualised assessment and treatment to individuals with ID who have previously been in prison or hospital for challenging and/or offending behaviour. With few inpatient beds, however, there are limited resources available and, as the authors note, inpatient services can be expensive.

PROGRAMME CONTENT AND DELIVERY

The risk-needs-responsivity (RNR) model is currently one of the most influential in the sex offender treatment field (Ward & Brown, 2004). The risk principle states that the most effective treatments are those which match an individual's identified level of risk, while the needs principle states that treatments should directly target criminogenic needs, that is those which are thought to directly reduce the probability of further sexual re-offending. The difficulty, as Keeling, Beech and Rose (2007) point out, is that assessments of risk for ID sex offenders are limited and, they state, no treatment programmes offering different levels of intervention according to individual risk have been identified for this client group.

There has been more work to identify criminogenic needs in sex offenders with ID, including the development of a dynamic risk assessment tool specifically for this client group (the Dynamic Risk Assessment and Management System, developed by Lindsay *et al.*, 2004) and measures of offence-supportive beliefs and attitudes (e.g., the Questionnaire of Attitudes Consistent With Sexual Offending, see Lindsay, Michie, Whitefield, Martin, Grieve & Carson, 2006). Other researchers have used measures designed to assess need in offenders without ID, or have adapted them for this client group (see Keeling, Beech & Rose, 2007, for a review). From this work, as well as that with sexual offenders without ID, researchers have been able to make recommendations for key treatment programme components. Craig, Stringer and Moss (2006) suggest that programmes for ID sex offenders commonly include work to address denial, cognitive distortions and victim empathy, raise awareness of the law and offending behaviour, prevent relapse, develop social and relationship skills, provide sex education and reduce inappropriate sexual arousal. Such components clearly represent a step forward from the pharmacological interventions which have previously been common or the only forms of intervention for ID offenders (Ashman & Duggan, 2002; Lambrick & Glaser, 2004). Aside from the question of whether such interventions are effective in reducing sexual re-offending, there are concerns in using these medications with ID offenders, who may lack the capacity to consent to such treatment and may be less able to report any side-effects (Leonard, Shanahan & Hillery, 2005). However, while there is progress in identifying particular treatment needs for this group, many of those listed above are similar to those for sex offenders without ID. While there may be important areas of overlap, there should be further consideration of whether there are specific needs for the ID group. This is discussed in more detail later in this chapter.

The final element of the RNR model is the responsivity principle. This states that in addition to level of risk and types of need, effective treatments are matched to the learning styles of the offender and take account of both external factors impacting on treatment effectiveness (such as the setting and therapist characteristics) as well as the internal characteristics of the offender that influence his ability to benefit from the intervention (Looman, Dickie & Abracen, 2005). Looman and colleagues state that, in comparison with assessment of risk and need, responsivity factors have received relatively little attention within mainstream sex offender work. Keeling, Beech and Rose (2007) note that some measures of internal responsivity factors for ID offenders are well developed, including those measuring intellectual and adaptive functioning, literacy and comprehension. However, other internal responsivity factors identified in mainstream offender research, such as treatment motivation or interpersonal style (Looman, Dickie & Abracen, 2005), or personality factors, emotional/mental health, or demographic factors (Blanchette & Browne, 2006) may be differentially applicable to ID offenders. Allam,

Middleton and Browne (1997) note that ID sex offenders have often lived in institutions, had limited education and few career opportunities, little or no sexual experience and are aware of their difference from others. As these authors state, 'some of these characteristics are shared by non-disabled sex offenders but facilitators have to be aware of the way in which a learning disability could have affected an individual's life experiences and perceptions as well as his ability to engage in and benefit from treatment' (ibid. p. 75). The learning style of ID sex offenders may also require greater assistance to generalise skills beyond the immediate treatment setting (Griffiths, Watson, Lewis & Stoner, 2004).

TREATMENT IN DIFFERENT SERVICE MODELS

The CJS

The UK prison service offers sex offender programmes to those with a sentence that is sufficiently long to complete the course. While diversion of ID offenders from the prison system has been recommended, it is apparent that some ID offenders are in UK prisons. Developing services to meet their needs is therefore important; as Hayes states, 'even one or two prisoners with ID need to receive appropriate health, education and rehabilitation programmes' (2005a, p. 6). An adapted programme is available for offenders who experience difficulty with the language and literacy skills required in the main core programme (National Probation Directorate, 2002), which would therefore include, but is not exclusively for, ID offenders. The adapted programme is broadly similar in length and frequency to the main programme and is based on CBT principles, although it differs slightly in its focus, concentrating more on increasing sexual knowledge, modifying offence-supportive thinking and recognising risk factors (National Probation Directorate, 2002) and less on victim empathy work. The central targets, then, include many key components identified by Craig, Stringer and Moss (2006), but it focusses less on other social or life skills that ID offenders may lack.

Factors within the prison setting may impact on its treatment programmes. Perhaps foremost of these is the prison ethos itself, in which the primary principles are those of punishment and deterrence while rehabilitation is a secondary aim. The prison environment is unlikely to provide many opportunities for the development, practice and generalisation of social and living skills and may even lead to deterioration in adaptive skills (Cockram, 2005a). Whether programme facilitators have the necessary knowledge and skills for working with ID offenders must also be considered. Researchers have highlighted the high risk of victimisation facing ID prisoners (see ibid.), a risk even higher, perhaps, if they are sex offenders. ID offenders may struggle to cope with prison regimes and rules and find themselves viewed negatively, or at best ambivalently, by other inmates and even prison staff (Glaser & Deane, 1999). Their response to threatening situations may be physical rather than verbal, potentially resulting in further difficulties and sanctions (Petersilia, 2000). Cockram (2005a) notes that most ID prisoners in Western Australia are moved to the only protective unit, which is located within a maximum security prison. If ID offenders are struggling to cope with these difficulties, it may adversely affect their ability to benefit from treatment.

It is perhaps on account of difficulties such as these that Looman, Dickie and Abracen (2005) suggest that appropriate community treatment is generally more effective than that in institutional settings. However, mandating offenders to receive treatment via the criminal justice route can at least ensure they receive intervention, and applying legal pressure to attend may not lead to poorer outcomes (Day, Tucker & Howells, 2004; Linhorst, McCutchen & Bennett, 2003), although research in this area has not specifically addressed those with ID, or those undertaking sex offender programmes. Charging and prosecuting ID offenders can increase the level of specialist support they receive (Jahoda, 2002) and may lessen some difficulties that might otherwise be present in financing long-term treatments for those not subjected to the due process of law (Rose, Jenkins, O'Connor, Jones & Felce, 2002). The question remains, however, whether some of these points could be addressed in a non-prison environment.

The UK prison service's adapted programme has been introduced in community settings with ID offenders on probation over recent years (National Probation Service for England and Wales, 2004). While community-based treatment provides increased opportunity for developing and generalising social and living skills, programme content remains centred around offence-related goals and a probation order still contains a punishment aspect, which may again detract from the development of daily life skills. Hayes (2004b), meanwhile, outlines the Special Offender Services programme in Pennsylvania, USA, which adopts a joint-working approach between the criminal justice and human services systems. Each offender receives intensive supervision, counselling and programmes for specific needs, such as substance abuse, as well as vocational training and placement assistance.

While a probation order can protect ID offenders from the difficulties of imprisonment, it may still pose problems for this group. These include difficulties in reading or understanding the contracts and letters used by the probation service; communication difficulties, either individually or in group treatment programmes; and difficulties in keeping appointments with probation officers, either because of difficulties in telling the time or a failure to understand the importance of these meetings (Mason & Murphy, 2002a). However, Mason and Murphy (ibid.) found that many ID offenders on probation were still living with relatives, suggesting that they may be able to access support and assistance from families in a way that would not be possible in prison.

Mental Health/Specialist Services

Theoretically, the ethos of these services is less focussed on punishment and more on rehabilitation. Community-based services are certainly better placed to teach skills in a more life-realistic setting and to thereby reinforce and generalise them across the individual's daily environment (Lambrick & Glaser, 2004). Rose, Jenkins, O'Connor, Jones and Felce (2002), for example, describe including residential and community staff in their group programme alongside the primary facilitators in order to provide support and facilitate generalisation to the home/work environment of group members. Garrett (2006) suggests that linking with families and carers is particularly important in working with ID offenders as they will be relied upon to help individuals practice and develop skills in their daily environments – something that is clearly less possible in institutions such as prisons or hospitals. Lindsay, Steele, Smith, Quinn and Allan (2006) describe the large number of day centres associated with their service, allowing the majority of clients to be treated in the community and to receive training in daily and community living skills and education or work placements.

However, McBrien and Murphy (2006) suggest that it is often difficult for general community-based services, with differing experience, competence and approaches, to meet the needs of ID offenders. Variations in experience and skills are important external responsivity factors, which may impact on the extent to which an offender benefits from treatment. While a high risk of victimisation and other difficulties have been identified for ID offenders in prison, such risks may also exist in other residential institutions. Hayes (2004b) describes findings from the Community Services Commission and Intellectual Disabilities Rights Service (2001) which states that in one institution almost half of all injuries received by residents came from assaults by other residents and also by staff.

PROGRAMME OUTCOMES

It is important to know what treatments 'work', particularly if we wish to divert ID offenders from prison into other programmes. While there is growing optimism in mainstream sex offender work that treatment can be effective, development of specialised programmes for ID offenders and evaluation of their outcomes has lagged behind (Courtney & Rose, 2004; Wilcox, 2004). Ashman and Duggan (2002), for example, found no randomised controlled trial studies of the effectiveness of interventions for ID sex offenders. Griffiths, Watson, Lewis and Stoner (2004) cite studies reporting lower recidivism rates following community-based, rather than institutionally-based, intervention, but Barron, Hassiotis and Banes (2002) suggest that the efficacy of interventions in different service settings has not been adequately examined. Hayes (2004b) cites work suggesting that detention within a secure hospital has little impact on offending behaviour. It is only recently that specialist units for offenders have undertaken stringent outcome evaluations (Keeling, Rose & Beech, 2006b, 2007). Some community-based programmes are beginning to evaluate outcomes. Rose, Jenkins, O'Connor, Jones & Felce (2002), for example, examined the outcome of a 16-week therapy group for referrals to a specialist ID psychology department. There were no known incidents of re-offending in a one-year period, an overall reduction in attitudes consistent with offending and increased knowledge in relation to the law and sexual behaviour. However, there was also an unexpected increase in locus of control (LOC) scores. Lindsay and Taylor (2005) document a number of case studies by Lindsay and colleagues, in which treatment has produced changes in offence-related cognitions and low rates of re-offending over various follow-up periods.

However, these and other studies suffer from methodological problems. These include small sample sizes and a lack of longitudinal research designs (Hayes, 2004a) as well as widely varying periods of follow-up (Barron, Hassiotis & Banes, 2002). Barron *et al.* outline a number of community-treatment outcome studies, in over half of which participants number 20 or fewer. There are also variations in the definition of ID, with some studies outlined by Barron *et al.* including those with an IQ over 80, as well as those with an IQ below 50 in the same sample, which may mask differential effects according to level of intellectual functioning.

Many studies rely on recidivism rates as their primary outcome measure. This is problematic as it indicates only behaviour that is detected and proceeded with, rather than reflecting all sexual offences actually committed. This is perhaps compounded for ID sex offenders who, as the first part of this chapter indicates, may sometimes find that there is no response to their offending. Whether this alters once an individual has a criminal record is not clear. Similarly, the variation in follow-up periods reduces the extent to which meaningful comparison between re-offence rates can be made across programmes. Barron, Hassiotis and Banes contend that evaluations of treatment efficacy should not be limited to recidivism but should also include assessment of, 'clinical, rehabilitation, humanitarian and public safety domains' (2002, p. 461). Definitions of 'successful outcome' are varied; Xenitidis, Henry, Russell, Ward and Murphy (1999), for example, defined discharge to a community setting as a good outcome from the inpatient MIETS service, although they acknowledge not recording how long patients remained in these placements following discharge. Programmes focussing primarily on offence-related factors may see reduction of these and low recidivism rates as primary indicators of effectiveness; other programmes which seek to develop and generalise life skills may wish to include these as measures of effectiveness. With different aims, approaches and outcome measures, comparison of efficacy across treatments is problematic.

Long-term outcome may also be influenced by factors outside the specific programme aims and setting. The theoretical principles on which ID treatment programmes are based are often drawn from mainstream sex offender work and then adapted. Tudway and Darmoody (2005), however, contend that there is little evidence for the effectiveness of adapting mainstream programmes for ID offenders and, when we do this, we may over-focus on certain elements and neglect other, potentially applicable, components. However, recent research suggests that adapted programmes can be effective for 'special needs' participants when compared to a mainstream group (Keeling & Rose, 2005, Keeling, Rose & Beech, 2007). The ID offender's experience upon completing a programme and returning to the community may also influence whether treatment is ultimately successful. Murphy (2000) noted that many ID individuals who have contact with the CJS are not well known to ID services and have not requested or received special services after leaving school. Cockram (2005a) found that the greatest proportion (59 per cent) of the ID offenders in her prison sample had not been in receipt of any disability services, had higher levels of unemployment than prisoners without ID, were more likely to report being single and more likely to have no educational/training qualifications. Green, Gray and Willner (2002) further noted that criminal convictions were significantly more likely for those with no structured daytime activities which, they comment, is noteworthy as day services form a key part of service provision for those with ID, suggesting that there is a group of individuals whose needs may have been neglected, although it is not known whether such activities were ever offered. Returning to these same difficulties after completing treatment may also impact on its long-term effectiveness.

IMPROVING SERVICE PROVISION

The above summary clearly highlights that improvements and developments are needed in services for ID offenders. The remainder of this chapter discusses these, from initial involvement with the CJS through to improving treatment services, and concludes with suggested developments for post-treatment/post-release provision.

Initial CJS Involvement

There are potential discrepancies and inequalities in initial responses to offending behaviour by those with ID, suggesting that the initial stages of this process need more detailed examination, particularly regarding whether or how offenders enter the CJS. As Cockram states, there is little point in debating 'new sentencing procedures if the greatest impact and inequity occurs at the point of apprehension' (2005b, p. 3). Petersilia (2000) lists a number of areas requiring improvement, including education/training, developing assessments for ID and increasing availability of appropriate disposal routes for ID offenders.

Education/Training

Education and training regarding ID and offending should perhaps have three main target groups. As the consequences for individuals depend in part on initial decisions of whether or not to report offending, education programmes need to be directed at those likely to be making such decisions, particularly, perhaps, care staff. Some challenging behaviours may be difficult to distinguish from offending (Lyall, Holland & Collins, 1995), and some staff might fear reporting sexual behaviour that is not clearly an offence to be a return to the past desexualisation and suppression of sexuality in those with ID (see Yool, Langdon & Garner, 2003). However, as described previously, staff may also be unwilling to report clear instances of sexual assault. Training about sexual behaviour and sexual offending may therefore be important. McConkey and Ryan (2001) found that while a large proportion of care staff had encountered sexually inappropriate behaviour during the course of their work only 22 per cent reported receiving training in sexuality issues, although neither their training or work experiences related specifically to sexual offending. Whether responding to allegations of sexual offending raises particular difficulties for staff should be investigated, including reasons for reporting or not reporting such behaviours. Training is unlikely to be a complete solution, however; McConkey and Ryan found that staff who had previously encountered their hypothetical sexual scenarios rated themselves as more confident in dealing with similar future scenarios and confidence ratings were not influenced by previous training. Of course, this gives no indication of the actual response of staff to incidents, and most of the research scenarios did not relate to sexual offending.

Care staff could be supported further by development of clear policies for dealing with allegations and routine training in implementing these. Such policies do not seem to be universally available; only 39 per cent of staff at care homes registered for those with ID but without mental disorder reported policies or guidance regarding offending by those with ID (McBrien & Murphy, 2006). Policy development may lessen the vagaries of individual decision-making but, more importantly, may help staff feel more supported in reporting; McBrien and Murphy (ibid.) found that nearly half (48 per cent) of the care staff in their sample feared some form of criticism for reporting rape.

A second group for whom education and training is important is CJS professionals. As they form the initial point of involvement, it is important that the police increase their ability to recognise ID, particularly acknowledging that ID may not be immediately physically apparent and that individuals may attempt to disguise their difficulties. It is also important to increase awareness of particular difficulties that those with ID may have in terms of understanding, responding to interview questions and in their tendency towards acquiescence. Petersilia (2000) suggests a need to routinely educate all CJS personnel about how to accommodate those with ID throughout the CJS process, to provide an enhanced availability of expert witnesses to give information about ID and to train appropriate adults to assist ID offenders through the process. Finally, Howard and Tyrer (1998) note that juries may also need assistance to recognise the potential unreliability of confessions made by those with ID. However, it is clear that in order for legal professionals to assist and advise juries in this way they will require sufficient knowledge and understanding themselves. This issue has been recognised in England and Wales, where criminal justice professionals now have best practice guidance to turn to when working with individuals who have a learning disability along with advice on how to support them effectively within the context of current legislation (Care Services Improvement Partnership, 2007).

Petersilia (2000) additionally suggests that those with ID and their families/carers need education about the justice system and what to do should they come into contact with the police. This could include education about their legal rights and ways of avoiding victimisation or becoming involved in criminal activities either through inadequate knowledge of unlawful behaviour or through pressure from others.

Assessing ID

The research literature suggests that pre-trial identification of ID is poor in the CJS (Murphy & Mason, 1999). While education and training could certainly help to raise awareness of important issues, they are not sufficient to improve identification and assessment. Screening tools have been developed to assist with this, although, as Mason and Murphy (2002b) note, this is not an easy task as these screens must be brief, practical, easy to administer/interpret and also accurate.

The HASI takes up to 10 minutes to administer and contains a small number of brief subtests. As Hayes (2005a) notes, the HASI does not give a diagnosis of ID but instead indicates individuals who require full-scale diagnostic assessments. Mason and Murphy (2002a) developed the Learning Disabilities in the Probation Service (LIPS) assessment to screen individuals' cognitive and social functioning. This tool uses one verbal and one non-verbal test of cognitive functioning and includes questions relating to social functioning, although only those that assess an individual's ability to cope with the CJS (Mason & Murphy, 2002b). The LIPS assessment was designed for the UK probation service and has so far been validated on a much smaller sample than the HASI. Furthermore, the LIPS has primarily been validated with adult male offenders while the HASI has been validated with males, females and adolescents (Hayes, 2005a). Construction of practical and accurate assessment measures is an important step and further development and refinement, alongside increased awareness of their rationale and importance may be important in improving our responses to ID offenders. More care with general assessment also needs to follow after individuals who may have ID have been identified; for example, more emphasis could be placed on assessing adaptive behaviour rather than concentrating on intellectual assessment alone (Keeling, Beech & Rose, 2007).

Response Rationales

There is a risk in assuming that 'if individuals with mental retardation were identified they would be appropriately served' (Petersilia, 2000, p. 9) as this is unlikely to occur until we determine appropriate responses for individuals identified by these assessments and place them in services that are likely to benefit them. This raises two issues. The first queries our understanding of what is beneficial; Simpson and Hogg (2001), for example, contend that there is an assumption in the UK that ID offenders should be diverted from the CJS, yet, they state, there is little empirical evaluation of whether diversion actually benefits individuals, either by enhancing quality of life or reducing re-offending. The second issue is how we decide which services offenders are placed in. Glaser and Deane (1999), for example, compared the characteristics of a small sample of ID offenders who had been either admitted to an intensive residential treatment programme or imprisoned. While acknowledging their small sample size, the authors reported that although these two settings should serve different populations there were in fact strong similarities between those in each setting. Furthermore, if individuals were transferred between settings the rationale for so doing tended 'to be arbitrary and ill-defined' (ibid., p. 347). Murphy (2000) suggests that decisions about care pathways are typically made at times of crisis, such as following a re-offence, and as such are reactions rather than considered plans for the future. The RNR model described earlier recommends allocating individuals to programmes according to risk level, but this is currently difficult with ID sex offenders.

Identifying ID offenders, then, is only the first step; we need to examine further possible disposal options and their likely benefit and to think more clearly about how to allocate services. It is also important to consider how to make service provision more consistent across regions and less ad hoc in nature. There could also be a role for a programme accreditation scheme, paralleling that for the UK prison and probation service non-ID sex offender programmes, to examine effectiveness and provide best practice guidelines.

Treatment

To improve treatment services, a number of areas need to be considered, which are outlined below. Limitations of space preclude complete discussion of each of these, but key areas are highlighted for further consideration and empirical study.

Programme Content and Assessment of Need

As the earlier discussion highlighted, many programme components suggested for ID offenders are broadly similar to those for offenders without ID. While there is evidence that these components are successful in reducing recidivism in ID offenders (see Lindsay, Steele, Smith, Quinn & Allan, 2006) there remains a need to further consider specific needs of ID offenders and whether needs assumed to be similar have different levels of importance for ID sex offenders.

LOC, for example, has been linked with the successful completion of treatment programmes in non-ID offenders (Fisher, Beech & Browne, 1998), and an external LOC at the end of treatment represents a non-positive outcome. However, some studies have indicated that a more external LOC is frequently found among those with ID (Langdon & Talbot, 2006), raising questions about whether LOC is related to treatment outcome for ID sex offenders. Langdon and Talbot's own study compared ID sex offenders (who had or had not undertaken treatment) and ID non-offenders on a measure of LOC and cognitive distortions. While the treatment group scored significantly lower on the cognitive distortion measure there were no significant differences among the three groups in terms of LOC, with all participants' scores indicating external LOC. Although their sample size was too small for firm conclusions to be drawn and, as the authors note, the treatment group received a variety of interventions, the fact that treatment appeared to have reduced cognitive distortions but not altered LOC, raises the question of whether LOC is related to treatment outcome for ID offenders in the same way as non-ID offenders and of its relevance as a treatment component. Similarly, Rose, Jenkins,

O'Connor, Jones and Felce (2002) found that LOC became more external over the course of their treatment programme, despite improvement on other outcome measures. However, it may be that LOC measures used in these studies are less appropriate for those with ID, although this would not necessarily explain the increased LOC in their study.

While LOC is therefore potentially a component of mainstream sex offender programmes which is of less relevance to outcome in ID offender treatment, the emphasis placed on increasing sexual knowledge among ID sex offenders appears greater than in mainstream programmes. Talbot and Langdon (2006) noted that poor sexual knowledge has been found in individuals with ID, and they reported that their small sample of non-ID participants scored significantly higher on a measure of sexual knowledge than those with ID. While it is in no way suggested that increasing sexual knowledge should not be a treatment goal, why this is a key aim in many ID programmes, while other life skills/knowledge are less central, is curious, perhaps indicating a belief that limited sexual knowledge contributes to sexual offending in ID offenders more specifically. Talbot and Langdon feel that the similarly low sexual knowledge scores in their untreated offenders and non-offender groups suggest that poor sexual knowledge is not a central risk factor for ID offending, although their small sample prohibits definitive conclusions. Perhaps we need to consider further why increasing sexual knowledge forms a key target when there is little investigation of how it impacts on outcome (Barron, Hassiotis & Banes, 2002; Talbot & Langdon, 2006). Such focus may be warranted, but at present there is little research to demonstrate this.

While there is evidence of the need to include some factors from mainstream work, such as cognitive distortions, into work with ID offenders, other aspects of mainstream treatment, such as LOC, may have different levels of relevance or importance. Important factors for both groups may still require slightly different focus in working with ID offenders. Work to address non-ID offenders' own experiences of victimisation, for example, is available in many treatment programmes but may be more important for ID offenders, as those with ID may experience higher levels of victimisation (Sobsey, 1994) and may receive less help if they report it. Wilcox (2004) notes that involvement in such groups has helped ID offenders to progress more effectively through their main treatment programme.

Ward, Mann and Gannon (2007) argue that the predominant RNR model advocates reducing, removing or modifying negative factors rather than attempting to positively equip offenders to lead better lives. Should programmes for ID offenders therefore place greater focus on developing skills for daily living, including those needed in relationships, employment and/or leisure, and how these could be promoted outside the treatment setting? This may require more than skills training. Steptoe, Lindsay, Forrest and Power (2006) reported that the social relationships of ID sex offenders were poorer than those of a non-offender group and that the offenders also made less use of leisure facilities. Interestingly, however, the offenders indicated that they were content with these poorer relationships, either, the authors suggest, because they have adapted to their situation or because they believe that there is little likelihood of improvement. Thus, work may have to go beyond simple skills-based teaching to address individuals' beliefs about themselves and their social situation.

Theoretical Underpinnings

Ward, Mann and Gannon (2007) additionally argue that the RNR model's focus on reducing negative factors risks a 'one-size-fits all approach to treatment' (p. 89), limiting consideration of whether all offenders have the same needs. This raises two questions: firstly, do ID offenders share the treatment needs of non-ID sex offenders and, secondly, do all ID sex offenders have similar needs, or are there differences across offender/offence types? Such questions need to be addressed in theories underpinning treatment programmes. The previous section has briefly considered whether sex offenders with and without ID have similar treatment needs, and further exploration of this issue is recommended.

Mainstream sex offender research is beginning to examine different needs across offender types. The self-regulation model (Ward, Hudson & Keenan, 1998) proposes that offenders follow different 'pathways' to a sexual offence according to their self-regulation style and their particular goals. Bickley and Beech (2002) tested this model with non-ID sex offenders and suggested that offenders following different paths have different treatment needs. This model has also been considered in relation to ID and special needs offenders; a review of the literature suggests that there should be some differences between ID and mainstream offenders (Keeling & Rose, 2006). The Good Lives model (Ward, Mann & Gannon, 2007) proposes even more individualised formulation, considering the specific internal skills/capabilities and external conditions that are required for each offender to achieve the outcomes important to him, which may previously have been achieved through offending. Both these models argue for more individualised treatment rather than assuming a common set of needs.

A noteworthy feature is the multifactorial nature of these models, compared with theoretical understanding of ID sex offending. In reviewing theories of sexual offending by men with ID, Lindsay (2004) describes factors such as mental illness, impulsivity, sexual abuse history, 'counterfeit deviance' or actual deviant preferences, mediated by cognitive distortions and inappropriate sexual arousal, all of which are primarily single-factor hypotheses and lack the complexity of theories of non-ID sexual offending. Research is required to determine whether models of non-ID offending sufficiently describe offending by those with ID or whether we need ID-specific models which are 'informed by, and sensitive to, unique developmental and socialisation influences to address the underlying motivation driving such behaviours' (Tudway & Darmoody, 2005, p. 285). These theories should drive the development of treatment programmes.

Researchers have examined the self-regulation model in an ID offender group. Keeling, Rose and Beech (2006a) used Bickley and Beech's (2002) methodology to classify 'special needs' sex offenders to one of the four possible pathways. However, as these special needs offenders share characteristics of sex offenders both with and without ID, it remains unclear to which group they are most similar and whether the self-regulation model has validity with ID offenders (for further detail see this volume, Chapter 4). The Good Lives Model (Ward, Mann & Gannon, 2007) may also have relevance for ID offenders, with its focus on developing the internal and external skills/capabilities required to obtain desired human 'goods'. Such 'goods', including sexual satisfaction, personal agency, or relatedness to others (see Ward & Brown, 2004), may often be lacking in disadvantaged groups, such as people with ID. Steptoe, Lindsay, Forrest and Power's (2006) research suggested that ID sex offenders may have poorer social relationships than non-offenders (good of 'relatedness to others'), while likelihood of conviction was related to poorer access to day activities (Green, Gray & Willner, 2002) (good of 'excellence in work and play'), suggesting that offenders may need assistance in developing capabilities and/or opportunities for achieving these goods. However, while areas of relevance for ID offenders can be identified in these theories it may yet be more beneficial to develop specific models for this group. This is an area for further research.

Finally, some work has focussed on developing the accounts of ID sex offenders and their therapists into a model of offending (Courtney, Rose & Mason, 2006). Using grounded theory, a qualitative approach, it has been possible to develop a model of offending behaviour. The process model developed has many similarities with models developed within the mainstream sex offending literature, suggesting considerable similarities and justifying the adaptation of treatment and other strategies to offenders with ID.

Outcomes

Further research is needed to identify which particular components of programmes are effective in treating ID offenders, to develop any which are not yet targeted and to incorporate these into clinical practice.

Process Variables

As part of the responsivity principle, researchers have outlined ways of adapting ID offender programmes to increase individual receptivity, including the use of drawings, videos and other visual aids, greater repetition of material and reduced content for each session (Allam, Middleton & Browne, 1997; Craig, Stringer & Moss, 2006; Keeling & Rose, 2005). Craig, Stringer and Moss report that most ID treatment groups run for at least one year, the minimum duration they recommend. However, Lindsay and Smith (1998) found that with only one year of treatment, offenders continued to hold offence-supportive attitudes and were more likely to re-offend. Those receiving two years of treatment, meanwhile, had much more positive outcomes on both these measures.

However, it seems important to go beyond these factors and consider other process variables that may impact on treatment effectiveness. That little emphasis has so far been placed on this in ID programmes may reflect both the nascency of many programmes, and the fact that consideration of these issues is only just beginning in mainstream sex offender work. However, engaging and motivating ID sex offenders may be particularly important if we are going to advocate lengthy periods of treatment. One element of this is the group process itself, which has long been the primary method for sex offender treatment but which is heavily influenced by the interactions within it. Clear differences have been found between groups in terms of their group climate, even when they are running the same programme (Beech & Hamilton-Giachritsis, 2005). Studying non-ID sex offenders in prisons, these authors found that cohesive groups (in which members felt involved, committed and concerned for other members) and groups which encouraged expression of feelings led to reductions in offence-supportive attitudes. Given the difficulties of some ID offenders with social skills, self-esteem and communication, dynamics within groups may be particularly important. As Rose, Jenkins, O'Connor, Jones and Felce note, many men declined to participate in group work as they did not want to discuss their problems in a group and even among those who did accept, 'there was a wariness (bordering on suspicion) and caution' (2002, p.149) in the initial sessions. Of course, this may not be very different to early sessions of non-ID offender groups, but social/communication difficulties may make this harder to deal with, particularly in short-term programmes, such as these authors describe. Craig, Stringer and Moss (2006) also report one ID group member whose anxiety appeared heightened in the group setting, who contributed little and was often unable to engage, even when prompted. This may have a negative impact on factors such as self-esteem. Rose *et al.* (2002) noted that men who had already undertaken individual work were more likely to accept a place in the group, which may become a prerequisite for future groups.

Programme staff bring another dynamic to the treatment process. Staff from a variety of backgrounds contribute to the development and delivery of programmes, potentially influencing their responses to and interactions with offenders. This raises the issue of whether group facilitators should be forensic specialists, experienced ID workers or both. Wilcox (2004) suggests that because ID sex offenders are dispersed throughout the CJS and mental health systems, no one professional group has the resources or expertise for working with them. Leonard, Shanahan and Hillery (2005) similarly advocate work being conducted by multidisciplinary teams with both forensic and ID expertise.

Perhaps more important, however, are the characteristics of staff and their interactions with offenders and the impact of this on treatment outcome. Marshall *et al.* (2003) outline some of the therapist characteristics they believe to be important in working with sexual offenders. While these are likely to be similar for offenders with and without ID, some characteristics may be comparatively more important in working with ID offenders, particularly if staff are not ID specialists. Therapist warmth and respect, for example, may be particularly important. As people with ID are typically a marginalised and undervalued group this, combined with a label of 'offender', may compound negative responses from others, including service providers. The need to be treated warmly, respectfully and genuinely, therefore, may assume additional importance in this group. Similarly, Marshall *et al.* advocate therapist qualities such as flexibility, appropriate directiveness and encouragement to participate. These may be particularly important for ID offenders in a group setting, in which level of functioning can vary considerably between members, in which more initial therapist direction may be needed and in which increased participation may be better achieved through methods that rely less on verbal strategies. Drapeau (2005) reported that non-ID child molesters undergoing a prison-based programme expressed a wish for greater 'mastery' – increased independence and opportunity to make some decisions on their own. It is worth considering whether similar feelings might occur in ID offenders; for those living in care homes, for example, limited independence and decision-making may be a daily fact of life. The question of whether there is a similar desire for mastery among ID offenders may benefit from further investigation as this could relate to the 'goods' they want to achieve and may have implications for the settings in which treatment takes place.

Post-Treatment/Post-Release Services

Long-term outcomes may depend not just on the treatment programme itself, but also upon the situation to which offenders return following completion of it. Hayes (2005a) states that post-treatment provision for ID offenders requires cooperation between services and long-term focus, including accommodation services, continuing life skills or other specialist programmes and appropriate healthcare. One of the biggest difficulties may be finding appropriate accommodation; Cockram (2005a) suggests that it is difficult to locate accommodation for a person who has an ID, more so if they have served a prison sentence, particularly for a sexual offence. Alexander, Crouch, Halstead and Piachaud (2006) emphasise the importance of appropriate placements upon release. While their sample was small and patients from a medium secure unit may not be representative of all ID offenders, they found that patients leaving a medium secure service who had to change residence during the follow-up phase were four times more likely to be readmitted to hospital. They argue that this adds empirical support to clinical impressions that placement difficulties and subsequent moves increase the likelihood of re-offending and re-admission, thereby highlighting the importance of aftercare. One difficulty involves identifying which services have responsibility for providing and monitoring long-term care needs and integrating the specific needs of each individual, which stresses the need for interagency working. This is achievable: Petersilia (2000) describes the 'Passports To Learning' programme in the USA, in which the prison programme is supplemented by post-release programmes, including continued counselling and skills programmes and attention to education and vocational needs. However, this is an independent scheme not run by the government. More thought should be directed to developing such working in the public sector. This suggests that services should be redesigned with the very specific needs of these clients in mind. For example in the UK, to serve populations of a reasonable size with an appropriately skilled group of staff, alternative service configurations need to be considered. Many residential treatment programmes serve relatively large geographical areas. In a similar way community treatment and follow-up services could be organised at a regional level to ensure that sufficient numbers of staff with appropriate experience are available to provide effective and efficient services and to develop new services and treatments for ID sex offenders.

CONCLUSIONS

There remains much to be done to manage and treat ID sex offenders effectively. Efforts need to be made to apply existing theory to this group of sex offenders in a systematic way and to use this to guide the development of services and interventions. Nevertheless, there are still a large number of actions that can be taken now to develop services. Improving education and training for staff and carers at all levels, particularly in relation to the recognition of ID in the CJS would seem to be an important goal. Hopefully this could lead to prevention and minimisation of offending and will lead to a more consistent approach to the provision of services and effective management of offenders. More resources are also needed to develop treatment approaches and monitor the outcome of treatments, particularly for offenders with more severe ID. However, developments are required not only in the area of therapeutic provision but also in the way treatment programmes are delivered and organised. It would seem important to provide more opportunities for treatment in community settings for this group.

Community services could provide effective treatment and supervision options for some offenders without the necessity of moving away to a residential treatment provision if sufficient support and expertise is available locally. Those who do need to be treated in residential settings will also benefit from the opportunity to develop new skills in the community after their residential treatment while it will be ensured that appropriate supervision is provided to minimise risk. Having stronger community services may also help local services develop specific skills in working with offenders with ID and may facilitate the development of the early intervention and prevention programmes that seem to be missing from the range of services currently available.

Developing a broader range of potential service responses should facilitate more person-centred responses to offenders with ID, from identifying who is at risk through managing the response to offenders and the provision of treatment in appropriate settings followed by the ongoing management of risk. These changes will not only require more research but also service developments that lead to innovative patterns of service delivery and ultimately less offending and effective rehabilitation of offenders.

REFERENCES

Alexander, R.T., Crouch, K., Halstead, S. & Piachaud, J. (2006). Long-term outcome from a medium-secure service for people with intellectual disability. *Journal of Intellectual Disability Research, 50* (4), 305–15.

Allam, J., Middleton, D. & Browne, K. (1997). Different clients, different needs? Practice issues in community-based treatment for sex offenders. *Criminal Behaviour and Mental Health, 7,* 69–84.

Ashman, L. & Duggan, L. (2002). Interventions for learning disabled sex offenders. *Cochrane Database of Systematic Reviews,* 2002, Issue 2.

Barron, P., Hassiotis, A. & Banes, J. (2002). Offenders with intellectual disability: The size of the problem and therapeutic outcomes. *Journal of Intellectual Disability Research, 46* (6), 454–63.

Beech, A.R. & Hamilton-Giachritsis, C.E. (2005). Relationship between therapeutic climate and treatment outcome in group-based sexual offender treatment programmes. *Sexual Abuse: A Journal of Research and Treatment, 17* (2), 127–40.

van den Bergh, P.M., & Hoekman, J. (2006). Sexual offences in police reports and court dossiers: A case-file study. *Journal of Applied Research in Intellectual Disabilities, 19,* 374–82.

Bickley, J.A. & Beech, A.R. (2002). An investigation of the Ward and Hudson pathways model of the sexual offence process with child abusers. *Journal Of Interpersonal Violence, 17* (4), 371–93.

Blanchette, K. & Browne, S.L. (2006). *The Assessment and Treatment of Women Offenders.* Chichester: John Wiley & Sons.

Care Services Improvement Partnership (2007). *Positive practice, positive outcomes: A handbook for professionals in the criminal justice system working with people with learning disabilities.* London: Department of Health.

Cockram, J. (2005a). People with an intellectual disability in the prisons. *Psychiatry, Psychology & Law, 12* (1), 163–73.

Cockram, J. (2005b). Justice or differential treatment? Sentencing of offenders with an intellectual disability. *Journal of Intellectual & Developmental Disability, 30* (1), 3–13.

Community Services Commission and Intellectual Disabilities Rights Service (2001). *Crime prevention in residential services for people with disabilities: A discussion paper.* Surry Hills, NSW: Community Services Commission and the Intellectual, Disability Rights Service.

Courtney, J. & Rose, J. (2004). The effectiveness of treatment for male sex offenders with learning disabilities. *Journal of Sexual Aggression, 10* (2), 215–36.

Courtney, J., Rose, J. & Mason, O. (2006). The offence process of sex offenders with intellectual disabilities: A qualitative study. *Sexual Abuse: A Journal of Research and Treatment, 18* (2), 169–92.

Craig, L.A., Stringer, I. & Moss, T. (2006). Treating sexual offenders with learning disabilities in the community: A critical review. *International Journal of Offender Therapy and Comparative Criminology, 50* (4), 369–90.

Day, A., Tucker, K. & Howells, K. (2004). Coerced offender rehabilitation – a defensible practice? *Psychology, Crime & Law, 10* (3), 259–69.

Department of Health (2001). *Valuing People: A new strategy for learning disability for the 21st century.* London: The Stationery Office.

Drapeau, M. (2005). Research on the processes involved in treating sexual offenders. *Sexual Abuse: A Journal of Research and Treatment, 17* (2), 117–25.

Fisher, D., Beech, A. & Browne, K. (1998). Locus of control and its relationship to treatment change and abuse history in child sexual abusers. *Legal and Criminological Psychology, 3,* 1–12.

Garrett, H. (2006). Development of a community-based sex offender treatment programme for adult male clients with a learning disability. *Journal of Sexual Aggression, 12* (1), 63–70.

Glaser, W. & Deane, K. (1999). Normalisation in an abnormal world: A study of prisoners with an intellectual disability. *International Journal of Offender Therapy and Comparative Criminology, 43* (3), 338–56.

Green, G., Gray, N.S. & Willner, P. (2002). Factors associated with criminal convictions for sexually inappropriate behaviour in men with learning disabilities. *The Journal of Forensic Psychiatry, 13* (3), 578–607.

Griffiths, D.M., Watson, S.L., Lewis, T. & Stoner, K. (2004). Sexuality research and persons with intellectual disabilities. In E. Emerson, C. Hatton, T. Thompson & T. R. Parmenter (Eds), *The international handbook of applied research in intellectual disability* (pp. 311–34). Chichester: John Wiley & Sons.

Hayes, S. (2004a). Interaction with the criminal justice system. In E. Emerson, C. Hatton, T. Thompson & T. R. Parmenter (Eds), *The international handbook of applied research in intellectual disability* (pp. 479–94). Chichester: John Wiley & Sons.

Hayes, S. (2004b). Pathways for offenders with intellectual disabilities. In W. L., Lindsay J. L. Taylor & P. Sturmey (Eds), *Offenders with developmental disabilities* (pp. 67–89). Chichester: John Wiley & Sons.

Hayes, S. (2005a). *Prison Services and Offenders With Intellectual Disability – The Current State of Knowledge and Future Directions*. Paper presented at the Fourth International Conference on the Care and Treatment of Offenders With a Learning Disability. Preston, UK, 6–8 April. Available from www.ldoffenders.co.uk/conferences/4thCon2005/4thConFiles/PrisonServicesSusanHayes.doc.

Hayes, S.C. (2005b). Diagnosing intellectual disability in a forensic sample: Gender and age effects on the relationship between cognitive and adaptive functioning. *Journal of Intellectual & Developmental Disability, 30* (2), 97–103.

Hayes, S., Shackell, P. & Mottram, P. (2006). Identifying intellectual disability in a UK prison. *Abstracts of the Second International Conference of IASSID Europe, Journal of Applied Research in Intellectual Disabilities, 19* (3), 256.

Howard, T.J. & Tyrer, S.P. (1998). Editorial. People with learning disabilities in the criminal justice system in England and Wales: A challenge to complacency. *Criminal Behaviour and Mental Health, 8,* 171–7.

Jahoda, A. (2002). Offenders with a learning disability: The evidence for better services? *Journal of Applied Research in Intellectual Disabilities, 15,* 175–8.

Keeling, J.A., Beech, A.R. & Rose, J.L. (2007). Assessment of intellectually disabled sexual offenders: The current position. *Aggression and Violent Behavior, 12,* 229–41.

Keeling, J. & Rose, J. (2005). Relapse prevention with intellectually disabled sexual offenders. *Sexual Abuse: A Journal of Research and Treatment, 17* (4), 407–23.

Keeling, J. & Rose, J. (2006). The adaptation of a cognitive-behavioural treatment programme for special needs sexual offenders relapse prevention with intellectually disabled sexual offenders. *British Journal of Learning Disabilities, 34* (2), 110–6.

Keeling, J., Rose, J. & Beech, A. (2006a). A comparison of the application of the self-regulation model of the relapse process for mainstream and special needs sexual offenders. *Sexual Abuse: A Journal of Research and Treatment, 18,* 373–82.

Keeling, J., Rose, J. & Beech, T. (2006b). A preliminary investigation into the effectiveness of an Australian custody-based cognitive-behavioural treatment for special needs sexual offenders. *British Journal of Forensic Psychiatry and Psychology, 17* (3), 372–92.

Keeling, J., Rose, J. & Beech, A. (2007). A comparison of the treatment efficacy of sexual offender programs for special needs and non-special needs sexual offenders. *Journal of Intellectual and Developmental Disabilities.*

Lambrick, F. & Glaser, W. (2004). Sex offenders with an intellectual disability. *Sexual Abuse: A Journal of Research and Treatment, 16* (4), 381–92.

Langdon, P.E. & Talbot, T.J. (2006). Locus of control and sex offenders with an intellectual disability. *International Journal of Offender Therapy and Comparative Criminology, 50* (4), 391–401.

Leonard, P., Shanahan, S. & Hillery, J. (2005). Recognising, assessing and managing offending behaviour in persons with intellectual disability. *Irish Journal of Psychological Medicine, 22* (3), 107–12.

Lindsay, W.R. (2004). Sex offenders: Conceptualisation of the issues, services, treatment and management. In W. L. Lindsay, J. L. Taylor & P., Sturmey (Eds), *Offenders with developmental disabilities* (pp. 163–85). Chichester: John Wiley & Sons.

Lindsay, W.R., Michie, A.M., Whitefield, E., Martin, V., Grieve, A. & Carson, D. (2006). Response patterns on the questionnaire on attitudes consistent with sexual offending in groups of sex offenders with intellectual disabilities. *Journal of Applied Research in Intellectual Disabilities, 19*, 47–53.

Lindsay, W.R., Murphy, L., Smith, G., Murphy, D., Edwards, Z., Chittock, C., Grieve, A. & Young, S.J. (2004). The Dynamic Risk Assessment and Management System: An assessment of immediate risk of violence for individuals with offending and challenging behavior. *Journal of Applied Research in Intellectual Disabilities, 17*, 267–74.

Lindsay, W.R. & Smith, A. H. W. (1998). Responses to treatment for sex offenders with intellectual disability: A comparison of men with 1- and 2-year probation sentences. *Journal of Intellectual Disability Research, 42* (5), 346–53.

Lindsay, W.L., Steele, L., Smith, A. H. W., Quinn, K. & Allan, R. (2006). A community forensic intellectual disability service: Twelve-year follow-up of referrals, analysis of referral patterns and assessment of harm reduction. *Legal and Criminological Psychology, 11*, 113–30.

Lindsay, W.R. & Taylor, J.L. (2005). A selective review of research on offenders with developmental disabilities: Assessment and treatment. *Clinical Psychology & Psychotherapy, 12*, 201–14.

Linhorst, D.M., McCutchen, T.A. & Bennett, L. (2003). Recidivism among offenders with developmental disabilities participating in a case management program. *Research in Developmental Disabilities, 24*, 210–30.

Looman, J., Dickie, I. & Abracen, J. (2005). Responsivity issues in the treatment of sexual offenders. *Trauma, Violence & Abuse, 6* (4), 330–53.

Lyall, I., Holland, A.J. & Collins, S. (1995). Offending by adults with intellectual disabilities and the attitudes of staff to offending behaviour: Implications for service development. *Journal of Intellectual Disability Research, 39*, 501–8.

McBrien, J. & Murphy, G. (2006). Police and carers' views on reporting alleged offences by people with intellectual disabilities. *Psychology, Crime & Law, 12* (2), 127–44.

McConkey, R. & Ryan, D. (2001). Experiences of staff in dealing with client sexuality in services for teenagers and adults with intellectual disability. *Journal of Intellectual Disability Research, 45* (1), 83–7.

Marshall, W.L., Fernandez, Y.M., Serran, G.A., Mulloy, R., Thornton, D., Mann, R.E. & Anderson, D. (2003). Process variables in the treatment of sexual offenders: A review of the relevant literature. *Aggression and Violent Behavior, 8*, 205–34.

Mason, J. & Murphy, G.H. (2002a). People with intellectual disabilities on probation: An initial study. *Journal of Community & Applied Social Psychology, 12*, 44–55.

Mason, J. & Murphy, G. (2002b). People with an intellectual disability in the criminal justice system: Developing an assessment tool for measuring prevalence. *British Journal of Clinical Psychology, 41*, 315–20.

Murphy, G. (2000). Policy and service development trends: Forensic mental health and social care services. *Tizard Learning Disability Review, 5* (2), 32–5.

Murphy, G. & Mason, J. (1999). People with developmental disabilities who offend. In N. Bouras (Ed.), *Psychiatric and behavioural disorders in developmental disabilities and mental retardation* (pp. 226–45). Cambridge: Cambridge University Press.

National Probation Directorate (2002). *The treatment and risk management of sexual offenders in custody and in the community.* London: National Probation Directorate.

National Probation Service for England and Wales (2004). *Sex offender strategy for the national probation service.* Retrieved from www.probation2000.com/documents/Sex%20Offender%20 Strategy%20Sep%202004.pdf on 4 December 2009.

Noble, J. & Conley, R. (1992). Towards an epidemiology of relevant attributes. In R. Conley, R. Luckasson & G. Bouthilet (Eds), *The criminal justice system and mental retardation: Defendants and victims* (pp. 51–62). Baltimore: Paul Brookes.

Petersilia, J. (2000). *Doing justice? Criminal offenders with developmental disabilities.* Berkeley, CA: California Policy Research Center.

Rose, J., Jenkins, R., O'Connor, C., Jones, C. & Felce, D. (2002). A group treatment for men with intellectual disabilities who sexually offend or abuse. *Journal of Applied Research in Intellectual Disabilities, 15,* 138–50.

Simpson, M.K. & Hogg, J. (2001). Patterns of offending among people with intellectual disability: A systematic review. Part II: Predisposing factors. *Journal of Intellectual Disability Research, 45* (5), 397–406.

Sobsey, D. (1994). Sexual abuse of individuals with intellectual disabilities. In A. Craft (Ed.), *Practice issues in sexuality and learning disabilities* (pp. 93–115). London: Routledge.

Steptoe, L., Lindsay, W.R., Forrest, D. & Power, M. (2006). Quality of life and relationships in sex offenders with intellectual disability. *Journal of Intellectual & Developmental Disability, 31* (1), 13–19.

Talbot, T.J. & Langdon, P.E. (2006). A revised sexual knowledge assessment tool for people with intellectual disabilities: Is sexual knowledge related to sexual offending behaviour? *Journal of Intellectual Disability Research, 50* (7), 523–31.

Tudway, J.A. & Darmoody, M. (2005). Clinical assessment of adult sexual offenders with learning disabilities. *Journal of Sexual Aggression, 11* (3), 277–88.

Ward, T. & Brown, M. (2004). The Good Lives model and conceptual issues in offender rehabilitation. *Psychology, Crime & Law, 10* (3), 243–57.

Ward, T., Hudson, S.M. & Keenan, T. (1998). A self-regulation model of the sexual offence process. *Sexual Abuse: A Journal Of Research And Treatment, 10* (2), 141–57.

Ward, T., Mann, R.E. & Gannon, T.A. (2007). The good lives model of offender rehabilitation: Clinical implications. *Aggression and Violent Behavior, 12,* 87–107.

Wilcox, D.T. (2004). Treatment of intellectually disabled individuals who have committed sexual offences: A review of the literature. *Journal of Sexual Aggression, 10* (1), 85–100.

Xenitidis, K.I., Henry, J., Russell, A.J., Ward, A. & Murphy, D. G. M. (1999). An inpatient treatment model for adults with mild intellectual disability and challenging behaviour. *Journal of Intellectual Disability Research, 43* (2), 128–34.

Yool, L., Langdon, P.E. & Garner, K. (2003). The attitudes of medium-secure unit staff toward the sexuality of adults with learning disabilities. *Sexuality and Disability, 21* (2), 137–50.

Index

Assessment and Treatment of Sexual Offenders with Intellectual Disabilities: A Handbook
Edited by Leam A. Craig, William R. Lindsay and Kevin D. Browne
© 2010 John Wiley & Sons, Ltd.

6225099R00221

Printed in Great Britain
by Amazon.co.uk, Ltd.,
Marston Gate.